D1462596

The Praeger Guide to Hearing and Hearing Loss

The Praeger Guide to Hearing and Hearing Loss

Assessment, Treatment, and Prevention

Susan Dalebout

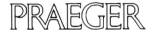

Westport, Connecticut
London

Library of Congress Cataloging-in-Publication Data

Dalebout, Susan.
  The Praeger guide to hearing and hearing loss : assessment, treatment, and prevention / Susan Dalebout.
  p.   cm.
  Includes bibliographical references and index.
  ISBN 978–0–313–36476–1 (alk. paper)
  1. Hearing disorders—Popular works.   2. Hearing—Popular works.   3. Deafness—Popular works.   I. Title.   II. Title. Guide to hearing and hearing loss.
  RF291.35.D35   2009
  617.8—dc22   2008036338

British Library Cataloguing in Publication Data is available.

Library of Congress Catalog Card Number: 2008036338
ISBN: 978–0–313–36476–1

First published in 2009

Praeger Publishers, 88 Post Road West, Westport, CT 06881
An imprint of Greenwood Publishing Group, Inc.
www.praeger.com

Printed in the United States of America

The paper used in this book complies with the Permanent Paper Standard issued by the National Information Standards Organization (Z39.48–1984).

10 9 8 7 6 5 4 3 2 1

For my father
who bears hearing (and vision) loss with incredible
grace and good humor.

And for my mother
who is the reason that he's always so cheerful.

Contents

Preface

I was inspired to write this book by my father and his friends with hearing loss (many of whom I have known all my life). Most of them—even those with hearing aids—understand surprisingly little about their hearing problems and what can be done about them. They are wary of exaggerated advertising claims, buying something that doesn't really help, and being overcharged. They are confused about whose advice they should trust, and sometimes they call on me. This book was written as a resource for them and so many others like them.

I had significant help along the way from two very special people. The first is Robert L. Shook, author of many books and mentor to many aspiring authors. Bob, whose late mother had a hearing loss, was tenacious in encouraging me to write this book. He went out of his way to be kind, and he has been remarkably generous with his valuable time.

The other person is my husband, Harry Levins, without whom this book would never have been finished. I know of no one with greater intellect, powers of analysis, and problem-solving ability, and I am grateful that he was willing to apply his exceptional talents to this endeavor. In addition to making an enormous investment of time, his patience, encouragement, and resolve have been steadfast. I am truly blessed to have a husband who is as capable as he is loving.

Abbreviations

AAA	American Academy of Audiology
ABA	American Board of Audiology
ABR	Auditory Brainstem Response
ADA	Americans with Disabilities Act of 1990
ALD	Assistive Listening Device
ALDA	Association of Late-Deafened Adults
ALD/S	Assistive Listening Device/System
ALS	Assistive Listening System
ASHA	American Speech-Language-Hearing Association
ASL	American Sign Language
ATA	American Tinnitus Association
AuD	Doctor of Audiology
BC-HIS	Board Certified in Hearing Instrument Sciences
BICROS	Bilateral CROS
BTE	Behind-the-Ear Hearing Aid
CA	Communication Assistant
CAN	Computer-Assisted Note-Taking
CART	Computer-Assisted Real-Time Transcription
CBT	Cognitive Behavioral Therapy
CCC-A	Certificate of Clinical Competence-Audiology
CD	Compact Disk
CIC	Completely-in-the-Canal Hearing Aid
CN	Cranial Nerve
CPA	Cerebellopontine Angle
CROS	Contralateral Routing of the Signal

DAI	Direct Audio Input
dB	Decibels
DSP	Digital Signal Processing
EEG	Electroencephalographic
ENT	Ear, Nose, and Throat
EPA	Environmental Protection Agency
FCC	Federal Communications Commission
FDA	Food and Drug Administration
FM	Frequency Modulated
HAC	Hearing Aid Compatible/Hearing Aid Compatibility
HAT	Hearing Assistance Technology
H.E.A.R.	Hearing Education and Awareness for Rockers
HEAR	Medicare Hearing Enhancement and Auditory Rehabilitation Act of 2007
Hz	Hertz
HLAA	Hearing Loss Association of America
IHS	International Hearing Society
IL	Induction Loop
IP	Internet Protocol
IR	Infrared
ITC	In-the-Canal Hearing Aid
ITE	In-the-Ear Hearing Aid
LACE	Listening and Communication Enhancement Program
LDL	Loudness Discomfort Level
NAC	N-acetylcysteine
NBC-HIS	National Board for Certification in Hearing Instrument Sciences
NIOSH	National Institute for Occupational Safety and Health
NPC	Noise Pollution Clearinghouse
NRR	Noise Reduction Rating
OAEs	Otoacoustic Emissions
OME	Otitis Media with Effusion
OSHA	Occupational Safety and Health Administration
PE	Pressure Equalization
RF	Radio Frequency
RITE	Receiver-in-the-Ear Hearing Aid
SHHH	Self Help for Hard of Hearing People (now HLAA)
SNR	Signal-to-Noise Ratio (also used here for Signal-to-Noise Relationship)
SRT	Speech Reception Threshold
TL	Tolerance Level
TMJ	Temporomandibular Joint Syndrome
TRS	Telecommunication Relay Services
TRT	Tinnitus Retraining Therapy
TTD	Telecommunication Device for the Deaf

TTS	Temporary Threshold Shift
TTY	Teletypewriter
UCL	Uncomfortable level
VBA	Veterans Benefits Administration
VCO	Voice Carry Over

PART I

Learning about the Problems

CHAPTER 1

Is This You or Someone You Love?

Oh you men who think or say that I am malevolent, stubborn, or misanthropic, how greatly do you wrong me. You do not know the secret cause which makes me seem that way to you.... For six years now I have been hopelessly afflicted...by the...sad experience of my bad hearing. Ah, how could I possibly admit an infirmity in the one sense which ought to be more perfect in me than others, a sense which I once possessed in the highest perfection, a perfection such as few in my profession enjoy or ever have enjoyed. Oh I cannot do it; therefore forgive me when you see me draw back when I would have gladly mingled with you. My misfortune is doubly painful to me because I am bound to be misunderstood; for me there can be no relaxation with my fellow men, no refined conversations, no mutual exchange of ideas. I must live almost alone, like one who has been banished; I can mix with society only as much as true necessity demands. If I approach near to people a hot terror seizes upon me, and I fear being exposed to the danger that my condition might be noticed....

Ludwig van Beethoven, October 6th, 1802

DO YOU RECOGNIZE YOURSELF OR SOMEONE YOU LOVE IN ANY OF THESE SITUATIONS?

You and your spouse have always been socially active. You enjoy concerts, plays, lectures, movies, religious services, dining out, and travel. But now you must work to understand what's being said, and sometimes the effort is exhausting. And, try as you might, there are times when you get only bits and pieces. Occasionally, you give yourself a break and let your mind wander. But then you lose track of the conversation. You feel self-conscious and worry that your problem will be discovered. Eventually, you decide that social activities just aren't as much fun as they used to be, and one by one, you give them up. You tell your spouse that you've lost interest in them—that you'd simply rather not go out. It's clear that he's disappointed about the changes in your lifestyle. You feel guilty about depriving him of activities you once enjoyed together, but it's no longer possible to *share* them in quite the same way. After all, your hearing loss makes it difficult for you to speak privately to one another in public places. As a result, your ability to experience an event *together* has been diminished. Your spouse worries that you're becoming withdrawn and perhaps depressed. Sadly, you realize that your hearing loss has changed his life as much as it's changed yours. And it's taking a toll on your relationship.

You're at a business dinner. You give your order to the waitress and return your attention to your dining companions. Then you realize that the waitress is still standing over you. Judging from the expectant look on her face, you suspect that she's asked you a question. You ask her to repeat what she has said. Apparently she does, but all that you hear is the din of multiple conversations, clattering dishes, and unwanted music. You ask her to repeat again. She mumbles something, but you still don't get it. Why doesn't she make some effort to help you understand? You feel upset. Your companions look anxious—not knowing whether to intervene and risk embarrassing you, or be polite and pretend not to notice. Eventually the meal is served, but you have to work at hearing throughout the evening. In the future, you'll think twice about having a business meeting in a restaurant. Although your hearing is adequate in the quiet of your office, attempting to have an important conversation in a noisy restaurant is just too stressful.

You're a baby boomer in your mid-fifties. You eat a healthy diet, run and weight train each day, and often bicycle 100 miles. You take good care of yourself, and you're in great shape. These days you're careful to protect your hearing while mowing the lawn, but you've enjoyed your share of loud music and rock concerts in the past. You were happy to learn that your hearing was normal when an audiologist tested it about 5 years ago, but lately you're having trouble understanding friends in noisy situations. You wonder if you're beginning to lose some hearing.

You're at a family gathering. You've been looking forward to the event for months, and you're eager to interact with your children and grandchildren. But suddenly it seems like everyone is talking at once. You hear their voices, but you can't make out their words. You ask people to repeat, but even then you have trouble understanding. You're aware that asking for repetition disrupts the conversation, and so you decide to just listen and catch whatever you can. As the conversation jumps from person to person, however, you can't keep up. Eventually, you become lost. You quit trying and let your mind drift to other things. Suddenly, someone asks you a question. Caught off guard, you make your best guess and give a vague response. The looks you receive suggest that your answer was off target, but no one bothers to pursue it. The conversation quickly moves on. You worry that people might think you're becoming senile. You wonder if they might be right. You're ready to go home—to a place where your hearing loss isn't a problem. Next time, you'll be less enthusiastic about attending an event with so many people.

Your spouse tells you that you don't hear well, but you refuse to believe it. After all, who can understand someone who talks with the water running, from behind a newspaper, or from another room? Your hearing is all right; it's just that your spouse—and everyone else—mumbles. You can hear them talking, but you don't catch *everything* they're saying. You hate asking them to repeat things—that only confirms what they already think about your hearing and makes you feel foolish. Most of the time, you just keep quiet. Sometimes you pretend that you heard what was said; other times you act as if you weren't paying attention. When forced to give a response, you bluff and hope that your answer doesn't give you away.

You're attending a meeting with a group of acquaintances, and the speaker isn't using the microphone. You raise your hand and politely ask that she do so. She replies, "I think everyone will be able to hear me if I speak up." You object and ask again that she use the microphone. Others in the audience react to your request with annoyance and sarcastically suggest that you get a hearing aid. Apparently, they're unaware that you already depend on hearing aids, but that hearing aids can't solve every listening problem. You feel humiliated and angry. You wonder how people can be so insensitive.

You and your spouse are meeting friends at a restaurant for dinner. You haven't seen these friends in a long time, and so there'll be quite a bit of catching up to do. Your spouse has been looking forward to the evening with enthusiasm, but you've been dreading it. Because this is a social event, she reminds you to wear your hearing aid. You try to remember where you put it, because you haven't worn it for some time. You bought it 5 or 6 years ago to please her—she thought it would make a world of difference. You don't wear it often, only on occasions when you know that hearing will be difficult. You arrive at the restaurant and—no surprise—it's a noisy place. You keep fumbling with your hearing aid, trying to adjust it to catch more of the conversation. Your spouse keeps telling you that it's whistling. Finally, looking embarrassed and irritated, she insists that you turn it off (which is a relief). As you tune out, you begin thinking about all of the things that your audiologist has told you over the years . . . like the more you used the aid, the more you would benefit from it . . . that your brain would need time to adjust to different sound input, and that adjustment would not occur unless you wore the aid regularly . . . that you should practice wearing the hearing aid in easy listening situations before using it in more challenging ones. She offered you and your spouse hearing rehabilitation sessions that she said would help, but you weren't interested. You figured it was just a marketing ploy. She said that you would hear better with two hearing aids than with just one, and that over time speech understanding in your unaided ear might deteriorate from lack of use, but you figured that was just another sales tactic. She told you about dramatic improvements in hearing aid technology over the last few years, but you refused to spend money on a new hearing aid. Leaving the restaurant, you can't help but notice how disappointed your spouse looks. Is it time to reconsider some of your audiologist's advice?

MY TURN

My mother is lying on a hospital gurney being prepped for surgery. I've traveled from another state to be there, and I wait with my father. Although my parents are vigorous and appear younger than their age, they've been married for nearly 60 years. They share and consult about everything. No experience, thought, or decision escapes thorough analysis and discussion between the two of them. This morning, my father and I wait nervously for an opportunity to see my mother before surgery. The institutional rooms we pass through are cold, with hard walls, hard floors, and hard ceilings that make listening conditions poor. In addition, people and machines are making noise everywhere. Finally, someone comes to tell us where to find my mother, what to expect, and what we're supposed to do next. I turn to my father and realize that he's missed much of what was said. We continue to receive instructions throughout the morning, and I watch my father struggle to hear them. We spend hours listening for our names to be called in the surgical lounge. Finally, it's time to speak with the surgeon about my mother's condition. Thankfully, she gives us her report in a small room intended for counseling, but even then, my father understands little of what is said. On this day, I am obviously very concerned about my mother, but I am also very concerned about my father. I realize that in difficult listening situations he's lost without my mother. As a daughter, it's painful to see my father looking vulnerable because he can't hear. In my case it's especially painful, because I've been an audiologist for more than 30 years.

THIS BOOK

If reading any of this makes you think of yourself or someone you love, then you probably have stories of your own to tell. The question is, are there solutions to these problems? The answer isn't simple. When it comes to hearing loss, there is no silver bullet. Unlike vision, which can usually be restored to normal with medical/surgical treatment or corrective lenses, most hearing losses can't be medically treated or restored to normal with amplification. Nonetheless, there are many things that you can do to minimize the negative impact of hearing loss and significantly improve the quality of your life. And that's what this book is about.

This book was written for my father and the millions like him, whose lives have been altered by hearing loss. In fact, I have used my father's hearing loss to illustrate information presented throughout the book. This book is also for my mother and the millions like her, whose lives have been changed by a partner's hearing loss. In truth, this is a book for adults of any age with *any* degree of hearing loss—from slight to profound—and the people who love them.

Could *You* Have a Hearing Loss?

Do your best to answer these questions *honestly*.

Do you

- Think that people mumble or don't speak clearly?
- Hear people talking but have trouble understanding their words?
- Find yourself asking people to repeat what they've said?
- Miss details in meetings, lectures, plays, or religious services?
- Get complaints about the television being too loud?
- Fail to hear the doorbell or telephone ring?
- Have trouble hearing over the telephone?
- Notice that it's more difficult to hear with one ear than the other?
- Have difficulty understanding when there are multiple conversations (or other background noise) in the room?
- Find that watching people's faces makes it easier to understand, especially in poor listening conditions?
- Have difficulty understanding conversations in restaurants?
- Get complaints about speaking too loudly?
- Feel tired or stressed after a conversation?
- Find understanding the words of women and children particularly difficult?
- Have difficulty following the dialogue in movies?
- Have trouble understanding speakers in public places?
- Have trouble understanding soft or whispered speech?
- Have difficulty hearing birds singing or a watch ticking?
- Have difficulty determining where sounds are coming from?
- Misunderstand what people are saying and respond inappropriately?
- Feel that people get annoyed because you've misunderstood them?
- Guess at what people have said because you're unable to catch all of the words?
- Pretend to understand when you don't?
- Feel anxious or avoid situations because you fear it will be difficult to hear?
- Find that music is no longer enjoyable?
- Have friends or relatives who've questioned your hearing?

If you answered "yes" to more than two of these questions, you need to have a hearing evaluation. Don't wait to invest in your relationships and improve the quality of your life. Help for hearing loss *is* available.

CHAPTER 2

The Sensual Ear: Hearing and Hearing Loss

Blindness cuts us off from things, but deafness cuts us off from people.
Helen Keller

By most estimates, more than 31 million Americans experience significant hearing loss—that's a whopping one in ten of us. Even that figure, however, fails to convey the real impact, because hearing loss never affects just one person. The family members, friends, and coworkers of every person with hearing loss are affected as well.

It's a myth that hearing loss affects only old people. Although it's more common among people who are older, more than half of all Americans with hearing loss are under the age of 50. And hearing loss is becoming evident in younger and younger people all the time. Among adults, the breakdown is something like this: one in twelve 30-year-olds, one in eight 50-year-olds, one in three 65-year-olds, and one in two 75-year-olds has a hearing loss.

The vast majority of people with hearing loss grew up with normal (or relatively normal) hearing and gradually began losing it as adults. If you're part of that large and ever-expanding group, this book is meant for you. The book is intended to help you minimize the negative impact of your hearing loss and maximize the quality of your life.

ALL HEARING LOSSES ARE NOT THE SAME

People with hearing loss may be considered hard of hearing, deaf, or Deaf. Those with measured hearing levels in the severe-to-profound hearing loss range are usually considered deaf. Those with lesser degrees of hearing loss are generally considered hard of hearing. People who are "Deaf" identify *themselves* as members of the Deaf community and are said to be culturally Deaf. Membership in the Deaf community is based less on the degree of hearing loss and more on the use of American Sign Language (ASL) as the primary mode of communication. ASL is not English that's signed; rather, it's a complete language unto itself, altogether different from English. Most members of the Deaf community have been deaf since birth or early childhood, or they come from Deaf families. Among the 31.5 million Americans with hearing loss, 95 to 98 percent are hard of hearing; a relatively small number are deaf (perhaps 1 million), and an even smaller number are culturally Deaf. It's estimated that about 300,000 Americans use ASL as their primary language.[1]

The term *hearing impaired* is sometimes used to describe all people with hearing loss. Although this is convenient, the term is not used here because many people who are culturally Deaf find it objectionable. Members of the Deaf community generally do not consider themselves impaired; rather, they consider deafness an essential part of their nature. Given a choice, most would not change their deafness any more than most people would change their race or gender. In contrast, people who once relied on hearing for communication miss it dearly when it's gone. Given a choice, they would enthusiastically choose normal hearing. The perspectives of these groups couldn't be more different. While both are perfectly valid, this book is intended for people who want to hear better.

THE IMPORTANCE OF HEARING IN OUR LIVES

In 1910, Helen Keller wrote, "I am just as deaf as I am blind. The problems of deafness are deeper and more complex, if not more important, than those of blindness. Deafness is a much worse misfortune. For it means the loss of the most vital stimulus—the sound of the voice that brings language, sets thoughts astir and keeps us in the intellectual company of man."[2] Ms. Keller expressed this sentiment on more than one occasion. In her words, " . . . after a lifetime in silence and darkness to be deaf is a greater affliction than to be blind. . . . Hearing is the soul of knowledge and information of a high order. To be cut off from hearing is to be isolated indeed."[3]

For most of us, connections to other people depend on hearing—and nothing could be more important. But our dependence on hearing goes beyond even that. Hearing connects us to the world in which we live. It's been suggested that this connection occurs on at least three levels: primitive, warning, and symbolic.[4]

At the *primitive level,* hearing provides a constant auditory background that gives us a sense of comfort and security. Even though we tune out many background sounds (for example, the refrigerator running, the computer fan humming, the clock ticking), our unconscious awareness of them makes us feel alive and part of a living world. Background sounds also become part of the "soundscapes" that enrich our lives (leaves crunching underfoot, birds singing in the trees, waves crashing on the shore, children laughing in the distance). The loss of these sounds can leave a listener feeling isolated and alienated, and may result in depression.

For most people, there's an unconscious expectation that actions will produce sound. To watch a glass fall to the floor without hearing it shatter is disconcerting—like living in a movie with the sound track turned off. And an inability to hear the sounds we make ourselves (like those associated with sneezing, laughing, chewing, or moving about) can be even more unsettling. People who experience sudden hearing loss often report that the world feels "dead" to them.

Fortunately, most listeners lose only part, rather than all, of their hearing, and they lose it very gradually. Although they miss many sounds of importance, they continue to hear enough of the auditory background to feel connected to the world. Even when hearing loss is quite severe, hearing aids and cochlear implants usually restore an auditory background—although a period of adjustment is sometimes required to actually appreciate that. It takes time for the brain to reorient itself to a world filled with sound and to become accustomed to hearing in a new way. In fact, new hearing aid users often find the auditory background annoying at first. Adjustment takes patience and practice. Similarly, when an experienced hearing aid user gets new hearing aids that process incoming sounds in a slightly different way, the brain requires another period of adjustment.

At the *warning level*, sounds provide information about what's going on around us, even in the dark, around corners, and through walls. We don't need to see the source of a sound to understand its meaning or know its location. A knock at the door signals the presence of a visitor. A car horn signals potential danger. The cry of a child signals an unmet need.

Naturally, an inability to hear warning sounds creates feelings of anxiety and insecurity. If you can't hear the alarm clock, you may not sleep for fear of being late for work. If you're a parent (or grandparent), you may worry constantly about not hearing your child cry out. If you're startled by people suddenly appearing without having heard them approach, you may find it difficult to concentrate. Fortunately, alerting devices are available to solve most of these problems.

Hearing at the warning level is never turned off; it works around the clock. The brain is always monitoring the sound environment, even when we're unaware of it. When a sound of potential significance is detected, the brain pushes it into our consciousness. For example, imagine yourself (with normal hearing) in a room where lots of people are talking. You're having a conversation with a friend when you hear your name mentioned across the room. Your attention was focused on the conversation with your friend, but your brain was monitoring sounds throughout the environment. The sound of your name could be important, so it gets flagged for immediate attention. This unconscious monitoring system allows us to remain vigilant, even while we rest. A sleeping mother can ignore dozens of sounds—even loud ones—yet awaken the moment her child cries. Hearing at this level also enables us to multitask. For example, a parent can be cooking dinner while monitoring the sounds made by a child playing in a nearby room and feel confident that he is safe.

At the *symbolic level*, sound becomes the primary means for communication, the most human of all experiences. Not only does hearing allow us to detect speech, it makes it possible for us to comprehend its meaning, even subtle nuances of meaning. Virtually all people with hearing loss have some difficulty at this level, especially when listening conditions are poor (for example, when there is background noise). Fortunately, hearing aids, cochlear implants, assistive listening devices, and hearing rehabilitation can, for the most part, restore the ability to detect speech and understand its meaning.

In addition to these three basic levels, hearing is a source of enjoyment. For some, the ability to appreciate music is deeply significant. For them, a loss of hearing can mean losing one of life's greatest pleasures. For others, it may be the ability to enjoy the sounds of nature that's critically important. There are people who actually mourn the loss of their favorite sounds.

Hearing affects the quality of our lives in more ways than we could possibly name, but above all, it contributes to the *easy* flow of communication between human beings. Although it's possible to communicate in other ways, most of us choose to hear and speak. And it is through hearing that we come to know the thoughts and feelings—the very essence—of the people in our lives.

THE TROUBLE WITH HEARING LOSS

It's hard to understand. People who would gladly go out of their way to help someone who's blind or physically disabled are likely to become impatient when talking with someone who's hard of hearing. If you doubt this, try asking someone to repeat more than a couple of times during a conversation. People seem to have less empathy for hearing loss than they do for other disabilities, perhaps because hearing loss is invisible—there's no white cane, no wheelchair to signal the disability. Or perhaps because hearing loss is so common people don't consider it a real disability—maybe they think it's something we all face sooner or later.

Whatever the reason, one thing is clear. People are more inclined to be helpful when they believe a person with hearing loss is doing everything possible to help himself—and most often that means wearing hearing aids. Refusal to use hearing aids can be a source of anger and resentment among family members ("she is so stubborn," or "he is so selfish"), and failure to wear hearing aids that have already been purchased is a common source of frustration ("I have to scream on the telephone; why isn't she wearing the hearing aids we bought her?"). However, it's important to understand that hearing aids cannot solve all hearing-related problems. Although hearing aids can be incredibly helpful, they cannot bring back normal hearing. There will be situations in which the wearer will continue to have difficulty, and learning to use good communication habits is essential.

People often are reluctant to acknowledge hearing problems, sometimes even to themselves. Because hearing loss is painless, invisible, and usually develops very gradually, it's easy to ignore—at least at first. But there are times when not acknowledging a hearing loss is about more than just missing the signs. Sometimes it's about denial, and sometimes denial is about the lingering stigma attached to hearing loss. Think about it. A person who wouldn't think twice about wearing eyeglasses to correct a vision problem is apt to deny a hearing loss. A loss of vision is acceptable; a loss of hearing is not. People fear that acknowledging a hearing loss will make them appear old or incompetent when, in reality, it's pretending *not* to have a hearing loss that's likely to make them appear confused (or aloof, indecisive, or otherwise befuddled). Attempting to conceal a hearing loss is more likely to make it apparent than wearing hearing aids ever would. When people attempt to bluff their way through conversations, awkward and embarrassing situations are bound to occur. Responses are likely to seem strange or off target, and sometimes rude or insensitive.

People who deny hearing loss sometimes blame others, believing there wouldn't be a problem if people would only speak clearly. They may be convinced that children are no longer taught to speak properly, or that people these days are too rushed, too lazy, or too disrespectful to do so. They may blame family members for talking to them when they're out of "earshot." They may even accuse people of deliberately excluding them from conversations or talking behind their backs. Admittedly, communication partners are imperfect. There's no doubt about that. But if you have an *untreated* hearing loss, your hearing loss is the real source of the problem.

Even people who recognize they have a hearing loss are likely to wait years before seeking help. The average wait is 7 years, but many people wait much longer. People delay for many reasons: they may not believe they have a hearing problem or they may wish to conceal it; they may be unable to afford help; they may be misinformed about the help that's available; or they may simply put off taking action. The truth is, most people *never* seek help. In this country, only 25 percent of the people who could benefit from hearing aids actually use them. In other words, only one in four adults with hearing loss is doing something about it.

Hearing loss affects our ability to function socially, emotionally, and intellectually. Not seeking help—whether because of denial, vanity, money, or procrastination—can take a heavy toll. Research studies have shown that *untreated* hearing loss can lead to embarrassment, fatigue, irritability, tension, stress, social isolation, loneliness, rejection, paranoia, anxiety, negativism, depression, endangered personal safety, impaired memory, and relationship stress. It can also degrade coping skills, the ability to learn new tasks, alertness to the environment, personal effectiveness, and general health.[5,6] A national task force recently described it as "a potentially devastating health condition if left untreated."[7] It seems that those who choose to do nothing about hearing loss do so at their own peril.

But it's not all doom and gloom. There's good news too. Several years ago, the National Council on Aging commissioned a major study in which more than 2,000 people with hearing loss (some used hearing aids whereas others did not) and nearly 2,000 of their significant others (mostly spouses) were surveyed.[8] The study's purpose was to examine the impact of hearing aids on quality of life; to date, it's the largest study of its kind. The results were striking. The use of hearing aids was associated with improved social, emotional, psychological, and physical well-being, regardless of the degree of hearing loss. Those who used hearing aids had higher scores for interpersonal relationships (including greater intimacy), emotional stability, sense of control, cognitive function, and health status. They were also more likely to interact with other people and to participate in organized social activities. Both hearing aid users and family members indicated significant improvement in nearly every area measured: relationships at home, feelings about self, social life, mental health, physical health, etc. Notably, *family members* reported greater benefits related to the use of hearing aids than the hearing aid users themselves.

If that's not enough, another important study has shown that working Americans with hearing loss earn far less than people with normal hearing—for those with the most severe hearing loss, up to $12,000 less per year.[9] However, for people who wear hearing aids, that difference is (on average) cut in half. Study results indicated that for each 10 percent increase in the severity of hearing loss, the decrease in average annual household income was $2,250 for people who did not wear hearing aids, but only $1,130 for those who did. These figures show that the financial benefit of wearing hearing aids far exceeds their cost.

Untreated hearing loss finds its way into virtually every aspect of our lives. Routine trips to the market, the drugstore, or the post office can become embarrassing experiences that create a sense of dread. Activities that once brought joy—like interacting at family gatherings, eating in restaurants, going to movies, or traveling—can become frustrating and unsatisfying. Interactions with loved ones can become stressful, making a family member with hearing loss feel tense and irritable, and then guilty and ashamed. Functioning in the workplace may require additional effort. It may be more difficult to hear on the telephone or in meetings, and communicating with coworkers, customers, clients, students, patients, or parishioners may become a challenge. The ever-present fear of missing something may create a constant sense of anxiety. The need to devote one's full attention to listening may make multitasking impossible. Feelings of inadequacy may overwhelm feelings of competence, and career advancement may seem hopeless.

Untreated hearing loss can lead to feelings of loneliness, isolation, or worse. Think about how much of what we know about the world comes from merely observing and overhearing. As "distance" senses, hearing and vision allow us to receive information not specifically directed to us. But hearing loss takes away the ability to hear from a distance—and the ability to overhear. This can make people with hearing loss feel confused or out of step with everyone else. They may feel anxious about not knowing what everyone else knows. Even worse, being unable to hear what other people are talking about can lead to feelings of distrust, alienation, and even paranoia. It's human nature to assume occasionally that conversations we cannot hear are about us.

All in all, it's not surprising that some people react to hearing loss with anger or resentment, that some feel anxious or fearful about their personal safety, or that some lose their self-confidence and sense of identity. In fact, it's not hard to understand why some who lose their hearing mourn its loss and wrestle with the stages of grief that Elizabeth Kübler-Ross first associated with the death of a loved one: denial, anger, bargaining, depression, and acceptance.[10]

Coping with hearing loss is made more difficult by a lack of understanding about its nature. Friends and family members often express frustration about what appears to be inconsistent hearing ability (the *he-hears-when-he-wants-to* problem). Inconsistent responses can be interpreted as disinterest, willfulness, even laziness. However, learning just a few things about the nature of hearing loss makes it easier to understand that inconsistencies in the ability to hear are very real. For example

- Hearing loss is not an all-or-nothing business. The continuum ranges from slight hearing loss to total deafness (although total deafness is very uncommon, which means that most people hear *some* things but not *all* things).
- Hearing loss rarely affects all pitches equally. This means most people *hear* speech, but with some of the information filtered out—and typically it's the most critical information that's missing. It's this "filter effect" that makes speech hard to understand. For example, instead of actually *hearing* the difference between "sat," "fat," "pat," and "that," people with hearing loss are likely to hear only /a/, /a/, /a/, and /a/. The important high-pitched consonant information has been filtered out, leaving only the low-pitched vowel sounds. Imagine trying to read this page with all of the consonants erased. The loss of the consonants makes it difficult to tell one word from another using hearing alone. The listener must fill in what's missing by watching speakers' faces and using contextual cues. People with hearing loss must constantly combine fragments of information from hearing, vision, and context to make sense of what's being said.
- Listeners with certain types of hearing loss also experience distortion. This means they can hear people talking, but they have difficulty understanding what's being said. Speech sounds mumbled or garbled, and speaking louder doesn't make it clearer. This highlights the difference between *audibility* (the ability to hear someone talking) and *intelligibility* (the ability to distinguish one

word from another). Think about listening to someone speak a foreign language. You can *hear* the words, but you can't decipher them, and asking the speaker to talk louder doesn't solve the problem.

- For a person with hearing loss, the ability to understand speech varies with the listening conditions. Someone who does well in quiet, one-to-one conversations may have a terrible time understanding when the speaker is far away, there's background noise, or the room acoustics are poor. If the effort required to understand is too great, the listener may "tune out" or avoid such situations altogether.

Using impaired hearing and other bits of incomplete information to understand speech is exhausting. It's similar to putting together a complex puzzle by trial and error; you try something that might fit, decide it doesn't, reject it, and try another. Unlike a puzzle, however, the stream of speech rushes on, and topics change constantly. That kind of effort is enough to tucker anybody out. Fortunately, a major benefit of using hearing aids, assistive listening technology, and other hearing rehabilitation strategies is that listening becomes easier and less tiring.

> **My Dad**
> My dad has always been gregarious, the life of the party; however, before he got his hearing aids I would see him "tuning out." Instead of watching, listening, and trying to make sense of fragments (which can be exhausting), I would see him staring into space and thinking about something else. Even with his hearing aids, he has to work to hear. I'm so happy to have him back in the conversation—I really missed him.

Finally, when a listener is older, inconsistent responses can be misinterpreted in a different way. When conversation is directed to an older person and she doesn't respond—or the response doesn't make sense—a hearing problem can be confused with senility. Unfortunately, hearing loss actually *can* contribute to cognitive decline. Untreated, it can cause a person to withdraw from conversations and social interactions. With less communication, the person becomes increasingly isolated. With less stimulation, the assumption of mental decline can become a reality.

> **Poor Etiquette for Communicating with Someone with a Hearing Loss**
> When talking with someone who has a hearing loss, *never*
>
> - Respond with annoyance when asked to repeat (or say things like, *"Turn up your hearing aids!"* or *"Never mind, it wasn't important."*)

- Begin talking without getting her attention first
- Talk without face-to-face contact
- Ridicule him for misunderstanding or giving inappropriate responses
- Talk to others under your breath or with your face turned away
- Talk about her as if she isn't there
- Treat him like a child
- Leave her out of conversations or activities because communication is too much work
- Accuse him of hearing only what he wants to hear
- Take over "hearing" without being asked

THE TROUBLE WITH LIVING WITH SOMEONE WHO HAS A HEARING LOSS

Hearing loss never affects just one person; it affects virtually everyone with whom a deaf or hard-of-hearing person communicates, and especially those with whom he communicates most. It probably comes as no surprise to hear that it places special stress on a marriage (or similar relationship). If one of you has a hearing problem, *both* of you have a hearing problem. And if you're really committed to minimizing the negative impact of hearing loss and maximizing the quality of your lives, *both* of you will have to work at it. *Both* of you will have to make adjustments, and *each* of you has a role.

If your partner has an untreated hearing loss, you already know that easy, spontaneous communication can become labored and difficult. Sweet nothings and comfortable small talk can all but disappear, leaving nothing but the exchange of essential information. You may find that sharing personal thoughts and feelings is a challenge—subtle (and not-so-subtle) nuances may be missed and what's been missed may be difficult to explain. There may be times when your partner is too tired to talk or to listen, making you feel rejected.

Over time, your partner may withdraw from social situations and want less interaction with other people. You may go out less as a couple because it's difficult to have private conversations in public places. Of course, this also changes *your* life. In fact, research suggests that it's the better-hearing spouse who's likely to feel greater disappointment about a shrinking social life. You may find that your partner is also less communicative at home. In other words, you may be staying home more and enjoying it less. It may feel like your partner is withdrawing from your social life *and* you at the same time. To make matters worse, your partner may be experiencing difficult emotions and struggling to hang on to her sense of self. She may be unable or unwilling to talk about these painful feelings or the changes that the two of you are experiencing. You may feel shut out.

If your partner has *not* withdrawn from social situations, he may be trying to compensate in ways that aren't helpful. For example, some people pretend they're not paying attention so they don't have to admit they can't hear. Many people bluff or pretend to understand when they really don't. Of course, it's only a matter of time until that house of cards collapses. Other people monopolize conversations—after all, there's no need to hear anyone else if you never give up the floor.

Blaming others is another inappropriate coping strategy. Spouses are often blamed for speaking while turned away, from too far away, from behind a newspaper, or with the water running. And it's probably true; you probably do all of those things on occasion, and you'll definitely need to develop communication habits that improve understanding if you want your relationship to work (see Chapter 10). However, you cannot accept responsibility for your partner's untreated hearing loss, nor should you be expected to make all of the accommodations. Your partner must be willing to take responsibility for the hearing problem and do everything possible to help himself. Seeking help for hearing loss is a sign of love and respect. Your spouse must understand that choosing to do nothing (when help is available) is a selfish choice.

If your spouse relies on inappropriate coping strategies, it may embarrass you. More likely, you find it painful to watch the person you love feel humiliated, vulnerable, or left out. In an effort to help, you may try to "hear" for your partner, or maybe your partner gives you that responsibility. Either way, you may find yourself constantly explaining things that were missed—during conversations with friends, at meetings, at the movies, in stores, or at restaurants. In other words, you may become your partner's interpreter. You may find yourself handling all of the telephone calls and taking responsibility for all of the business transactions. At best, this can make shared activities less enjoyable; at worst, it can change the relationship dynamic and cause resentment. In any case, it's not a long-term solution for hearing loss.

Untreated hearing loss can also affect romance. It can cause feelings of inadequacy, low self-esteem, and diminished self-worth—and these feelings can affect intimacy and sexuality. Although getting help for hearing loss is the very thing that will turn these feelings around, it's also the very thing people resist. People fear that acknowledging hearing loss will mean getting hearing aids, and that hearing aids will make them less feminine, less masculine, less sexy. To be sure, our society places tremendous value on attractiveness that's unattainable and youth that's unsustainable. Women are expected to be beautiful and alluring. Men are expected to be strong and virile. Sexy means young, and hearing aids say *old*. Any expert will tell you, however, that a healthy sex life is actually built on intimacy, and intimacy is based on communication. Instead of inhibiting romance, hearing aids can actually encourage it. Sergei Kochkin, President of the Better Hearing Institute, put it this way: "The best aphrodisiac in the world is effective communication. When you can listen to another person and respond to that person as a unique individual, you affirm their existence. When you affirm your significant other's existence, this facilitates intimacy. You might say then that modern hearing instruments are Viagra for the ears!"[11]

Hearing Aids and Romance

My friend told me about his fear that his wife, who is 9 years younger, would see him as an "old man" when he got hearing aids. For the most part, he feels that fear was unfounded; however, he admits that he still wonders if his hearing aids make her feel that he's growing old.

That being said, hearing loss does present practical challenges when it comes to romance. A partner with hearing loss may be too tired for intimacy, or he may miss cues that are intended to lead to intimacy. Timing can be thrown off, and spontaneity may be lost. Pillow talk may be impossible in a dark room without hearing aids. Some of these problems can be discussed ahead of time. Both partners, however, must be willing to talk honestly about their feelings—with compassion, mutual respect, and a sense of humor. Talking with a counselor who understands the implications of hearing loss can also be helpful for couples who are struggling to adjust.

There's no doubt about it; living with hearing loss can be difficult. But living with someone who has a hearing loss can be difficult too. Without meaning to, people who don't hear well may *appear* thoughtless or inconsiderate. Because they haven't heard correctly, they may do the very thing that you've just asked them not to do, they may appear to ignore your questions or requests for assistance, they may seem oblivious to feelings that you've shared, or they may unknowingly interrupt you. You may grow weary of repeating what you've said (as well as what everyone else has said), speaking loudly, hearing your partner speak loudly, stopping what *you're* doing and going to face your partner when you want to communicate, or hearing the blare of the television. You may grow weary of living with a partner who gets tired and irritable or worry about your partner's safety when you're not around. It's easy to understand why better-hearing spouses often perceive greater difficulty *before* and greater benefit *after* a hearing aid fitting than do their partners with hearing loss.

Of course, spouses aren't the only ones affected by a family member's untreated hearing loss. If you have young children, you know that getting them to talk about sensitive issues or confide in you about their feelings can be difficult. These important conversations can be even harder for a parent who cannot hear well. There are times when every youngster is reluctant to repeat what he has just said, to look a parent in the eye, or to use a strong, clear voice. Adult children may have different concerns. They may worry about the safety of a parent who's unable to hear the doorbell, the telephone, the smoke alarm, or an intruder. They may feel disappointed that phone calls, once pleasant times for sharing and catching up, have become times for shouting and repeating bits and pieces of information. Communicating with grandchildren can be especially challenging. Small children have high-pitched voices, making it particularly difficult for most adults with hearing loss to hear them. Their speech is also immature, and they can be shy. A grandparent's inability to communicate with his grandchildren can cause disappointment for all three generations.

How to Help Your Partner with Hearing Loss

- Encourage her to accept hearing loss as a fact of life—let her know that the problem affects both of you and that together you'll find solutions.
- Learn how to improve communication between the two of you (see Chapter 10).
- Don't let him give up or withdraw.
- Encourage your partner to have a hearing evaluation (see Chapter 4) and go with her to all audiology appointments (another pair of eyes and ears can be very helpful).
- Encourage him to follow the audiologist's recommendations for treatment.
- If the recommendations include a trial with hearing aids (see Chapter 7), listen carefully to the audiologist's advice about realistic expectations and adjustment to hearing aids. Use this information to encourage your partner to give hearing aids a fair chance during the trial period.
- Learn about hearing assistance technology (see Chapter 9) and hearing rehabilitation (see Chapter 10).
- To the extent possible, accept your partner's emotional responses to hearing loss and hearing aids. Understand the challenges and fatigue that she is likely to experience. Like anything else, using hearing aids becomes easier with practice.
- Read on for much more advice.

STAYING IN THE GAME

If you want to live life to the fullest, you're going to have to find ways to live with your hearing loss. This book tells you how to do that.

Some of the information in this book can't be explained without discussing auditory structures and their functions; therefore, the next chapter provides very basic information about auditory anatomy and physiology.

Reading it makes the chapters that follow easier to understand. However, if that prospect strikes you as painful, you can always refer to the Subject Index to locate the information you need in Chapter 3.

The first step toward addressing your hearing loss is to have a qualified audiologist thoroughly evaluate your hearing. You should choose an audiologist as carefully as you would choose a physician. You need an audiologist you can trust, in whom you have confidence, and with whom you feel comfortable communicating. Information about what to look for in an audiologist is included in Chapters 4 and 7.

After your hearing evaluation, the audiologist will explain your test results and make recommendations. It's possible that the explanation will be too fast, too technical, or just too much at one time, making you feel a little overwhelmed. If you can, read the information in Chapter 4 *before* your hearing test. Doing so will make it easier to understand the results and ask good questions. *During* your appointment, ask if you can take a copy of the test results with you. *After* the hearing evaluation, use the information in Chapter 4 to review the results at your own pace. If new questions arise, you can always follow up with your audiologist at that time. If you've already had a hearing evaluation, contact your audiologist now and ask for a copy of the report. Use the report and the information in Chapter 4 to gain a better understanding of your hearing loss.

Your audiologist will tell you if it's necessary or advisable to see a physician about your hearing loss. Five to ten percent of all hearing losses are caused by medical conditions that can be diagnosed and treated by a physician (for example, an ear infection). When no medical condition exists, your audiologist can explain the probable cause of your hearing loss based on your test results and the history you provide (for example, hearing loss due to aging or noise exposure). If you're like most people, you'll want to learn more about the condition(s) responsible for your hearing problem. Chapter 5 provides information about common causes of hearing loss in adults.

Many people with hearing loss (and some without it) are plagued by noises in their ears (often described as high-pitched ringing). Such noise is called *tinnitus*. Everyone experiences tinnitus on occasion, but for some people it's constant and nearly unbearable. Chapter 6 contains information about tinnitus and the techniques being used to manage it.

Based on the results of your hearing test and the information that you share with your audiologist, he will make recommendations about the steps that should be taken next. These recommendations may or may not include a trial with hearing aids (see Chapter 7). The audiologist's recommendations are based on the nature of your hearing loss, the demands that your lifestyle places on your hearing, your feelings about wearing hearing aids, and other factors. When talking with your audiologist, it's important to be honest about your motivation, preferences, and expectations. Not everyone is driven to hear.

What Are Your Listening Needs?[12]
At home . . .

- What is your current living situation? Dormitory? Apartment? House? Retirement community? Assisted-living facility? Nursing home?
- Do you live alone? With another person? With children? With grandchildren?
- Is there a need to communicate from upstairs to downstairs, or across several rooms?
- Do you watch television?
- Do you spend a lot of time on the telephone?
- Are there people in your life who are more difficult to hear than others?
- Do you have difficulty hearing the doorbell? The telephone? The smoke alarm?
- What is your most challenging hearing problem at home?

At work . . .

- What is your work environment like? Noisy? Quiet? Large office? Small office? Vehicle? Outside?
- How much interaction with people does your job require?
- How much telephone use does your job require? Which type of telephone do you use? Landline? Speakerphone? Cell phone?
- Do you handle voice messages?
- Do you take dictation from a phone or recorder?
- Do you attend meetings? Lectures? Seminars?
- Do you give presentations?
- Do you run meetings?
- Do you work with small children?
- Is it necessary for you to hear noises and signals produced by machinery?
- Are there situations (or people) in your work environment that make communication especially difficult?
- Is your employer aware that reasonable accommodations are required by the Americans with Disabilities Act (for example, telephone amplifiers or assistive listening devices for meetings)?
- What is your most challenging hearing problem at work?

During social and recreational activities . . .

- Do more of your social activities involve one-to-one interactions or interactions with larger groups?
- Do you attend movies, lectures, concerts, or plays?
- Have you ever used an assistive listening system in a public place?
- Do you go to dinner parties? Restaurants?
- Do your recreational activities involve sporting events? Listening to music? Bird-watching?

- Are there activities that you avoid because you can't hear well?
- What is your most challenging hearing problem in social or recreational situations?

You'll be relieved to know that today's hearing aids are not your father's hearing aids. No longer do they simply make all sounds louder. Instead, state-of-the-art hearing aids use digital technology to process sounds in ways that could be only imagined a few short years ago. For example, most hearing aids include circuits that make soft sounds audible but keep louder sounds from becoming uncomfortable. Many include multiple microphones and other programmable features that enable them to automatically adapt to the listening environment. For instance, a microphone that picks up sounds coming from all directions might work best in a quiet setting, but a directional microphone that picks up sounds coming only from the front might work better in a noisy setting. Contemporary hearing aids are smart enough to understand the environment and choose the best combination of features. Today's hearing aids are even smart enough to nearly eliminate the whistling (acoustic feedback) that's always plagued hearing aid users. All this is accomplished by an extremely tiny computer housed within the hearing aid. Believe it or not, the processing power of a desktop computer is now contained inside an instrument no bigger than the top of a pinky finger (along with its own energy source in the form of a tiny battery).

Digital technology is indeed state of the art, enabling the audiologist to customize a hearing aid to fit your particular hearing loss and to reprogram the aid should your hearing change in the future. Digital technology also offers sophisticated technical features and signal processing strategies. Whether you actually *need* those features and processing strategies depends on the nature of your hearing loss and the demands on your hearing. "Entry-level" digital hearing aids—and even nondigital hearing aids—are perfectly suitable for some hearing losses and lifestyles, and they can be much less expensive. Your audiologist can guide you through those decisions.

Hearing aids come in a variety of styles, some of which are virtually invisible. Among those that are visible, some are now small, sleek, and fashionably high-tech looking. Hearing aid features and styles are described in Chapter 7. Also included in that chapter is nuts-and-bolts information about the cost of hearing aids, where to buy them (and where not to buy them), trial periods, service fees, insurance coverage, warranties, batteries, and other useful information. Chapter 7 also explains why two hearing aids really *are* better than one (in almost all cases).

If your hearing loss is quite severe, the help that hearing aids can provide may not be enough. You may be a candidate for a *cochlear implant*, a surgically implanted device that bypasses damaged parts of the ear and stimulates hearing nerves with electrical current. Training is often required to teach the brain to interpret this new type of stimulation as "sound." People of all ages, including many who lost their hearing as adults, have had great success with implants. Implant technology and candidacy requirements are explained in Chapter 8.

Hearing aids and cochlear implants, although very helpful, have limitations, particularly across distance and in poor listening conditions. The use of hearing assistance technology (HAT) can improve speech understanding in many of these situations. Some of these devices rely on remote microphone technology to improve the signal-to-noise relationship (SNR). With remote microphone technology, a microphone is placed near the desired sound source (for example, a television, a teacher, the stage, a passenger in a car), and sound is transmitted directly to a receiver worn by the listener—without wires or cords. This reduces the effect of speaker–listener distance and makes the desired sound louder than the background noise (improving the SNR and speech understanding). Hearing aids alone cannot accomplish this.

HAT includes systems that are used in public places like auditoriums, theatres, and places of worship, but it also includes personal devices that go practically anywhere. This technology can make it easier to converse in a restaurant, hear at meetings, talk on the telephone, communicate in the car, and watch television without driving everyone else in the house crazy. Assistive listening technology helps people participate more fully in all aspects of their lives and should be considered by every listener with hearing loss. Chapter 9 covers various aspects of hearing assistance technology.

If your hearing loss is quite severe, you may have difficulty hearing things like an alarm clock, the doorbell, a smoke alarm, the telephone, or a child crying in another room. Alerting devices are available to solve many of these problems. Most use flashing lights or vibration to make a listener aware of sound in the environment. Information about these devices is also included in Chapter 9.

Despite the remarkable technological advances of the past decade, there's still nothing that you can buy that's as good as the human auditory system—and that's unlikely to change in the foreseeable future. Fortunately, there are skills and strategies that—when combined with technology—can help to minimize the negative impact of hearing loss. Some of these are things that you can do; others are things that your significant other(s) can do. Teaching these skills and strategies is called *hearing rehabilitation*. Chapter 10 describes the full array of hearing rehabilitation services. Some services help listeners take full advantage of their hearing aids (adjusting to new hearing aids, learning to operate and care for them, etc.). Others involve instruction on important topics related to hearing and hearing loss (how hearing loss affects communication, the benefits and limitations of hearing aids, etc.). Still others involve practicing new skills (combining speechreading with aided hearing, "stage managing" your surroundings to improve communication, etc.). Additional components may include personal adjustment counseling or family instruction and support.

Most people take their hearing for granted—at least until something goes wrong with it. The information in Chapter 11 can help you protect the precious hearing you have left and enable you to educate friends and family members about the importance of life-long hearing conservation. After all, who's in a better position to educate others about the value of protecting their hearing than someone who's already lost some of hers? Chapter 11 discusses the causes of hearing loss that are preventable—primarily exposure to occupational and nonoccupational noise (including iPods and other personal music players) and ototoxic medications. The chapter also covers information about various types of wearable hearing protectors (earplugs and earmuffs), actions that *you* can take to combat noise, and future trends in hearing restoration and hearing loss prevention.

Finally, a section at the end of the book provides resource information for a variety of hearing-related topics. The Resources section is followed by a Subject Index.

My Dad

Sometimes after my family has been discussing something for several minutes, my dad will bring up the very thing we've been talking about—unaware that it's not new to the conversation. It isn't until then that I realize how much he's missing, sometimes even with his hearing aids.

CHAPTER 3

How We Hear: How the Ears and Brain (Should) Work

The hearing ear and the seeing eye, the Lord has made them both.

Proverbs 20:12

Understanding how the ears work fascinates some people, which is not surprising, because the auditory system is utterly amazing. For everyone else, the best reason to read this chapter is that it will help you to understand the chapters that follow. Nevertheless, if you're really not up to reading about hearing anatomy and physiology, it's okay to move on. When you come across unfamiliar terms later in the book, you can always use the Subject Index to locate explanations in this chapter. Before we can talk about how we hear, however, we need to talk just a bit about sound.

JUST A BIT ABOUT SOUND

You may already know that all sound is created by vibration. Pluck a guitar string, and you cause it to vibrate. Strike the head of a drum, and you set it into vibration. Speak and you cause your vocal apparatus to vibrate (you can feel the vibration by placing your fingers on your throat while you talk). Vibrating objects cause disturbances in the air around them that ultimately become sound.

When an object vibrates, the air molecules close to it are pushed away. Displaced molecules bump into neighboring molecules, which bump into *their* neighboring molecules, and so on. Molecules stay in their own "neighborhoods," but the chain reaction of disturbance moves farther and farther away from the vibrating object. In some ways, this disturbance is like "The Wave" moving through a stadium. Fans stay in their places, but the movement gets passed along. In the case of sound, molecules stay in their places, but the disturbance gets passed along. It's this moving disturbance, or pressure wave, that becomes sound when it reaches an eardrum and can be perceived. Both sound and The Wave need something to carry them along. For The Wave, the medium is people; for sound, the medium is often air.

About 300 years ago, a British philosopher asked if a tree falling in the woods makes a sound if there's no one around to hear it. Perhaps you've heard this question before. It's mentioned here to demonstrate that sound is both a physical event and a perceptual experience. Physical events can be measured; perceptual experiences cannot. Physically, sound is nothing more than a disturbance of molecules traveling through air. Arguably, the disturbance doesn't become *sound* until the pressure wave hits an eardrum, causing someone to hear it. Hearing is the experience of perceiving the pressure wave. A tree falling in the woods might disturb molecules over the surface of a huge sphere that expands for miles in every direction, but it doesn't make a *sound* unless there's someone around to hear it. And even then, only the minute fraction of energy that strikes an area the size of an eardrum (about the diameter of a pencil eraser) actually becomes sound.

Every sound has physical characteristics that make it different from other sounds. For example, each sound has a frequency and intensity that can be measured. The concepts of frequency and intensity take on more importance when we talk about hearing testing in Chapter 4. We perceive a sound's frequency as its pitch and its intensity as its loudness.

The *frequency* of a sound is determined by the speed of vibration, and we measure it in hertz (Hz). For example, the sound produced by a piano string vibrating 250 times per second would have a frequency of 250 Hz. We would perceive it as having a pitch close to that of middle C. A sound produced by a piano string vibrating 500 times per second would have a frequency of 500 Hz and would be perceived as having a pitch higher than middle C. Each speech sound is made up of energy that varies in frequency. For example, the energy that forms a low-pitched sound like /m/ is concentrated at about 250 Hz, whereas the energy that forms a high-pitched sound like /s/ is concentrated at about 5,000 Hz. We produce different frequencies (and therefore make different sounds) by varying the way we use our vocal apparatus (vocal folds) and *articulators* (tongue, lips, teeth, nasal cavity, and palate).

The *intensity* of a sound is determined by the strength of vibration, and it's measured in decibels (dB). A *decibel* is a special type of number called a *logarithm* (log). Most of us are unfamiliar with (and intimidated by) logs and logarithmic scales. We're more comfortable with linear scales like rulers and thermometers, in which each step is equal to all the others. But a linear scale isn't a practical way to represent human hearing. The loudest sound the human ear can tolerate is 10 million times greater

Table 3.1. Decibels Compared with Linear Measures of Sound.

Linear Measure of Sound	Logarithmic Measure of Sound (dB)	Common Sounds
1	0	Threshold of normal hearing
10	20	Rustling of leaves
100	40	A quiet library/whispered speech at 3 ft.
1,000	60	Conversational speech at 3 ft.
10,000	80	Vacuum cleaner/shouted speech at 3 ft.
100,000	100	Pneumatic jack hammer at 6 ft.
1,000,000	120	Rock concert
10,000,000	140	Jet engine at 9 ft.

The numbers in each row are ten times greater than the numbers in the previous row.

than the softest sound a (normal) ear can detect. Converting to a logarithmic scale allows this enormous range to be squeezed into a manageable scale and makes it easier to work with the numbers. Unlike a linear scale, each step on a decibel scale is larger than the one that comes before it. Twenty dB is ten times greater than 0 dB, 40 dB is 100 times greater than 0 dB, 60 dB is 1,000 times greater than 0 dB, and so on. In Table 3.1, the numbers in each row are ten times greater than the numbers in the previous row.

WHAT DOES THE BRAIN HAVE TO DO WITH HEARING?

We make sense of sound with our brains, not with our ears. Let's consider our "ears" to be all the parts of the auditory system leading up to the brain (this is known as the *peripheral* auditory system; *peripheral* meaning distant from the brain). It's the responsibility of our ears to pick up and change vibrations traveling through air into mechanical energy—then into hydraulic energy—and finally into neural energy that can be interpreted by the brain as meaningful sound. In addition to making these energy conversions, our ears pass critical information about the frequency and intensity of incoming vibrations along to the brain. But our ears can't integrate tiny bits and pieces of information into a meaningful whole; only the brain is capable of accomplishing that miracle.

The peripheral auditory system can be defined as the auditory structures from the outer ear through Cranial Nerve (CN) VIII. The cranial nerves are twelve pairs of specialized nerves (one member of each pair for each side of the body) that send instructions from the brain to the muscles of the head and neck and/or bring back sensations of hearing, vision, taste, smell, and touch for interpretation. Carrying sound information from the ears to the brain is the responsibility of CN VIII.

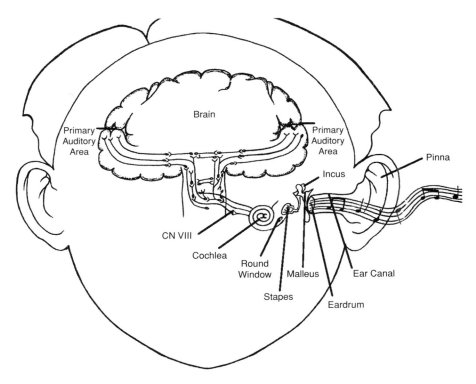

Figure 3.1. The Human Auditory System.

The *central* auditory system (*central* meaning having to do with the brain) can be defined as the neural pathways and neural centers important to hearing within the brain. Problems affecting the central auditory system can also cause hearing difficulty. However, because this book is intended for the typical adult who has acquired *peripheral* hearing loss, the focus will be on the peripheral portion of the auditory system rather than the brain.

Typically, we divide the peripheral auditory system into three major sections: the outer ear, middle ear, and inner ear. In reality, the three sections function as a whole, processing incredibly complex sounds almost instantaneously. This discussion will start with the outermost structure and work inward.

THE PERIPHERAL AUDITORY SYSTEM

The Outer Ear

The outer portion of the ear consists of two structures: the appendage attached to the side of the head that some of us use for wearing earrings and eyeglasses (called the *pinna*) and the ear canal.

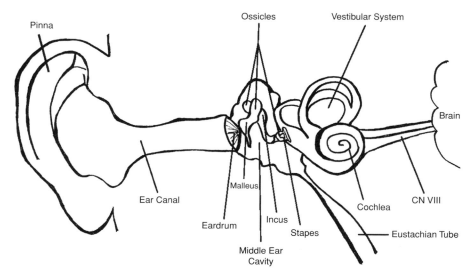

Figure 3.2. The Peripheral Auditory System: Outer Ear, Middle Ear, and Inner Ear.

The Pinna

The pinna is made of cartilage covered by skin. It has crevices, folds, ridges, and depressions. Just like a fingerprint, each pinna is unique. In fact, "earprints" criminals left behind when they pressed their ears against a surface to eavesdrop have been used to solve crimes. The pinna works like

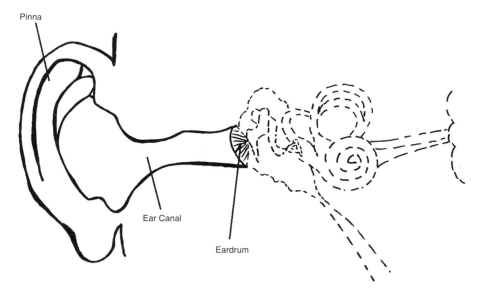

Figure 3.3. The Outer Ear.

a satellite dish, collecting sound waves traveling through air and funneling them into the ear canal. Although many species of animals can actually move their pinnae to catch sounds, that ability has been lost in most humans. The pinnae also help us to locate the source of sounds (above versus below, front versus back). However, in humans, loss or absence of the pinnae does not have a disabling effect on hearing.

The Ear Canal

In adults, the ear canal is about an inch long, with a diameter about the size of a pencil eraser. After taking several sharp turns, it ends at the eardrum (*tympanic membrane*). It's the only cul-de-sac lined with skin in the human body. The eardrum has at least two important functions: protection and resonance.

The ear canal *protects* the more delicate middle ear and inner ear from foreign bodies and abrupt changes in temperature. The outer portion of the canal is formed of cartilage and covered by skin that contains hairs and glands. These glands secrete earwax (*cerumen*). Contrary to popular belief, earwax is a good thing. Earwax makes the ear canal unfriendly to bacteria and fungi that otherwise would grow in this dark, warm, moist environment, and it lubricates the skin, keeping it from cracking or feeling itchy. Along with hair follicles, earwax traps dead skin, dust, and debris. The outer portion of the canal is actually self-cleaning. Tiny hairs sweep earwax and other debris outward so that it can fall out of the ear. In contrast, the inner portion of the canal is formed of bone and tightly covered by skin that does not have hairs or glands. This portion is not self-cleaning. Earwax or debris forced into the bony portion (for example, with a cotton-tipped swab) is difficult to remove. Look for more information about impacted earwax and the dangers of using cotton-tipped swabs in Chapter 5.

> **My Dad**
> My dad has always had trouble with earwax, and he often asks me why. I tell him it's just an individual difference; some people's eyes make more tears, some people perspire more, some people have drier (or oilier) skin, and some people just produce more earwax. A build-up of earwax is often a problem for hearing aid users because the earmold/hearing aid disrupts the ear canal's self-cleaning mechanism.

The second function of the ear canal is to provide *resonance*. Remember that sound is vibration traveling through air. *Resonance* means that some vibrations get a greater boost (or are made larger) than others. This is how it works: the air that fills a cavity (any cavity, open or closed) has a resonant frequency (pitch) at which vibrations are naturally largest. Remember the famous TV commercial in which the opera singer hits a high

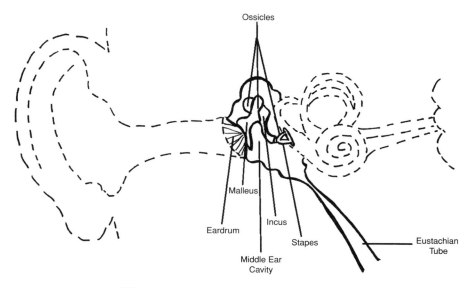

Figure 3.4. The Middle Ear.

note and shatters a wine glass? The wine glass contains air. When the singer hits a particular note—the resonant frequency of the air contained within the glass—vibrations in the air increase enough to shatter the glass.

Together, the cavities formed by the ear canal and pinna have a resonant frequency *range*. It just so happens that the very frequencies that are most important for understanding speech—and those that are most difficult to hear—get a substantial boost as a result of this resonance. Pathologic conditions affecting the ear canal will minimize the boost provided by ear canal resonance (see Chapter 5).

Finally, A protrusion of the lower jaw rests just below the ear canal when the jaw is closed. Occasionally, when teeth are missing or worn, the jaw is misaligned, or a person clenches or grinds his teeth, the protrusion can press against the ear canal and cause pain. This pain is referred to as *temporomandibular joint syndrome* or TMJ. Because TMJ pain often feels as if it is coming from the ear, patients sometimes seek the advice of audiologists or ear, nose, and throat (ENT) physicians (also known as otolaryngologists). However, this condition is best treated by dentists, orthodontists, or oral surgeons with a special interest in this type of problem.

The Middle Ear

The middle ear is a closed, air-filled space about the size of a plain (nonpeanut) M & M. The boundary in the direction of the outer ear is formed by the eardrum. The boundary in the opposite direction is formed by the bony shell of the cochlea, part of the inner ear.

The Tympanic Membrane (Eardrum)

The ear canal ends at the eardrum, which stretches across it like a drum-head. The eardrum forms the boundary between the outer ear and the middle ear and is considered part of both. When vibrations traveling through the ear canal hit the eardrum, they set it into vibration. At that instant, vibrations traveling through air (acoustic energy) are changed into mechanical vibrations (mechanical energy). Although the eardrum is composed of several layers (for strength), it's extremely sensitive. To cause the sensation of hearing in a normal ear, the eardrum needs to move only 1/100,000,000 of an inch—that's one/one-hundred-millionth of an inch—a movement too slight even to imagine.

To see the eardrum, we shine a light into the ear canal from a magnifying instrument called an *otoscope*. The eardrum is semitransparent, so light from the otoscope allows some of the structures on the other side (within the middle ear) to be seen.

The Middle Ear Cavity and Ossicles

The middle ear and the structures inside it form a critical link between the ear canal, which is filled with air, and the inner ear, which is filled with fluid. This link is necessary because opposition to the flow of energy (impedance) is much greater for fluid than it is for air. Without the middle ear, much of the sound energy traveling through air would bounce off the fluid-filled inner ear and be lost. That means our ability to hear soft sounds would be lost as well. To illustrate, try to imagine yourself sitting in a boat and shouting at someone who's underwater. Most of the energy in your voice (traveling through air) bounces off the water rather than reaching the diver below the surface. Without the middle ear, the same would be true of airborne sound trying to reach the fluid-filled inner ear.

The critical link is formed by the three tiniest bones in the body (called the *ossicles*), which mechanically transmit sound energy from the eardrum to the inner ear. The outermost ossicle, the malleus (commonly known as the hammer), is attached to the eardrum. In the other direction, it's attached to the incus (commonly known as the anvil) which, in turn, is attached to the stapes (commonly known as the stirrup), the smallest bone in the body. Together they form the ossicular chain. The stapes fits inside an opening in the bony shell of the cochlea called the *oval window*. The oval window is covered by a thin membrane that separates the air-filled middle ear from the fluid-filled inner ear. When the ossicular chain is set into motion by movement of the eardrum (to which the malleus is attached), the stapes vibrates in the oval window, disturbing fluids inside the inner ear.

Here's how the process goes: vibrations traveling through air hit the eardrum, causing it to vibrate. Because the eardrum is attached to the ossicles, they vibrate as well. The ossicles form a bridge between the eardrum and the inner ear. Movement of the stapes in the oval window passes the vibrations on to fluids inside the inner ear.

Because the eardrum is considerably larger than the stapes (about seventeen times larger), the vibrations are delivered with greater force at the oval window. This boost helps to compensate for the increased resistance that fluid has to vibration. You or someone you know may have some experience with this principle of physics. Think about wearing high heels at a garden party. You step into the grass, and your heel sinks into the soft earth. Your weight is distributed over your whole shoe, but it's concentrated over a smaller area at the heel, and this gives it greater force. As a result, your heel sinks into the grass, but the rest of your shoe does not (if you haven't had the pleasure of wearing high heels on soft ground, ask a friend). Conditions that affect the ability of the ossicles to transmit energy from the eardrum to the inner ear are likely to cause hearing loss (see Chapter 5).

The Eustachian Tube

Air inside the middle ear cavity is constantly absorbed by the tissues that line it. It is resupplied by the Eustachian tube, which connects the middle ear space with the back of the nose and upper throat. At rest, the Eustachian tube (about the size of a pencil lead) is closed; it opens now and then to allow fresh air to replace air that's been absorbed. Normally, this happens about 1,000 times a day when we swallow, sneeze, yawn, and chew.

The eardrum vibrates best (and therefore we hear best) when the air pressure on either side of it is equal (that is, when air pressure in the middle ear is the same as air pressure in the ear canal and outside world). The sensation of unequal pressure is familiar to all of us. For example, your ears have probably felt plugged when you were riding on a fast elevator, driving in the mountains, or ascending/descending on an airplane. That sensation results when pressure inside the middle ear is greater or less than pressure in the ear canal (and outside world). Normally, swallowing opens the Eustachian tube (you feel a "pop"), allowing pressure to equalize and the plugged sensation to be relieved. When the Eustachian tube isn't working properly (because of a head cold, allergies, or infection), it may be impossible to open it by swallowing or moving the jaw. When pressure can't be equalized, it's uncomfortable—even painful. Anatomically, infants and children are more prone to this type of problem than adults—ever wonder why babies scream when the airplane takes off or lands?

In addition to providing middle ear ventilation and pressure equalization, the Eustachian tube permits fluids in the middle ear to drain into the back of the nose (where we can get rid of them) and protects the middle ear from being infected by secretions going in the opposite direction. When the Eustachian tube is not working properly, fluid can fill the middle ear space or an infection may develop (see Chapter 5).

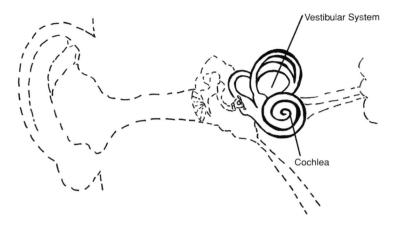

Figure 3.5. The Inner Ear.

The Inner Ear

Mechanical energy is transmitted from the middle ear into the inner ear when the stapes moves in and out of the oval window like a piston. The brain, however, can make sense only of neural energy. Structures inside the inner ear are responsible for converting the mechanical energy coming from the middle ear into neural energy that can be sent to the brain for interpretation.

Two different sensory systems share the inner ear: the *cochlea*, which is dedicated to hearing, and the *vestibular system*, which helps us to maintain balance and posture. The vestibular system contains structures that convert information about the body's position and movement into a neural code that can be interpreted by the brain. (If you're interested in learning more about the vestibular system, refer to the Resources section at the end of the book.)

The Cochlea (The "Snail")

The cochlea (the Latin word for "snail") is extremely complex, incredibly sensitive, and very efficient. It has more than 100,000 moving parts, yet it's the size of a pea. It's a snail-shaped tunnel hollowed out of the hardest bone in the body. Within the bony tunnel are smaller tunnels formed of membranes and filled with fluids. To make the snail shape, the cochlea coils around itself nearly three times. If it could be uncoiled, it would be approximately 1 inch long.

Uncoiled, the cochlea would look like it has three chambers (although two of them are actually connected). The oval window opens into the uppermost chamber, the *scala vestibuli*. A second window located below the oval window, called the *round window*, opens into the lowermost chamber,

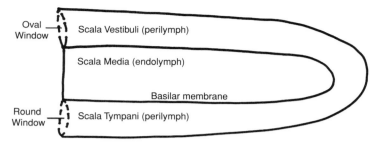

Figure 3.6. The Cochlea Uncoiled.

the *scala tympani*. Both windows are covered by thin, flexible membranes. The scala vestibuli and the scala tympani are connected like a prongs on a horseshoe and filled with a fluid called *perilymph*. When the stapes pushes *in* at the oval window, a wave of vibration travels through the perilymph and pushes *out* at the round window.

Between the scala vestibuli and the scala tympani lies a third chamber called the *scala media*. The scala media is filled with a different fluid called *endolymph*. The "floor" of the scala media is formed by the basilar membrane. Sitting on the basilar membrane are thousands of sensory cells. These are called *hair cells* because each one has more than 100 tiny, bristly hairs sticking up on top. Below the sensory cells are auditory neurons.

Vibration of the stapes footplate against the membrane covering the oval window causes the fluids in all three chambers to be disturbed. A traveling wave forms on the basilar membrane, which runs the entire length of the cochlea. Hair cells sitting atop the basilar membrane ride the wave and brush against a structure situated above them, which causes the bristly hairs on top to bend. Bending the hairs triggers a specific change in the hair cells that, in turn, causes the auditory neurons located immediately below them to send *neural* impulses to the brain. Voilà! Acoustic energy (sound waves traveling through air) has been converted into mechanical energy, and mechanical energy has been converted into hydraulic energy (which is really a special type of mechanical energy), and hydraulic energy has been converted into neural energy. Remember, only neural energy can be interpreted by the brain.

Hair cells in the cochlea are arranged and tuned like keys on a piano (except that there are 15,000 to 16,000 keys instead of 88). This arrangement enables the cochlea to perform a frequency analysis on incoming sounds and to pass that information along to the brain. Hair cells that respond to high-frequency sounds are located in the end of the cochlea closest to the middle ear (the base), whereas those that respond to low-frequency sounds are located in the end farthest from the middle ear (the apex). The traveling wave on the basilar membrane peaks when it reaches the hair cells tuned to the frequency of the incoming sound, and then fades away. This means that

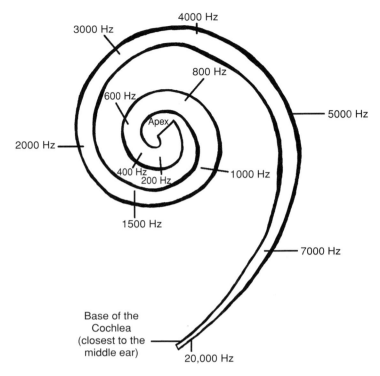

Figure 3.7. Frequency Organization of the Cochlea.

damage to a specific place in the cochlea results in a hearing loss that affects specific frequencies. For example, damage to hair cells in the base of the cochlea (closest to the middle ear) results in a high-frequency hearing loss.

Hair cells are extremely sensitive. Bending the hairs that stick out on top by a distance as small as an atom—the equivalent of moving the top of the Eiffel Tower half an inch—causes a normal hair cell to trigger a neural impulse. But hair cells are also very fragile. Nearly all hearing losses acquired in adulthood occur as a result of hair cell damage. In addition to causing a loss of loudness, damage to hair cells may diminish the cochlea's ability to analyze the frequency, intensity, and time characteristics of incoming sounds. This can cause distortion and affect the ability to understand speech. Hair cell damage can also cause an uncomfortable sensitivity to loudness. There are many causes of hair cell damage, including general wear and tear (aging), the use of toxic medications, and disease (see Chapter 5). A preventable cause is exposure to excessive noise (see Chapter 11). Repeated exposure to loud sounds wears hair cells out; like blades of grass that have been trampled too many times, eventually they no longer recover.

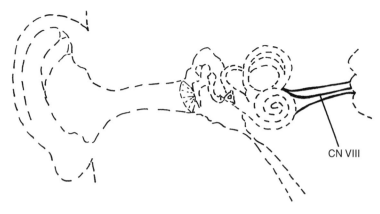

CN VIII

Figure 3.8. Cranial Nerve (CN) VIII.

My Dad
The hearing losses in my dad's right and left ears were caused by different conditions (both of which are discussed in Chapter 5); however, *both* conditions originate in the cochlea. The cochlea is the most common site of damage among people who lose their hearing as adults.

Cranial Nerve VIII

Auditory nerve receptors are located just beneath the hair cells in the cochlea. These receptors send impulses through fibers that join together to make the auditory branch of CN VIII. The auditory branch joins the vestibular branch, and CN VIII travels through a bony canal toward the brainstem—all hearing information enters the brain through this thick band of nerve fibers. CN VIII joins the brainstem at the point where several parts of the brain come together to form the cerebellopontine angle (CPA). It's in the bony canal and the CPA that acoustic tumors are most likely to develop (see Chapter 5).

THE CENTRAL AUDITORY SYSTEM

Once in the brainstem, auditory information (now in the form of a neural code) is analyzed and modified at various processing stations (called *nuclei*) before being sent "upstream" to other stations for further analysis and modification. As an example, information coming from the two ears is analyzed and compared at various stations; the comparisons help us to locate the source of sounds and to suppress background noise in the presence of multiple conversations (we're meant to hear with two ears;

that's why two hearing aids are usually better than one). The brain is able to synthesize and interpret the coded information contained within many neurons, resulting in the perception of sound.

There are many alternative and overlapping pathways within the central auditory system. Ultimately, they all lead to specialized auditory areas located in the temporal lobes of the brain (just above the ears). Because there's so much duplication, damage to the central auditory pathways does not always result in a hearing loss, at least in the conventional sense. Instead, central auditory disorders tend to be more subtle (for example, an inability to locate the source of sounds) and may not be revealed without special auditory tests.

SUMMARY

The powers of the human auditory system are nothing short of awesome. The human ear is capable of perceiving an enormous range of frequencies and intensities. The highest sound that can be heard is a thousand times higher (in frequency) than the lowest. The range of intensities that the ear can handle is even greater. The human ear can tolerate a sound 10 million times greater than the softest sound it can detect. This staggering range accounts for the use of a logarithmic scale (decibels or dB) to express intensity—the numbers would be too large to manage using a linear scale (like a ruler). Remarkably, in addition to being sensitive to a vast range of sounds, the human ear can detect minute differences in frequency, intensity, and time. It's this sensitivity to tiny differences between sounds that enables us to understand speech.

Our ears process extremely complex sounds in real time, around the clock, and often under extremely poor conditions. Sound waves traveling through air are collected by the pinna and funneled to the eardrum by way of the ear canal. The eardrum faithfully reproduces the sound waves that hit it, setting the ossicular chain into motion. The mechanical movement of the ossicular chain sets the fluids of the cochlea into motion, causing hair cells to be stimulated. This stimulation triggers neural impulses that are sent by means of the CN VIII to auditory stations in the brainstem. In the brainstem, networks of neurons act on the auditory information and send signals to specialized auditory locations in the brain. Approximately 30,000 nerve fibers coming from the inner ear communicate with about 100,000 neurons in the brainstem, and tens of millions of neurons in the auditory cortex. Neural information from the auditory system is combined with neural information from other sensory systems and neural information stored from past experiences to produce a meaningful interpretation of sound—all in an instant. In other words, it takes only an instant for the auditory system to transform molecular disturbances traveling through air into the words, "I love you."

CHAPTER 4

Assessment of Hearing: Understanding the Results of Your Hearing Test

Knowledge...is power.
Francis Bacon

This chapter is important because it discusses the ways in which hearing losses are characterized. In particular, reading the sections toward the end of the chapter (beginning with "Understanding Your Hearing Loss") will help you to learn about the nature of hearing loss—a necessary step if you hope to minimize its negative impact.

The tests and procedures described throughout this book are considered "best practices." Although not every test described in this chapter is required in every hearing assessment, *sometimes* practices proven to be helpful are ignored. One example from this chapter would be testing speech perception in background noise. Other examples will become apparent when hearing rehabilitation is discussed in Chapter 10. Nonetheless, knowledge is power. Because better-informed consumers insist on better products and services in the marketplace, educating readers about what they should expect is an important goal of this book.

Like some of the other chapters to come, this one assumes some knowledge about the anatomy and physiology of hearing. (If you haven't done so already, you may want to read Chapter 3.) In this chapter, if a paragraph or section seems too technical, skip it and keep reading. You needn't understand everything to benefit from material that comes later in the chapter.

THE FIRST STEP

If you suspect that you may have a hearing loss, the first step is to arrange for a thorough evaluation by a professional—but whom should you see first—a physician or an audiologist?

Physicians treat *medical* conditions affecting the ear: infections, diseases, tumors, and other problems. However, only 5 to 10 percent of the hearing problems that affect adults are medically or surgically treatable. In contrast, audiologists are hearing specialists trained in the prevention, diagnosis, and *nonmedical* treatment of hearing (and balance) disorders. Their job is to define the nature of a hearing loss and provide appropriate nonmedical treatment in the form of hearing technology (for example, hearing aids, cochlear implants, and assistive listening devices), counseling, and therapy. In other words, audiologists are trained to help people maximize the hearing that they have left (this is called *residual hearing*) and cope with hearing loss. Audiologists see patients with or without a physician's referral; however, they're quick to refer patients to physicians when hearing (or balance) problems suggest the need for medical evaluation. (*Note*: As of June 2008, Medicare beneficiaries currently need a physician's referral to see an audiologist; however, bipartisan legislation before the U.S. Congress would eliminate that requirement, giving them "direct access" to audiologists.)

Criteria for Medical Referral[1]

In accordance with guidelines issued by the U.S. Food and Drug Administration (FDA) in 1977, your audiologist will refer you to a physician if you have any of the following conditions. (Unfamiliar terms are explained later in the chapter.)

- A visible deformity of the ear
- Active drainage or a history of drainage from the ear during the previous 90 days
- Sudden or rapidly progressive hearing loss within the previous 90 days
- Acute or chronic dizziness
- Unilateral or asymmetric hearing loss within the previous 90 days
- Untreated conductive hearing loss (as evidenced by an air–bone gap of 15 dB or greater at 500, 1,000, and 2,000 Hz on the audiogram)
- Earwax or foreign body blocking the ear canal
- Pain or discomfort in or around the ear

In addition, your audiologist will make a medical referral if you have

- Growths in the ear canal
- Lesions (sores) in the ear canal
- Unusual redness of the ear canal or eardrum

- Perforation of the eardrum
- A persistent feeling of fullness in the ear
- Tinnitus of recent or sudden onset, especially in just one ear
- An unexplained difference in speech perception between ears
- A rapid deterioration in speech perception

Physicians and Hearing

Otologists, otolaryngologists, and otorhinolaryngologists are physicians with special training in the treatment of disorders involving the ear, nose, and throat. All three are more commonly known as ear, nose, and throat specialists, ENT physicians, or simply ENTs. An otologist is the most specialized, concentrating exclusively on disorders of the ear. An ENT is knowledgeable about the medical treatment of hearing loss. She should also be familiar with *nonmedical* treatments; in fact, many ENTs are affiliated with audiologists, and in some cases, audiologists are members of their practices. If you see an ENT first, he will likely refer you to an audiologist for an evaluation of your hearing and nonmedical treatment of your hearing loss.

You may feel more comfortable seeing your family physician first, and that's perfectly reasonable. However, your physician may not fully appreciate the significance of your hearing loss, because the typical medical examination involves conversation in a quiet room about fairly predictable topics. Your physician may also be unfamiliar with nonmedical treatment options and might not be in the habit of referring patients to audiologists. If your hearing loss is not among the 5 to 10 percent that can be medically treated, it may be dismissed as a natural consequence of aging. You may be advised to learn to live with it. If your hearing loss isn't medically treatable, ask your family physician for a referral to an audiologist. Alternatively, remember that you can seek the advice of an audiologist on your own (check with your insurance plan first).

AUDIOLOGISTS

The audiology profession emerged at the end of World War II, when tens of thousands of men and women returned from military service with permanent hearing losses. Today, every audiologist earns a graduate degree in audiology from an accredited university program. New professionals entering clinical practice are required to earn a doctoral degree; most of them hold the Doctor of Audiology (AuD) degree. There are also many audiologists with excellent qualifications and exceptional experience who continue to work with master's degrees (usually MA, MS, or MEd). In addition to rigorous coursework, all audiology students are required to complete a variety of clinical experiences and an intensive clinical internship. Your audiologist should be a member of the American Academy of Audiology (AAA) and/or the American Speech-Language-Hearing Association (ASHA). Both require members to abide by a strict code of ethics, ensuring that the services you receive are provided in an ethical manner. Both organizations also have continuing education requirements. A license to practice audiology is required in all states. This is different from a license to dispense hearing aids, which is discussed later.

Choose your audiologist with care. The first step is to check credentials. These usually appear on the audiologist's business card, letterhead, or website, but you can also call her office and ask. The audiologist's name should be followed by her graduate degree (for example, MA, MS, MEd, AuD, or PhD) and certification from the American Board of Audiology (ABA) and/or ASHA (CCC-A). Her state license number may also be included.

Graduate Degrees in Audiology

The audiologist you see has one (or more) of these degrees:

- Master's (four years undergraduate + two years graduate + 9–12 month internship)
- AuD (doctoral level: four years undergraduate + three years graduate + one-year internship). The AuD is a *professional* degree similar to those held by dentists (DDS), optometrists (OD), podiatrists (DPM), and veterinarians (DVM). A *clinical* PhD is similar to an AuD.
- PhD (doctoral level: four years undergraduate + four or more years graduate). This degree is usually held by audiologists who wish to teach and conduct research.

Beyond credentials, you should look for someone with whom you'd want to have a long-term relationship—someone you can trust, in whom you have confidence, and with whom you feel comfortable communicating. This should be someone who takes the time to learn about your hearing problems and how they make you feel. If you think that you might try hearing aids at some point, it's best to start with an audiologist who's licensed to dispense them. In this case, there are more questions to ask, and these are included in Chapter 7.

Audiologists most often work in hospitals, medical centers, and private practices. There are several ways to locate an audiologist in your area:

- Contact AAA or ASHA for a referral (see the Resources section at the end of the book for contact information).
- If you see an ENT physician, ask her for a recommendation.

- If you live near a university, check to see if it has a graduate training program in speech and hearing (you can ask AAA, ASHA or the university); if so, audiology services might be available through a university clinic (this is distinct from the audiology services that are provided at the university's hospital). Services at university clinics are very thorough and allow plenty of time for discussion and questions. However, because they're provided by audiology interns (graduate students in audiology working under the supervision of fully qualified, licensed audiologists), they may take a little more time. University clinics are probably the best places to find comprehensive hearing rehabilitation services (see Chapter 10).
- Audiology services are also available at most hospitals (including university hospitals); call your hospital's information number to inquire.
- Ask friends and acquaintances about their experiences with local audiologists (some of whom are probably in private practice).
- If all else fails, check the yellow pages under "Audiologists."

Other Hearing Aid Dispensers

Not all hearing aid dispensers are audiologists, who must have university degrees and a license to practice audiology. According to the U.S. Food and Drug Administration, the minimal requirements for a license to dispense hearing aids are (1) a high school diploma, and (2) at least 6 months of training under a licensed hearing aid dispenser. Typically, applicants must also pass both written and practical examinations.

Non-audiologist hearing aid dispensers who belong to the International Hearing Society (IHS) are known as Hearing Instrument Specialists. Hearing Instrument Specialists test hearing; select, fit, and dispense hearing aids; and provide on-going follow-up care and counseling. They must abide by the IHS Code of Ethics and maintain professional competency through continuing education.

Some (non-audiologist) hearing aid dispensers are certified by an independent certification board, the National Board for Certification in Hearing Instrument Sciences (NBC-HIS). To become board certified and use the NBC-HIS credential, applicants must have at least 2 years' experience as a dispenser and pass a national competency examination. To maintain certification, certified members must meet continuing education requirements.

When discussing hearing aid dispensers, this book refers to audiologists, in part, because they dispense most of the hearing aids in this country.[2] In some states, audiologists who dispense hearing aids are required to be licensed as audiologists *and* hearing aid dispensers. Always ask about a dispenser's education, experience, certification, licensure, and other credentials.

THE GOALS OF A HEARING EVALUATION

The most basic goal is to determine if your hearing is normal. If it's not normal, it's important to determine where in the auditory system the problem lies and, whenever possible, its cause. If there's any chance that the cause is a medical condition that could be treated, you will be referred to a physician. Other important goals include establishing the type, symmetry, configuration, and severity of your hearing loss (more about those terms later); assessing how much difficulty the hearing loss creates in your life; and determining the steps that should be taken to minimize it.

Each evaluation should be customized to fit the needs of the individual person. That means that it's not always necessary to do *all* of the tests described here; it also means that your audiologist may include tests that are not described here. In any case, this overview will give you a good idea of what to expect. The order in which tests and procedures are done varies from one audiologist to another.

NONMEDICAL EXAMINATION OF YOUR EARS (OTOSCOPY)

The audiologist examines each ear canal and eardrum with a lighted instrument called an otoscope. He's looking for things that could interfere with a complete and accurate hearing test (for example, a foreign body, earwax, or infection in the ear canal; or a hole in the eardrum). If something out of the ordinary is found, you will be referred to a physician—the hearing evaluation may or may not proceed that day. Some audiologists have equipment that allows you to watch a video image of your ear canal and eardrum during the examination. This is fun and much less stressful than looking at images of other body parts during medical examinations!

CASE HISTORY INFORMATION

Audiologists ask many questions; some will be about your general health and the medications you take regularly, so you should be prepared to supply that kind of information. You'll also be asked questions about your hearing: When did you first notice a hearing problem? Did it start suddenly or develop gradually? Has it become worse over time? Do you hear better in one ear than the other? In what types of situations do you find it most difficult to hear? Is there a history of hearing loss in your family? Have you been exposed to loud noise? Do you hear ringing or other noises in your ears? Do you have balance problems? You may also be asked questions about your vision, your ability to manipulate small objects with your fingers, and the type of support available to you at home. There's no need to worry about privacy; your audiologist is legally and ethically bound to keep all patient information confidential.

Because your audiologist is interested in knowing how your hearing loss affects you and your family on a daily basis, you may be asked to complete a self-assessment questionnaire. This information helps to determine the steps that should be taken to treat your hearing loss. If it turns out that a trial with hearing aids is in your future, the audiologist might ask you to complete other questionnaires *before* and *after* the trial period (and perhaps periodically thereafter). This can provide a measure of the improvement that amplification and hearing rehabilitation have made in your life. Audiologists are interested in accountability—or the effectiveness of their treatments—and this is one way to quantify that. Your spouse (or another significant other) may also be asked to complete questionnaires. You should answer the questions independently and then discuss them together. This usually makes for an interesting (and sometimes lively!) discussion.

TEST ENVIRONMENT

The following tests should occur in a commercially manufactured chamber designed to minimize unwanted sounds. The listener is seated in the chamber, and the audiologist is seated at a control panel on the other side of a window. They're able to see one another through the window and talk through a two-way communication system.

HEARING EVALUATION: BEHAVIORAL TESTS

Behavioral tests require responses from the person being tested. For example, the audiologist presents a tone and the listener raises a hand when he hears it, or the audiologist says a word and the listener repeats it. Five behavioral tests and one test procedure (masking) are described in this section.

Pure Tone Air Conduction Thresholds

This is the most basic hearing test. By systematically raising and lowering the loudness of pure tones (*pure tones* are tones of a single frequency), the audiologist measures the softest levels at which you just begin to hear at different pitches (frequencies). Those levels are called your *hearing thresholds*. If you have ever heard people say that someone is "on the threshold of a new life," you know that they are referring to the point at which something ends and something different begins. A *hearing threshold* refers to the loudness level at which the inability to hear a sound (because it's too soft) ends and the ability to hear it (because it's loud enough) begins.

The audiologist uses a calibrated, electronic instrument called an *audiometer* to present tones of various frequencies (pitches) at different intensities (loudness levels). You hear the tones (and speech) through traditional earphones or earphones that look and feel like expandable foam earplugs. You are then asked to signal in some way each time you hear a tone (for example, by raising your hand or pressing a button). You should respond every time you hear a tone (as soon as you hear it), even if it's very faint. You have several chances to hear tones at each frequency (some are loud enough for you to hear, others are too soft), so don't be upset if you think you missed one or if you responded by mistake. The audiologist has a system for taking that sort of thing into account; simply do the best you can.

Although the healthy human ear is capable of hearing across a wide range of frequencies (20–20,000 Hz), only those in the range that's most important for speech understanding are tested. The audiologist measures thresholds at five or six different frequencies in each ear and plots them on a graph called an *audiogram*. Your audiogram is a map of the softest sounds you can hear at different pitches (frequencies) in each ear. Looking at the audiogram, frequencies are shown by the vertical lines (think of keys on a piano), with low pitches on the left side (for example, 125 Hz) and high pitches on the right side (for example, 8,000 Hz). Loudness (intensity) levels are shown by the horizontal lines, with very soft levels at the top (for example, −10 dB) and very loud levels at the bottom (for example, 120 dB). Thresholds are plotted using Os (that might be in red) to represent the right ear and Xs (that might be in blue) to represent the left ear. If you forget those symbols (or any others used on the audiogram), there's usually a symbol key. If, for example, the audiologist determines that your threshold for the right ear at the frequency of 1,000 Hz is 30 dB, a (red) circle will be placed where the vertical line for 1,000 Hz and the horizontal line for 30 dB cross. When all of your air conduction thresholds have been measured and plotted, the audiologist can tell you about your degree of hearing loss (severity), how the hearing in your right ear compares with the hearing in your left ear (symmetry), and the shape (configuration) of your hearing loss (that is, which pitches are affected most and which are affected least). All of this is discussed in greater detail later in this chapter.

Pure Tone Bone Conduction Thresholds

Pure tone *bone* conduction testing is much like pure tone *air* conduction testing (as just described), except that the tones come from a small box (called a *bone vibrator*) that's placed on the bony bump behind your ear (or occasionally on the forehead). If you hold the box in your hand, you can feel vibration when a (low-frequency) tone is presented. Place the box against your head, however, and the vibration becomes sound!

We hear mostly by air conduction in everyday life. Air conduction testing (through earphones) tests the entire auditory pathway (see Chapter 3). The sound wave enters the ear canal from the earphone. When the wave hits the eardrum, the eardrum and the bones to which it's attached (the ossicles) vibrate. Movement of the innermost ossicle, the stapes, causes waves in the cochlear fluids. Disturbance of the cochlear fluids causes tiny hairs on top of the hair cells to bend. This effect triggers neural impulses

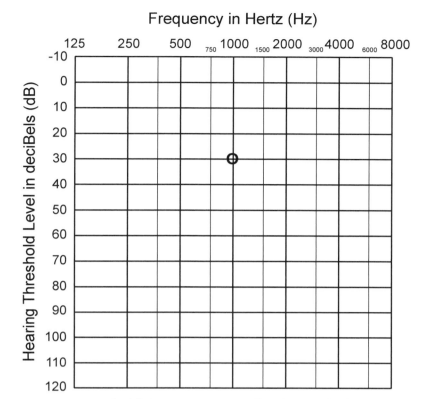

Figure 4.1. Example of an Audiogram. (Courtesy of Brad Ingrao, AuD.)

which are transmitted by Cranial Nerve (CN) VIII and the central auditory pathways to auditory areas in the brain. Voilà! Air conduction thresholds reflect the healthiness of the entire auditory system.

When we hear by bone conduction, the outer ear (pinna and ear canal) and middle ear (eardrum and ossicles) are bypassed, and the cochlea is stimulated directly. This is how it works. Instead of the stapes disturbing the cochlear fluids when it vibrates in the oval window, as happens during air conduction hearing, the cochlear fluids are disturbed when the bone vibrator (worn on the head) sets the bones of the skull into vibration. Because the cochlear fluids are contained in crevices within the bones of the skull, it's somewhat like jiggling a bowl that holds liquid. Fluids inside *both* cochleae are disturbed equally. (No need to worry—you aren't able to feel the bones of your skull vibrating.) As with air conduction hearing, disturbance of the cochlear fluids by bone conduction causes the tiny hairs on top of the hair cells to bend and trigger neural impulses.

Bone conduction thresholds are plotted on the audiogram using the symbols < and > for the right and left ears, respectively (again, red may be used for the right ear and blue may be used for the left ear). Comparing air conduction thresholds to bone conduction thresholds allows the audiologist to determine the *type* of hearing loss you have, whether or not it's treatable, the kinds of problems you're likely to experience, and the steps that should be taken next.

Speech Reception Thresholds

Speech reception thresholds (SRTs) are used to cross-check the accuracy of air conduction thresholds. As with any threshold, an SRT is expressed as a decibel (dB) level. In this case, it's the softest decibel level at which you can repeat very familiar two-syllable words (for example, hotdog, ice cream, sidewalk, popcorn, airplane). The words are spoken at different loudness levels, and some will be too soft for you to hear—that's how the test works. Other times, you'll be able to make very good guesses because the words have become so familiar during the test. Again, that's the way the test is supposed to work. There will be no visual cues (that is, you won't be able to watch the audiologist's face).

Speech Perception Testing

You may also hear speech perception testing called *speech recognition* or *speech discrimination* testing. The threshold tests described so far tell us about hearing sensitivity, or how much *loudness* is missing as a result of the hearing loss. In contrast, speech perception testing tells us about the *clarity* of hearing. Clarity and loudness are distinct qualities. For example, imagine yourself listening to the radio as you drive your car. As you travel beyond the range of your favorite station, the signal becomes garbled. You can turn the volume up as high as it will go, but that won't make the signal any clearer. This is similar to the difference between audibility and intelligibility mentioned in Chapter 2, and it accounts for a common complaint among listeners with hearing loss. These listeners often report that they can hear people talking but they can't make out what they're saying—and talking louder doesn't necessarily help. Sometimes speech is *loud* enough, but it isn't *clear* enough.

Speech perception testing can be performed in several different ways. You might be asked to repeat a list of one-syllable words (for example, up, down, in, out) presented at a comfortable listening level to each ear. Unlike SRT testing, in which two-syllable words become very faint, the words in this test should be easy for you to hear (although not necessarily easy for you to understand). Each word will probably come at the end of the sentence, "Say the word ____." The words are spoken into a microphone by your audiologist or by someone on a recording. In either case, there will be no visual cues (that is, you won't be able to see the speaker's face). Unlike the results of threshold tests, which are always expressed as the lowest *decibel levels* at which you just begin to hear tones or easily recognizable words, the results of speech perception testing are often expressed as percent correct scores (ranging from 0 to 100 percent). Generally speaking, scores between 90 and 100 percent are considered excellent, those between 80 and 90 percent are considered good, those between 70 and 80 percent are considered fair, those between 60 and 70 percent are considered poor, and those below 60 percent are considered very poor.

With the test just described, the words are presented at a listening level loud enough to overcome your hearing loss (often the level is equal to your SRT plus about 40 dB). If you have a significant hearing loss, that level could be quite loud. Using an audiometer, the audiologist can present words at any level without creating the distortion that comes with shouting. Scores obtained under these conditions represent the best case scenario: you are in a very quiet room, listening through high-fidelity earphones, and the words are presented at listening levels loud enough to overcome your hearing loss. Measuring your best performance is essential, but these scores don't reflect the hearing problems that you experience in real life. Therefore, testing should also be performed in ways that are more realistic. For example, testing might also be performed with the words presented at a level more typical of normal conversation.

The difference between scores obtained at an "ideal" listening level and those obtained at a conversational level may be considerable. For example, the ideal presentation level for you may be 85 dB, and your speech perception score at that level may be 90 percent. In contrast, your score at a conversational level (say, 50 dB) may be only 60 percent. This suggests that you're missing a lot at a conversational level (about 40 percent), but that you do very well (90 percent correct) when the volume is turned up. That's encouraging, because turning up the volume is exactly what hearing aids do. This result gives *some* indication of how successful you might be with hearing aids. A less encouraging result would be a score of 60 percent at a conversational level with little or no improvement at a louder listening level.

In addition to testing speech perception at more than one listening level, testing your understanding of words or sentences in background noise also provides information about the difficulties you experience in real-world listening conditions. For example, you may be asked to repeat one-syllable words while you're also hearing people talking in the background. Alternatively, you may be asked to repeat short sentences while you're hearing background noise. The sentences become louder and softer, but the noise level remains the same. In this case, the test result tells us how much louder (in dB) the sentences had to be than the noise for you to achieve a target score of 50 percent correct. This difference between the loudness of the sentences and the loudness of the noise is also known as the *signal-to-noise ratio* (SNR) (see Chapter 9). If you're a candidate for hearing aids, learning about your ability to understand speech in the presence of background noise can help your audiologist decide if special features that are designed to help you understand in difficult listening situations should be considered.

Ideally, speech perception ability is tested at more than one listening level and in the presence of background noise. When you look at your results, be sure that you understand how they were obtained (for example, at an ideal level versus a conversational level, in quiet versus in background noise) and what they mean (percent correct in quiet at an ideal level, percent correct in quiet at a conversational level, percent correct in background noise, the SNR [in dB] necessary to achieve 50 percent correct, etc.).

Finally, if your hearing loss is very severe, open-set speech perception tests (that is, tests in which the answer does not come from a closed set of possible answers) might be too difficult using your hearing alone (that is, without being able to see the speaker's face). In this case, other types of speech perception measures are available and may be more appropriate.

Masking

During testing you may (or may not) be asked to respond to tones and speech in one ear, while ignoring a static-like noise in the other ear. The static is called masking. An important goal of any hearing evaluation is to determine the hearing ability of each ear separately. In some situations, that's not possible without masking. For example, let's say you have normal hearing in one ear and a profound hearing loss in the other. When the audiologist tests your poorer ear, sounds have to be made very loud for you to hear them. As sounds get louder, however, there's a point at which they cross over and are heard by your better ear (actually, they cross over and are heard by bone conduction). When you hear the sound you respond, but your response is for the wrong ear; that is, it's really your better ear that heard the sound, but you respond while your poorer ear is being tested. Without masking, the test results would be inaccurate, making the hearing in your poorer ear look better than it really is. In this situation and many others, the audiologist puts masking noise in one ear to keep it "busy"— that is, to keep it from responding while the other ear is being tested.

When thresholds are obtained with masking in the opposite ear, the symbol on the audiogram changes. For example, a △ is used instead of a O for the right ear, and a □ is used instead of an X for the left ear. Os and △s are interchangeable (both represent pure tone air conduction thresholds for the right ear), and Xs and □s are interchangeable (both represent pure tone air conduction thresholds for the left ear). The same is true of bone conduction thresholds. When thresholds are obtained with masking in the opposite ear, a [is used instead of a < and a] is used instead of a >. When bone conduction thresholds are obtained for only one ear without masking, a ⊓ is used.

Loudness Discomfort Levels

The loudness level at which a sound becomes uncomfortably loud often is referred to as your *loudness discomfort level* (LDL). You may also hear it called your *tolerance level* (TL) or *uncomfortable level* (UCL). Typically, the listener is instructed to signal when a sound becomes so loud that it's uncomfortable—as if a further increase would be unbearable even for a few seconds.

You can use your LDL to find your *dynamic range*. Speech is used as our example, but the same can (and should) be done with tones. Choose an ear and subtract your threshold for speech (the SRT) from your LDL for speech. The difference is your dynamic range. The dynamic range represents the limits of useful hearing. Sounds must be loud enough to be heard (that is, greater than your threshold) but not so loud as to cause discomfort (less than your LDL).

People with hearing loss originating in the cochlea often have a reduced dynamic range. Sounds must be made louder to be heard (because of the hearing loss), but even moderately loud sounds can be uncomfortable. A reduced dynamic range makes fitting a hearing aid challenging because it sets the limits within which a hearing aid must operate. The hearing aid must amplify sounds enough to exceed threshold (so they can be heard) but not enough to exceed the loudness discomfort level. Traditionally, too much loudness has been a common cause of dissatisfaction with hearing aids. Today, most hearing aids have circuitry that allows loud sounds to be amplified less than softer sounds (see Chapter 7).

HEARING EVALUATION: PHYSIOLOGIC TESTS

In addition to traditional behavioral tests in which the listener provides responses, a basic hearing evaluation may include some physiologic measures of auditory function. Physiologic tests rely on *automatic* responses produced by the body rather than voluntary responses from the listener. Although these tests are extremely useful, they do not measure hearing in the perceptual sense. Physiologic measures simply tell us whether "the hearing hardware" is working properly. Four physiologic tests are described in this section.

Tympanometry

Tympanometry provides information about the healthiness of the middle ear. When a problem exists, tympanometry provides information about the type of pathology causing it (for example, fluid in the middle ear, poor

Eustachian tube function, perforation of the eardrum; see Chapter 5). To do the test, the audiologist seals your ear canal with a plug that feels very snug. The plug is connected to an instrument that changes the air pressure in your ear canal. You feel some pressure during the test (as when riding in an elevator), but it lasts for only a second or two. All you need to do is sit still; the instrument does all the work.

Acoustic Reflex Testing

While the plug is still in your ear, you might hear several loud tones. The audiologist is looking to see if a tiny muscle inside your middle ear, called the *stapedius* muscle (the smallest in the body), contracts in response to loud sounds. Believe it or not, that tiny muscle contraction, called the *acoustic reflex*, gives the audiologist information about the healthiness of the entire peripheral auditory system. It even provides information about auditory pathways in the lower brainstem. The audiologist uses the pattern of acoustic reflex results to help sort out different pathologies. Once again, the test should only take a few seconds, and all you have to do is sit still.

Otoacoustic Emissions

Remember the hair cells inside the cochlea? Those are the cells that have tiny, bristly hairs on top that are bent when the cochlear fluids are disturbed; this bending creates an effect that triggers neural impulses that are sent to the brain for interpretation. There are actually two different types of hair cells: outer hair cells and inner hair cells. It's the inner hair cells that actually trigger most of the neural impulses. Outer hair cells work to make inner hair cells more sensitive to sounds by expanding and contracting—or making themselves larger and smaller. Scientists call this the *hair cell dance*. Doing the hair cell dance creates sounds that travel back through the middle ear and out into the ear canal, where they can be measured with a tiny microphone. These sounds, once called *cochlear echoes*, are now referred to as *otoacoustic emissions* (OAEs). The presence of measurable OAEs suggests normally functioning outer hair cells and hearing that's probably normal or nearly normal. Although a problem could still be lurking further "upstream" in the auditory system—for example, a problem with the inner hair cells or CN VIII—these problems are considerably less common.

The test is performed by putting a plug into the ear canal, similar to the one used for tympanometry and acoustic reflex testing. The test is so quick and simple, it's used to screen the hearing of newborn babies before they leave the hospital. Because it evaluates outer hair cell function, and most of the things that cause hearing loss later in life are due to outer hair cell damage, it also has clinical uses for adults.

Evoked Potentials

It's less likely that evoked potential testing will be done as part of your hearing evaluation, but—just in case—here are the basics. The brain constantly generates spontaneous, random, electrical activity (*brain waves*). A portion of this activity can be recorded on the surface of the head using electrodes on the skin. This is referred to as *electroencephalographic activity*, or EEG. In addition to EEG, it's also possible to record brain waves generated in response to sounds that are presented to the listener. These responses are extremely small; therefore, we use very sophisticated techniques to find them in the much larger EEG noise. For example, we record many responses to the same sound (maybe thousands) and add them all together. A single response could never be seen in the EEG noise, but the same response multiplied by 1,000 can be.

The *auditory brainstem response* (ABR) is the evoked potential test most commonly used with patients. Like OAEs, the ABR is sometimes used to screen the hearing of newborn infants. In adults, it can be used to evaluate the function of CN VIII (and in some cases, the cochlea).

Before the test, the audiologist applies a few electrodes to the face or head and in or around the ears. It's necessary to prepare the skin to get a good result. During the test, sounds—probably clicks—are presented in rapid succession through earphones. You don't need to respond to the clicks in any way; the brain responds automatically. The more you relax, the faster the test goes and the clearer the results will be.

UNDERSTANDING YOUR HEARING LOSS

After testing, the audiologist will explain the results to you and, if you like, your significant others. Sometimes these explanations can be a little technical, so don't hesitate to tell the audiologist exactly what you want to know. You should learn about the *type* of hearing loss you have, its *symmetry* (that is, how the hearing in one ear compares with the hearing in the other), its shape or *configuration*, and its *severity*. All of these characteristics are explained later in this chapter. The audiologist will make recommendations about the steps that should be taken next. Recommendations could include a visit to your physician, hearing rehabilitation services, a trial with hearing aids, an assistive listening device, or other options.

Before you leave your audiologist's office, you should know . . .

- If you have a hearing loss
- If you should see a physician about your hearing loss
- The type of hearing loss that you have

- If you have a better ear
- If your hearing loss is worse at some frequencies than others
- The severity of your hearing loss
- If hearing aids can help you
- If there are other treatment options (for example, assistive listening devices or hearing rehabilitation services)
- How the hearing loss affects your ability to communicate
- What you can do on your own to improve communication
- How to prevent further hearing loss

Read on for information that can help you to understand the answers to all of these questions.

DESCRIBING A HEARING LOSS

Looking at the air conduction thresholds on your audiogram tells us whether any hearing loss exists. For adults, thresholds that fall between –10 and 20 dB on the audiogram are considered normal. Thresholds greater than 20 dB indicate some degree of hearing loss. When a hearing loss exists, it can be characterized by its type, symmetry, configuration, and severity.

Describing the Type of Hearing Loss

To determine the type of hearing loss (and therefore where in the auditory system the problem lies), we compare air conduction thresholds to bone conduction thresholds from the same ear. The comparison tells us whether the hearing loss is conductive, sensorineural, or mixed.

Conductive Hearing Loss

Remember that air conduction testing uses the entire auditory pathway. Sound waves from an earphone are sent into the ear canal. When sound waves hit the eardrum, the eardrum and the bones to which it's attached vibrate. Movement of the stapes (the last of the three bones) in the oval window sets up waves in the cochlear fluids. Waves traveling through the cochlear fluids cause tiny hairs on top of the hair cells to bend, triggering neural impulses that are transmitted by CN VIII to auditory areas in the brain. Air conduction thresholds reflect the healthiness of the entire auditory system. In contrast, *bone* conduction testing (in which the bone vibrator is placed behind the ear) bypasses the outer ear (pinna and ear canal) and middle ear (eardrum and ossicles) and stimulates the cochlea directly.

The outer ear and the middle ear conduct sound information to the cochlea, where it's analyzed and turned into a neural code that's sent to the brain. For this reason, the outer ear and the middle ear are called the

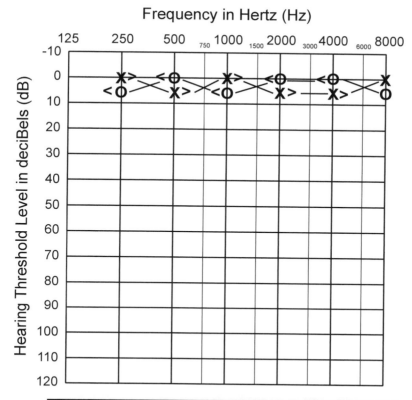

Figure 4.2. Example of Normal Hearing. (Courtesy of Brad Ingrao, AuD.)

conductive mechanism. If there's a problem in the conductive mechanism, bone conduction thresholds are normal, because bone conduction testing bypasses the part of the auditory system where the problem lies. Air conduction thresholds will *not* be normal because air-conducted sound must travel through the entire auditory system, including the conductive mechanism where the problem lies. Therefore, when an audiogram shows normal hearing by bone conduction (thresholds less than 20 dB) and a hearing loss by air conduction, *the hearing loss is conductive.* The difference between air conduction and bone conduction thresholds (in the same ear) is referred to as an *air–bone gap.* In a purely conductive hearing loss, the remaining parts of the ear (the cochlea, CN VIII, and beyond) are perfectly normal. An example of a purely conductive hearing loss would be one caused by an infection in the middle ear.

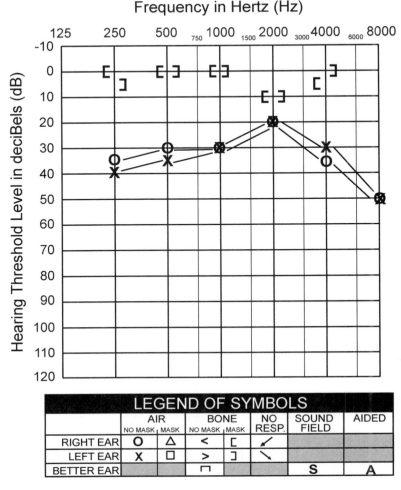

Figure 4.3. Example of a Conductive Hearing Loss. (Courtesy of Brad Ingrao, AuD.)

Sensorineural Hearing Loss

The cochlea is the sensory portion of the auditory system, and CN VIII is the neural portion. Together, the cochlea and CN VIII make up the *sensorineural mechanism*. Although strictly speaking, problems affecting only the cochlea cause a sensory hearing loss, and those affecting only CN VIII cause a neural hearing loss, we say that problems affecting either (or both) cause a *sensorineural hearing loss*. Sensory loss is far more common than neural loss. The term *nerve deafness* is almost always used incorrectly; people mean sensorineural hearing loss (which is almost always sensory rather than neural) when they use the term *nerve deafness*.

Remember that bone conduction testing bypasses the outer ear and middle ear and stimulates the cochlea and CN VIII directly. If there's a problem in the sensorineural portion of the auditory system, bone conduction

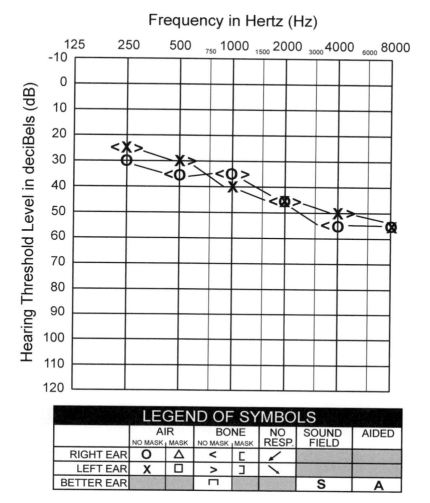

Figure 4.4. Example of a Sensorineural Hearing Loss. (Courtesy of Brad Ingrao, AuD.)

thresholds show a hearing loss, because the bone conduction pathway includes the damaged cochlea or CN VIII. Likewise, air conduction thresholds show a hearing loss because the air conduction pathway also includes the damaged cochlea or CN VIII. Air conduction and bone conduction thresholds will be similar; there will be no air–bone gap. In a purely sensorineural hearing loss, the conductive mechanism is perfectly normal. An example of a purely sensorineural hearing loss is one caused by prolonged exposure to loud noise.

Mixed Hearing Loss

When both air conduction and bone conduction thresholds are outside the normal range (>20 dB), *and* there's an air–bone gap (that is, bone conduction thresholds are better than air conduction thresholds), a conductive hearing loss *and* a sensorineural hearing loss exist in the same

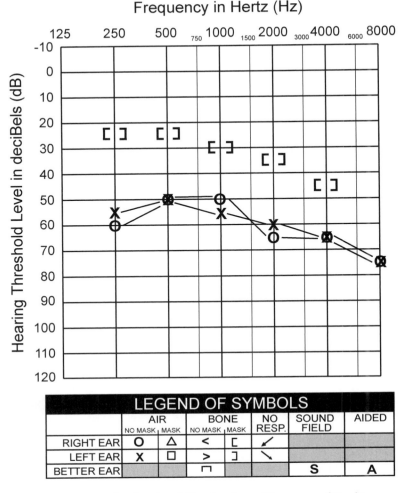

Figure 4.5. Example of a Mixed Hearing Loss. (Courtesy of Brad Ingrao, AuD.)

ear. The result is a *mixed hearing loss*. In this case, neither the conductive mechanism nor the sensorineural mechanism is normal. An example of a mixed hearing loss is one caused by prolonged exposure to loud noise *and* an infection in the middle ear.

Functional Differences between Conductive and Sensorineural Hearing Loss

Conductive and sensorineural hearing losses are caused by different problems affecting different parts of the auditory system. Anatomic and physiologic differences result in important *functional* differences. Functional differences mean that living with a conductive hearing loss is different than living with a sensorineural loss. Generally speaking, the hearing problems caused by sensorineural hearing loss are worse than those caused by conductive hearing loss.

A mixed hearing loss "behaves" like a sensorineural loss (the more troubling type) made worse by a conductive problem. The conductive loss adds to the reduction in volume but generally does not add distortion. It's sometimes possible to resolve the conductive portion of a mixed loss with medication or surgery. In this case, hearing can be improved, but only to the level of the permanent sensorineural loss. A mixed loss doesn't have any functional characteristics of its own. This means that we need to worry only about the differences between conductive and sensorineural losses. Here are some of the ways in which these two types of losses are functionally different:

- In many cases, conductive hearing loss can be corrected with medication or surgery. In contrast, sensorineural hearing loss is almost always permanent.
- In general, conductive hearing loss is more common among children, and sensorineural hearing loss is more common among adults; however, there are many exceptions to that rule.
- A hearing loss that's purely conductive has a maximum; it can't be worse than moderate or perhaps severe. In contrast, sensorineural hearing loss can be much more severe. This means that a profound hearing loss, for example, cannot be the result of conductive hearing loss alone; a loss that severe would have to be sensorineural or mixed.
- Listeners with conductive hearing loss are often able to tolerate sounds that are uncomfortably loud for listeners with normal hearing. In contrast, many listeners with sensory (cochlear) hearing loss find even moderately loud sounds painful. In this case, audiologists say that the listener's dynamic range (the range between the softest level at which a sound can be heard and the loudest level at which it can be tolerated) is reduced compared to normal. This makes fitting a hearing aid more challenging, although state-of-the-art hearing aids can usually overcome this problem with special circuitry.
- Listeners with conductive or sensorineural hearing loss may suffer from tinnitus (noises in the ears or head without an external source). In fact, some people with *normal* hearing suffer from tinnitus for which there is no explanation. Tinnitus tends to be a greater problem for listeners with sensorineural hearing loss, however. Chapter 6 provides more information about the causes of tinnitus and treatments that are available.
- In the case of conductive hearing loss, sound information reaching the cochlea is essentially unchanged except for a reduction in loudness. This means that all sounds are softer, but they are not distorted. If sounds can be made louder (as with hearing aids or an assistive listening device), they're usually quite clear. Sensorineural hearing loss is different. With sensorineural hearing loss, the signal is likely to be distorted to some degree. Even when sound can be made loud enough, it may not be perfectly clear (and in extreme cases, it may be too garbled to understand).
- Conductive hearing loss tends to affect all pitches (frequencies) more or less equally. In contrast, sensorineural hearing loss is likely to be worse at the higher frequencies. When this is the case, the hearing loss acts as a high-frequency

filter, reducing (or eliminating) important high-frequency information. This is an important issue because high-frequency information is more important to speech understanding than low-frequency information. High-frequency sounds contribute roughly 80 percent of the *information* necessary for speech understanding, whereas low-frequency sounds contribute roughly 20 percent. In contrast, low-frequency sounds contribute about 80 percent of the *volume* that allows us to detect speech, whereas high-frequency sounds contribute only 20 percent. When high-frequency hearing is poorer than low-frequency hearing, powerful, low-frequency vowels tend to overpower the weaker, high-frequency consonants needed to distinguish one word from another. So, instead of *hearing* "sit," "fit," and "hit," a listener with high-frequency hearing loss is likely to hear the vowel /i/, /i/, and /i/. In this case, the listener must depend on other cues to fill in what she has missed through hearing. The high-frequency filter effect, combined with the distortion that often accompanies sensorineural hearing loss, creates considerably more difficulty than a simple reduction in loudness. This is the reason why someone with sensorineural hearing loss might say, "I can hear you talking, but I can't understand what you're saying." In poor listening conditions, the problem is even worse.

Characteristics of the Speech Signal as Related to Hearing Loss

Speech is a *broadband signal,* meaning it's made up of energy at many different frequencies; however, the information that's most important for speech understanding is concentrated between 1,000 and 4,000 Hz. Typically, hearing is tested at six frequencies. According to the American National Standards Institute (ANSI), the distribution of speech information across those frequencies is as follows:

250 Hz	8%	2,000 Hz	33%
500 Hz	10%	4,000 Hz	23%
1,000 Hz	22%	8,000 Hz	0%

For most people, hearing is poorer at the high frequencies (1,000–8,000 Hz) than at the low frequencies (250–500 Hz), making speech difficult to understand.

My Mother's Friend, Eve

My mother asks me why her friend Eve seems to hear perfectly well with her hearing aids and my dad struggles to understand with his. She wonders if Eve's hearing aids are better than my dad's. In this case, the difference lies not with the hearing aids, but with the type of hearing losses involved. Eve has a *conductive* hearing loss, and my dad has a *sensorineural* hearing loss.

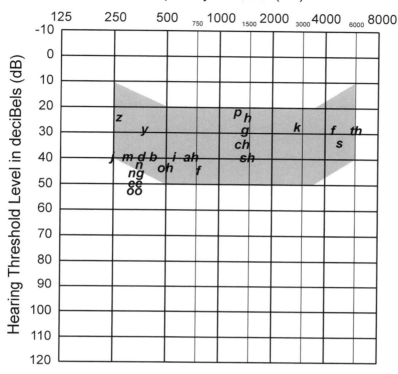

Figure 4.6. Average Frequencies and Intensities of Various Speech Sounds. The shaded area is known as the *speech banana*. The speech banana shows the frequency range (low to high pitch in hertz) and the intensity range (soft to loud in decibels) into which most speech sounds in the English language fall. If hearing thresholds fall within the speech banana or below it on the audiogram, it will be difficult to hear some (or all) speech sounds without amplification. Speech sounds must be made louder to exceed thresholds and be heard. (Courtesy of Brad Ingrao, AuD.)

My Dad
When wax fills my dad's ear canal (a common occurrence for him), it causes a *conductive hearing loss* on top of his permanent *sensorineural hearing loss*, and that results in a *mixed hearing loss*. Removal of the wax eliminates the conductive component of his hearing loss and improves his hearing, but only to the level of his permanent sensorineural loss (that is, to the level of the bone conduction thresholds on his audiogram).

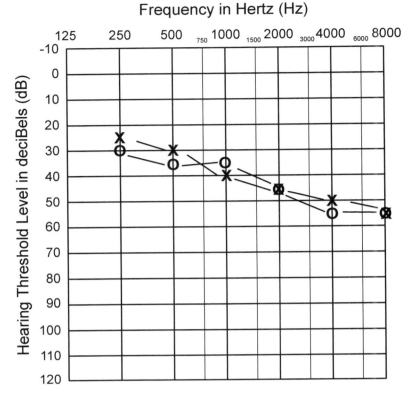

Figure 4.7. Example of a Bilaterally Symmetrical Hearing Loss. (Courtesy Brad Ingrao, AuD.)

Describing the Symmetry of a Hearing Loss

Comparing the air conduction thresholds for your right ear (Os) to the air conduction thresholds for your left ear (Xs) tells us how the hearing in your right ear compares with the hearing in your left. Remember, the farther down on the graph the symbols appear, the louder sounds had to be made before you could hear them. The ear with thresholds higher on the graph has better hearing.

A hearing loss that's (more or less) the same in both ears is bilaterally *symmetrical*. A hearing loss that affects both ears—but is worse in one ear than the other—is bilaterally *asymmetrical*. A hearing loss that affects just one ear is *unilateral*.

A unilateral hearing loss might *seem* unimportant, but it can cause significant difficulty (for example, school-aged children with unilateral hearing loss are ten times more likely to fail a grade than children with normal hearing[3]). The ability to localize (or locate the source of a sound through hearing) takes two ears, making it a problem for listeners with unilateral hearing loss. Unilateral hearing loss also makes it more difficult

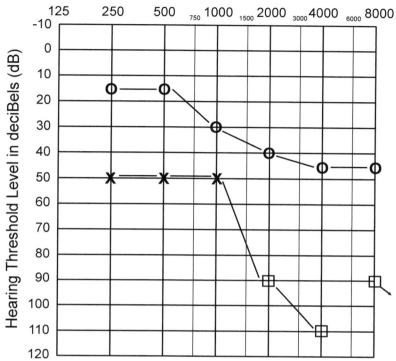

Figure 4.8. Example of a Bilaterally Asymmetrical Hearing Loss. (Courtesy of Brad Ingrao, AuD.)

to hear one conversation in the midst of many, making group situations especially stressful. As the conversation jumps from one person to another, the listener must search for the talker with his eyes; by the time the talker is located, the conversation may be moving on to someone else. In addition, listeners with unilateral hearing loss are often unaware when someone is talking to them on their "bad" side, and they fail to respond. People who are unaware of the hearing loss might form the wrong impression, and think that the listener is being rude.

Describing the Configuration of a Hearing Loss

Hearing loss configuration tells us how much hearing loss there is at each frequency. If you connect the thresholds for your right ear (Os) with a line (like connecting the dots), you'll see that your hearing loss is not the same at all frequencies. For example, thresholds at the low frequencies (250 and 500 Hz) might be normal, whereas thresholds at the high frequencies (4,000 and 8,000 Hz) might fall into the severe hearing loss range. For every hearing loss, thresholds form a shape or a configuration.

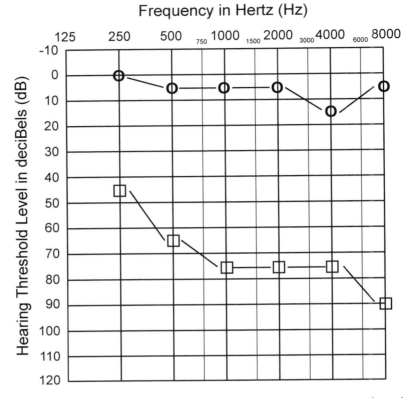

Figure 4.9. Example of a Unilateral Hearing Loss. (Courtesy of Brad Ingrao, AuD.)

Some causes of hearing loss (for example, noise-induced hearing loss or Ménière's disease) are associated with particular configurations, whereas others are not. Some common hearing loss configurations are shown here. Real hearing losses will not match these examples perfectly, and there are many less common configurations that will not match the few that are shown.

- A flat configuration means that thresholds are more or less the same at all frequencies (with perhaps no more than a 20-dB difference between the best and the poorest threshold across all the frequencies).
- A sloping configuration means that hearing is poorer at the high frequencies than at the low and middle frequencies. This is the most common configuration among people who lose their hearing as adults. Because hearing for low-frequency sounds like vowels is good, speech might be loud enough. However, because high-frequency consonant information is missing, it's difficult to distinguish one word from another. People with high-frequency hearing loss often complain that people mumble.
- A precipitous configuration is similar to a sloping configuration, but the difference between good hearing at the low frequencies and poor hearing at the high frequencies is more extreme (this shape is sometimes called a *ski slope*

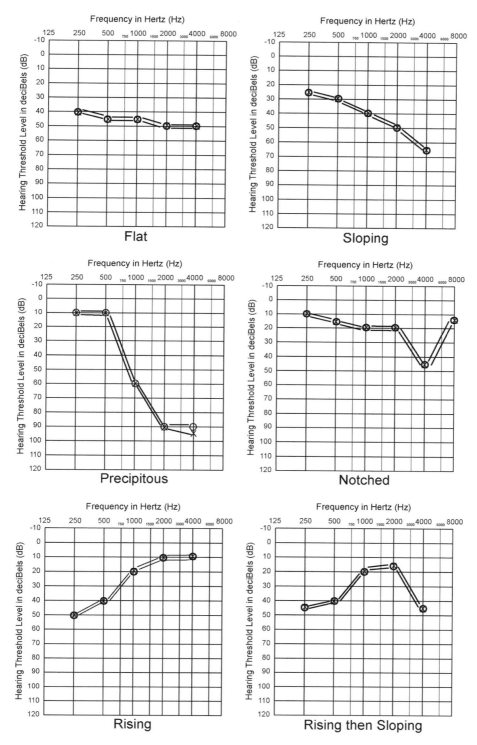

Figure 4.10. Examples of Common Hearing Loss Configurations (Courtesy of Brad Ingrao, AuD.)

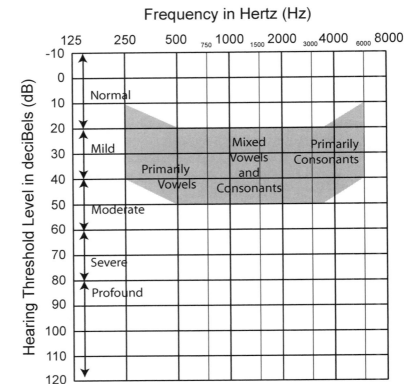

Figure 4.11. Categories of Hearing Loss Severity. Typically, all of the hearing thresholds for one ear do not fall into a single category. For convenience, the category in which the threshold at 500 Hz and the category in which the threshold at 4,000 Hz fall can be used to describe the "big picture." Hearing losses can be described as *mild to moderate, mild sloping to severe,* and so forth. (Courtesy of Brad Ingrao, AuD.)

configuration). This means that problems with speech perception are more extreme as well.

- A notched configuration means that hearing is essentially normal at most frequencies, but there's a hearing loss centered at about 4,000 Hz (alternatively, there may be hearing loss at other frequencies, with a notch indicating poorer hearing at 4,000 Hz). This configuration is typical of the hearing loss caused by exposure to loud noise. Hearing may be adequate in favorable listening conditions, but the inability to hear high-frequency consonants in less-favorable conditions may cause trouble. With continued exposure to noise, more frequencies will be affected, and speech perception may suffer. Avoiding exposure to noise and using hearing protection are absolutely essential.
- A rising configuration is unusual but not rare. It's sometimes associated with Ménière's disease or conductive pathologies. The listener notices a reduction in loudness.
- A rising-then-sloping configuration means that a rising hearing loss affects the low frequencies and a sloping hearing loss affects the high frequencies, with better hearing at the midfrequencies. This configuration is also less common.

Describing the Severity of a Hearing Loss

Air conduction thresholds (represented by Os and Xs) provide information about hearing sensitivity, or how loud a particular sound has to be for you to hear it. In other words, compared with a person who has normal hearing, how much extra volume do you need to be able to hear a sound? This comparison tells us about the *severity* of your hearing loss.

Contrary to what you may have heard, hearing loss is not measured in percentages. Average normal hearing is represented by 0 dB on the audiogram, and the *range* of normal hearing extends down to 20 dB (see Table 4.1). The farther from the top of the graph your thresholds are, the louder sounds have to be for you to hear them. You'll be unable to detect sounds that are higher on the graph than your thresholds.

It's important to understand that any degree of hearing loss can cause problems. In reality, effects vary depending on many factors, including the configuration of the hearing loss, speech perception ability, fatigue, distance from the speaker, and the level of noise in the listening environment. For example, someone with a mild hearing loss in a noisy environment might experience greater difficulty than someone with a more severe hearing loss in a quiet environment.

Table 4.1. Severity of Hearing Loss (for Adults)

Thresholds in dB[a]	Category	Likely Effect[b]
<20 dB	Normal	Even with normal hearing, may experience difficulty in poor listening conditions
20–40 dB	Mild	Trouble hearing soft sounds; with a 40-dB loss, might miss 50% of conversation, especially in poor listening conditions (if it's noisy, if there's distance between speaker and listener, if it's not possible to see speaker's face, etc.)
40–60 dB	Moderate	Trouble hearing soft and moderately loud sounds; with a 60-dB loss, might miss 80–100% of conversation, especially in poor listening conditions
60–80 dB	Severe	Can hear only very loud sounds; might not hear voices unless they are very loud and less than 1 foot away; might miss 100% of conversation, even in favorable listening conditions; communication without a hearing aid is extremely difficult, if not impossible
>80 dB	Profound	Might perceive sound as vibration; probably must rely on vision rather than hearing for communication

[a] A threshold is the loudness level at which the ability to hear a sound begins.
[b] These effects are very general and will vary widely from one person to another.

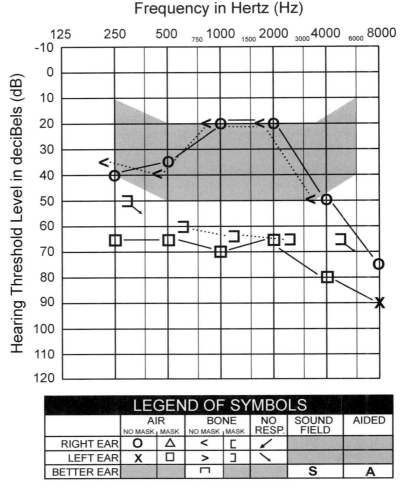

Figure 4.12. My Dad's Audiogram (Courtesy of Brad Ingrao, AuD.)

My Father's Hearing Loss

There's no standard way to describe a hearing loss; however, a complete description should include information about the type, symmetry, configuration, and severity of the loss. Sometimes it can be helpful to include information about speech perception ability and dynamic range as well.

My dad has a bilaterally asymmetric hearing loss. In his right ear, he has a rising-then-sloping sensorineural loss that's mild to moderate in severity. Speech perception ability in the right ear is excellent under ideal conditions. In his left ear, he has a flat, severe, sensorineural loss. Speech perception ability in the left ear is extremely poor (poor enough to make the hearing in that ear unusable). The dynamic range is also severely reduced. A conventional hearing aid is not helpful in the left ear.

CHAPTER 5

What Can Go Wrong: Causes of Hearing Loss and Auditory Disorders in Adults

The music in my heart I bore,
Long after it was heard no more.
Rob Roy's Grave,
William Wordsworth

This chapter includes brief descriptions of many of the conditions that cause hearing loss in adults. These descriptions are arranged according to the structures that are affected, going from outermost (starting with the pinna) to innermost (ending with the central auditory system; see Figures 3.1 and 3.2 in Chapter 3). You can choose to read the whole chapter, or only the sections that relate specifically to you and your hearing problems.

Once again, this chapter assumes some knowledge of the anatomy and physiology of hearing. If you come across terms with which you're unfamiliar, use the Subject Index to locate the information that you need in Chapter 3.

A QUICK REVIEW: CONDUCTIVE, SENSORINEURAL, AND MIXED HEARING LOSS

The pinna, ear canal, and middle ear system form what's called the *conductive mechanism* (see Figures 3.3 and 3.4 in Chapter 3). The middle ear system includes the air-filled middle ear cavity; the eardrum; the ossicles; several tendons, ligaments, and muscles; the Eustachian tube; and the oval and round windows. The pinna, ear canal, and middle ear structures are responsible for *conducting* sound energy from the air that surrounds us to the cochlea, where it's converted into a neural code that can be interpreted by the brain. Problems affecting outer or middle ear structures cause a conductive hearing loss. In a purely conductive hearing loss, the cochlea, Cranial Nerve (CN) VIII, and the central auditory pathways are normal.

The cochlea and CN VIII make up the *sensorineural mechanism* (see Figures 3.5 and 3.8 in Chapter 3). Problems affecting either (or both) cause a sensorineural hearing loss. In a purely sensorineural hearing loss, the conductive mechanism is normal.

When problems involving the conductive *and* sensorineural mechanisms occur in the same ear, a mixed hearing loss results. Neither the conductive mechanism nor the sensorineural mechanism is normal.

You may wish to review Chapter 4 for information about the functional differences between these types of hearing loss and how they are distinguished on an audiogram.

Causes of Conductive Hearing Loss

In many cases, problems affecting the outer and middle ear structures are medical conditions that can be remedied. With medical treatment, hearing can often be restored to normal. Some of the problems included here, for example skin cancers that occur on the pinna, do not necessarily cause hearing loss. They're mentioned because they're fairly common and require prompt medical attention.

Carcinomas (Cancers)

Skin cancer is the most common form of cancer. The three main types, from least dangerous to most dangerous, are basal cell carcinoma, squamous cell carcinoma, and melanoma. Basal and squamous cell cancers are far more common than melanoma, particularly on or around the ears. Melanoma is considerably more dangerous because it can quickly spread (metastasize) to other parts of the body.

Most skin cancers are caused by exposure to the sun (or tanning lights and lamps). People who have fair skin or greater exposure (for example, those who sunbathe or work outdoors) are at increased risk. With early detection, treatment is usually successful—but prevention is the best cure. Prevention includes minimizing exposure to the sun and monitoring the skin for new or changing lesions.

Basal cell carcinoma is the most common form of skin cancer. These tumors are most commonly found on sun-exposed areas such as the face, neck, chest, back, and scalp. Although they rarely spread to other parts of the body, they can cause damage when they grow and invade nearby tissues and structures. Left untreated, they can cause disability and disfigurement (especially when located near the nose, eyes, and ears).

Squamous cell carcinomas are less common, but they often occur on the pinna and in the ear canal. This type of tumor can spread to the middle ear, mastoid, or other areas of the head and neck (for example, the lymph nodes) and have serious consequences if not removed. Call your physician if you notice changes in an existing lesion or you discover a new one. Lesions that bleed easily or don't heal well are highly suspicious. If a cancer is identified, your doctor will discuss treatment options with you. With early detection, the prognosis is excellent; however, additional occurrences are common, so it's important that both you and your doctor check your skin regularly. Remember, if you're suspicious about a lesion of *any* sort, have it evaluated.

My Husband, Harry

Harry had what looked like a small sore with a scab in the bowl of his pinna. It didn't heal, and it often bled when he washed his ears. We visited a dermatologist, who told us that it was nothing to worry about. Months passed, and I insisted that he go back. When he finally did, we learned that it was a basal cell carcinoma. Although the part that was visible was still quite tiny, the cancer had advanced beyond the stage in which it could be removed with a simple surgical procedure performed in the office. The tumor was removed at a surgical center using the Mohs technique. Afterward, the dermatologist warned us not to wait so long before having something suspicious checked in the future (apparently, he had no memory of our earlier visit). Obviously, it pays to be persistent. Because additional occurrences are common, Harry has to visit the dermatologist every 6 months—or sooner when something suspicious turns up.

Earwax (Cerumen) in the Ear Canal

Only when the ear canal becomes completely blocked (impacted) by wax does a conductive hearing loss result (like water, sound will find any opening and pass through it). In addition to hearing loss, impacted wax can cause discomfort, a feeling of fullness, dizziness, or tinnitus (noises in the ear; see Chapter 6).

Earwax is produced by glands located under the skin that lines the outer portion of the ear canal. In that part of the canal, earwax is beneficial. It repels water, acts as a lubricant, and protects the eardrum from dust, dirt, and insects—even bacteria. The outer portion of the ear canal is self-cleaning; tiny hairs constantly sweep wax and debris outward. Picture wax (and the dirt it takes with it) on a conveyer belt working its way to the edge of the ear canal, where it falls out or can be wiped away. Unfortunately, some people have problems with wax. Perhaps they produce too much, it doesn't work its way out of the ear canal the way it should, or they actually *create* problems by overzealous cleaning (too little wax can make the ear canal dry and itchy).

Wax impaction is most likely to occur when something (like a cotton-tipped swab) is used to clean the ear canal. This disrupts the canal's self-cleaning mechanism by pushing wax and debris in the wrong direction (farther into the ear). Although cotton swabs will remove some of the wax, they can push the rest into the inner portion of the canal where there's no self-cleaning mechanism and it's far more difficult to remove. With continued pushing and packing, the canal can become blocked. Wax can become lodged against the eardrum, affecting its movement and causing hearing loss. In some cases, the eardrum can be punctured (perforated), and the ossicles can be damaged (discussed later in this chapter). Using "tools" like cotton swabs (or hair pins, paper clips, pencils, pens, matchsticks, toothpicks, or tweezers) to "clean" the ear can also injure the skin lining the canal, leaving it open to infection. The old adage that you should never put anything smaller than your elbow into your ear is absolutely true. The best way to clean your ear is to put a washcloth over your finger and gently wash the part of the ear you can reach.

Removing wax with instruments should be left to professional healthcare workers. However, you can try removing wax at home using a few drops of mineral oil, baby oil, or glycerin or by using one of the earwax-removal products available at your local drug store or supermarket. In either case, be sure to check with your doctor first, because using these products would be dangerous if you had a hole in your eardrum. If home treatment doesn't work, see your physician or an audiologist who's qualified to do wax removal.

Ear Candling

Ear candling involves using the heat produced by a lighted candle to soften earwax, making it easier to remove. This home remedy has been shown to be ineffective, and it can be dangerous. People have been burned.

Wax build-up is a particular problem for hearing aid users because the presence of something in the ear canal prevents wax from moving outward. When a hearing aid (or earmold) is pushed into the canal, wax clings to it. Wax often clogs hearing aid components and keeps them from working properly. In fact, wax is the most common reason for hearing aid repair. If you're a hearing aid user, you should check for wax in your hearing aid (or earmold and tubing) every day.

My Dad

My dad has always had trouble with wax build-up in his ear canals, and the problem is worse now that he's a hearing aid user. Recently, he complained that his voice sounded "hollow." I suspected that this was due to wax in the ear canal (causing the occlusion effect; see Chapter 7) and suggested that he use an over-the-counter wax removal product. It did the trick. He uses the small wax removal tool that came with his hearing aids to clean the wax out of his earmolds every day.

Foreign Bodies in the Ear Canal

A similar problem can be caused by a foreign body in the ear canal. It's a safe bet that anything that can fit into a human ear canal has already been put there by a child. Adults are more likely to get things stuck in their ears by accident, although there are some interesting exceptions to that generalization. In any case, the ear canal can become irritated or infected (discussed later in this chapter). When swelling caused by irritation or infection closes the canal, conductive hearing loss results. More serious damage occurs when amateurs attempt to remove foreign objects with "tools" (like hair pins or paper clips) and injure the canal. In addition to causing swelling and making the canal vulnerable to infection, the foreign object may be pushed into the inner portion of the canal, where it becomes more difficult to remove (sometimes requiring surgery under general anesthesia). Worse yet, the object can be pushed right through the eardrum, damaging the ossicles and sometimes even the cochlea.

Occasionally, insects become trapped in the ear canal; very small ones can get caught in the wax, and larger ones may not have enough room to turn around and fly out. Resist the temptation to put your finger into your ear, because the insect might sting, causing the ear canal to swell. Keep the ear pointed upward, as insects naturally fly or crawl up to escape. If you're certain that you don't have a hole in your eardrum (discussed later), you can suffocate the insect by filling the ear canal with oil (for example, baby oil, olive oil, or mineral oil). Don't use oil to remove other foreign bodies, however, because the oil might cause them to expand. Instead, see your physician for removal.

Furuncle in the Ear Canal

A *furuncle* is a boil usually caused by a "staph" (staphylococcal) infection of a hair follicle. Furuncles can occur anywhere on the body, but they're most common on the face, neck, armpit, buttocks, and thighs. They're especially painful when they occur in the nose and ear canal. A furuncle begins as a red, tender swelling that later oozes pus. It may drain and heal on its own, but it's best to have it evaluated by a physician. In the meantime, dry heat applied to the side of the head can help to relieve the pain and encourage healing.

External Otitis (Infection of the Ear Canal)

External otitis is an infection of the skin that lines the ear canal. The most common form is *swimmer's ear*, a bacterial infection that typically occurs in people who swim a lot, particularly in hot, humid weather. When earwax becomes wet, it absorbs water and swells, trapping moisture behind it in the ear canal. This creates a dark, moist environment that accelerates the growth of bacteria that typically live on the skin.

Initially, the ear may feel itchy and full. Itchiness is likely to be followed by inflammation, pain, and drainage. The ear canal can actually swell shut (which causes a conductive hearing loss); in some cases, the side of the face or lymph nodes may become swollen as well. The inner portion of the ear canal is the only place in the body where skin lies directly over bone with no subcutaneous tissue, which makes swelling in the ear canal especially painful. The pain usually gets worse when the ear canal is moved (for example, when chewing or if the pinna is manipulated), something that distinguishes an infection of the ear canal from a middle ear infection.

Trapped water is not the only cause of external otitis. As previously mentioned, another cause is infection of a scratch caused by a cotton swab or another "tool" inserted into the ear canal. Infection can also be caused by exposure to industrial chemicals or chemicals in products like hair spray and hair color.

Infection of the ear canal is more common among hearing aid users. Plugging the ear with a hearing aid (or earmold) results in less air and more moisture in the canal, and that increases the risk of infection. Hearing aids that are vented (have a small hole in them; see Chapter 7) allow air into the canal, keeping it dryer. Hearing aids should be disinfected daily and should not be worn during an infection.

It's important that an infection of the ear canal receive prompt medical attention. In the meantime, try using dry heat (for example, a heating pad or a warm cotton cloth) against your ear and an over-the-counter pain reliever. Because these infections have a tendency to recur, be sure to ask your doctor about preventive measures. She might recommend using over-the-counter drops after swimming or showering. Another remedy is to use a few drops of rubbing alcohol and white vinegar mixed together in equal parts. Alcohol keeps the ear dry and vinegar discourages bacterial and fungal growth. However, never use drops of any kind without checking with your doctor first. Under some circumstances, using drops could be painful and harmful. Another common solution is to dry your ears—very briefly—with a hair dryer. Recently, a product especially designed to dry ear canals has become available. The device delivers a gentle flow of warm air for 80 seconds and runs on a rechargeable battery. Check the Resources section at the end of the book for more information.

Itchy Ears[1]

Many people complain of itchy ears, which are often accompanied by dry, flaky wax (similar to dandruff on the scalp). Sometimes the condition can be improved by decreasing the intake of foods that aggravate it (for example, greasy foods, sugar, starches, and chocolate). For relief, doctors often prescribe a cortisone eardrop at bedtime.

Necrotizing (Malignant) External Otitis

Necrotizing external otitis is a relatively rare complication of external otitis that occurs most often in elderly patients with diabetes. It's a dangerous, aggressive condition that can spread to other structures (including the bones of the skull) and become life-threatening—even fatal. Once again, it often begins with an attempt to clean the ear canal with an implement like a cotton-tipped swab. The symptoms are generally similar to those associated with external otitis, except that the infection doesn't respond to conventional treatment. This condition typically requires extensive, long-term medical care.

Eardrum Perforations

An eardrum perforation is a hole in the eardrum. There are three main causes. Eardrum perforations can occur as part of an acute middle ear infection (otitis media, which is discussed later in this chapter). In this case, infected material (pus) trapped inside the middle ear causes the eardrum to bulge outward until it ruptures, allowing the infected material to drain. The perforation is preceded by pain, which is relieved by the rupture. A second cause is trauma with an object (for example, a cotton swab, hairpin, or other instrument). A third cause is a violent pressure change in the ear canal (for example, an explosion at close range, a slap on the ear, an accident in which the ear smacks against a hard surface). In this case, the column of air normally contained in the ear canal is pushed inward, rupturing the eardrum. Less common causes include temporal bone fracture (discussed later) and failure of an incision to close after surgical placement of a ventilating tube (also discussed later). Regardless of the cause, a perforation is usually associated with pain, which should go away quickly, and bleeding, which should stop spontaneously. The severity of the conductive hearing loss varies, depending on the size and location of the hole. Tiny perforations may cause no hearing loss at all. A perforation with significant hearing loss and vertigo (the sensation of spinning or that the room itself is spinning) constitutes a medical emergency, because this suggests possible damage to the inner ear.

Perforations often heal by themselves without complications, but medical evaluation is necessary. The ear must be kept dry, because infection can occur if water enters the middle ear through the hole. Unhealed perforations invite infection and increase the risk that a pseudotumor called a *cholesteatoma* will develop (discussed later). Perforations that don't heal spontaneously may require patching or more extensive reconstructive surgery.

Adults often believe that they've had a perforation for years, often since childhood. Although there might have been a perforation at one time, in many cases it's long since healed. Your doctor can tell you if a perforation exists.

Otosclerosis

Otosclerosis is a disease in which normal bone is replaced with new, abnormal bone. Initially, the new bone is soft and spongy, but over time it becomes hard and dense. The primary site of the disease is the oval window. (Remember, the stapes fits into the oval window. Vibration of the eardrum and ossicles causes the stapes to vibrate against the membrane covering the oval window, transmitting vibration to the cochlear fluids.) As otosclerosis progresses, the stapes eventually becomes stuck in the oval window. A conductive hearing loss results when the stapes can no longer transmit vibration to the cochlea.

Otosclerosis appears to be inherited in about 60 percent of cases, although not all people who inherit the gene develop the disease. It may be that the disease develops when genetic factors interact with certain environmental factors (for example, the measles virus). However, those environmental factors have yet to be identified. The disease process begins in childhood, but the hearing loss usually doesn't become noticeable until the listener reaches 20 to 30 years of age. Otosclerosis is twice as likely to occur in women. Often, women first become aware of the hearing loss during or immediately after pregnancy.

The conductive hearing loss is typically bilateral, but the disease can progress at different rates in the two ears (causing a bilaterally asymmetric hearing loss; see Chapter 4). Generally, hearing at the low pitches is affected first (this is called a *rising configuration*; see Chapter 4). Hearing may become progressively worse until the maximum conductive hearing loss is reached (a severe hearing loss). Over time, a sensorineural hearing loss may also develop, resulting in a mixed loss that can be severe or profound. Tinnitus and dizziness are not uncommon.

A surgical procedure called a *stapedectomy* has a high rate of success. Patients with the best surgical prognosis have normal sensorineural function (normal bone conduction thresholds; see Chapter 4) and good speech perception ability. Only one ear is operated on at a time, and the worst ear is done first. Stapedectomy is performed through the ear canal (no incisions are made outside the ear). The procedure involves removing part or all of the fixed stapes and replacing it with a prosthetic (artificial) device. The prosthesis reestablishes a connection between the eardrum and the cochlea, allowing vibration to be transmitted to the cochlear fluids.

A hearing loss can recur after surgery. This may be caused by a regrowth of otosclerotic bone or displacement of the prosthesis. With a first surgery, normal hearing is restored in approximately 90 percent of cases. Subsequent surgeries are less successful. Additional or alternative treatments can include sodium fluoride or biophosphonates, a class of drugs used to treat osteoporosis by inhibiting the breakdown of normal, healthy bone. Hearing aids can be useful instead of surgery or at some point following surgery. Because the loss is primarily conductive, patients with otosclerosis tend to be excellent hearing aid users.

Otitis Media (Infection or Inflammation of the Middle Ear)

Otitis media is the medical term for infection or inflammation of the middle ear. This condition often results in conductive hearing loss and when left untreated can result in permanent, sensorineural loss—but that's rare. Otitis media is most common among infants and young children; in fact, it's the most common diagnosis for children visiting a physician. There's concern that repeated episodes can negatively impact a young child's development. Otitis media also occurs in adults but much less often.

In adults, the cause of otitis media is a poorly functioning Eustachian tube (see Chapter 3). Remember, the Eustachian tube connects the air-filled middle ear cavity with the back of the nose and throat (the nasopharynx). The tube is normally closed but opens briefly when we swallow, yawn, or open our jaws. The tube has several important functions. First, it allows ventilation of the middle ear cavity. Air inside the cavity is constantly absorbed by the tissues that line it. Opening the Eustachian tube allows fresh air to replenish air that's been absorbed. Second, the Eustachian tube acts as a pressure valve, allowing pressure in the middle ear cavity and pressure in the ear canal (and outside world) to be equalized. Third, the Eustachian tube allows secretions from inside the middle ear to drain into the nose and throat (where they can be eliminated). In adults, the most common cause of Eustachian tube dysfunction is inflammation caused by infection (colds) or allergies. The tube becomes swollen and doesn't always open when we swallow, yawn, or chew.

There are several types of otitis media. More elaborate classification systems and different labels are sometimes used, but generally they involve variations on three interrelated types: acute, noninfectious (with effusion), and chronic.

Acute otitis media is an ear infection of relatively short duration (<3 weeks) that either gets better or develops into otitis media with effusion (discussed later). Symptoms generally include intense pain, fever, and loss of appetite and can also include vomiting and diarrhea. Many times infections develop during a common head cold, when bacteria from the nose and throat move into the middle ear through the Eustachian tube. As the infection progresses, the Eustachian tube becomes clogged and swollen (as does everything inside your head when you have a cold). With the Eustachian tube unable to open and ventilate the middle ear, bacteria multiply and create pus. The growing accumulation of secretions causes the eardrum to bulge outward, stretching it, and causing pain. Without treatment, the eardrum is likely to rupture, allowing the infected material to drain into the ear canal. With pressure on the eardrum relieved (by the rupture), the pain subsides and the perforation (usually) heals on its own. However, most ear infections are treated with antibiotics, making the natural progression to eardrum rupture unlikely. The antibiotic kills the bacteria in the secretions and stops the infection, but it doesn't eliminate the fluid that remains in the middle ear. Fluid trapped inside the middle ear causes a conductive hearing loss. This condition is *otitis media with effusion* (OME), commonly known as *fluid in the ear*.

Unlike acute otitis media, OME is noninfectious. It's characterized by thin, watery fluid in the middle ear cavity (remember, the middle ear space *should* be filled with air). OME often follows an episode of acute otitis media treated with antibiotics. The antibiotic kills the bacteria, but the noninfected fluid can remain in the middle ear for weeks or months. With the infection gone, the patient is no longer sick, but the conductive hearing loss remains. Although this can be a problem for young children who are at a critical stage of development, it usually doesn't cause a significant communication problem for adults (although most find it quite unpleasant).

Otitis media with effusion can also develop *without* a prior episode of acute otitis media. When the Eustachian tube cannot ventilate the middle ear (usually because of inflammation and swelling caused by a cold or allergies), the air inside the cavity is absorbed. As the air is absorbed, the pressure inside the middle ear becomes negative compared to normal, and a vacuum is created. The vacuum causes the eardrum to be pulled inward (retracted). Because the pressure inside the middle ear isn't equal to the pressure in the ear canal (and the outside world), the eardrum doesn't vibrate the way it should, and a slight conductive hearing loss can result. But remember when your grade school teacher told you that "Nature abhors a vacuum"? To relieve the vacuum, a thin, watery fluid is sucked out of the tissues that line the middle ear. This fluid cannot drain because the Eustachian tube doesn't open. As fluid accumulates, it causes a greater conductive hearing loss. If the fluid remains, it can become infected. Occasionally, acute otitis media treated with antibiotics alternates with OME in a repeating pattern, especially in children.

Chronic otitis media is an infection that can persist for months or years despite vigorous and appropriate medical treatment. Over time, infection causes irreversible damage to the middle ear tissues and underlying bone.

The condition is often defined by the presence of a persistent eardrum perforation, drainage, and hearing loss. The disease can be considered active or inactive at any point, but the perforation, drainage, and hearing loss remain.

Complications beyond eardrum perforation and conductive hearing loss can result when otitis media recurs often or progresses to the chronic stage. Today, these complications are the exception rather than the rule. *Adhesive otitis media* (sometimes called glue ear) can result after repeated cycles of inflammation and healing have occurred in the middle ear. Noninfected fluid thickens and becomes gel-like (imagine the consistency of oatmeal), sticking to the ossicles, reducing their movement, and causing conductive hearing loss. *Mastoiditis* is the extension of an infection from the middle ear into the surrounding bone (mastoid). Before antibiotics were available, mastoiditis was a common and serious complication of ear infections (acute otitis media). A surgery called *radical mastoidectomy* was often performed, resulting in the maximum conductive hearing loss in the affected ear. The purpose of the surgery was (and is) to preserve life rather than to preserve hearing. A *cholesteatoma* is a cystlike growth of skin in the middle ear. It sometimes develops when prolonged negative middle ear pressure sucks the eardrum in, causing severe retraction and stretching. A pocket or pouch can form in the eardrum. Old skin cells trapped in the pocket form the cholesteatoma. Infection of those cells (usually when contaminated water finds its way into the pouch) causes the cholesteatoma to grow by shedding and reencapsulating its own debris. As it grows inward, it causes serious infection and destroys bone and other tissues in its path. The ear may drain, sometimes with a foul odor, and there may be hearing loss, a feeling of fullness, earache, dizziness, and weakness of the facial muscles on the affected side (CN VII, the Facial Nerve, which carries information from the brain to the muscles of the face, runs through the middle ear). This is a serious condition that requires medical attention; most cholesteatomas must be surgically removed. Unfortunately, regrowth is not uncommon. *Tympanosclerosis* results from a pathologic scarring process. Tympanosclerotic plaques can cover the ossicles, reducing their movement and causing conductive hearing loss. Surgery is not indicated, because the abnormal scarring will be repeated. *Labyrinthitis* is an infection that spreads from the middle ear into the inner ear. The most common route is through the round window. Symptoms include fluctuating sensorineural hearing loss and vertigo during an episode of otitis media. This condition is a medical emergency that can cause a permanent loss of hearing or vestibular (balance) function on the affected side. *Facial paralysis* is a complication of acute otitis media that usually resolves with antibiotic treatment. When it occurs in conjunction with chronic otitis media, antibiotics are less likely to be effective, and the prognosis is not as good.

Otitis media is generally treated with antibiotics or a surgical procedure called *myringotomy* (see later discussion). With antibiotic treatment, symptoms usually improve in 48 to 72 hours but it's very important that all of the prescribed antibiotic be taken. When infections occur often, treatment options include using antibiotics to treat each episode, using antibiotics to prevent future episodes, or surgical treatment (myringotomy). Because of the increasing resistance of bacteria to antibiotics and the possibility that antibiotic treatment can predispose children to recurrent infections and episodes of otitis media with effusion, many physicians have become more conservative about using them to treat ear infections.

A *myringotomy* is a surgical incision in the eardrum that allows fluid to be suctioned out of the middle ear. In adults, the procedure can usually be performed in the office of an otolaryngologist (ENT physician). The return of hearing is immediate. Often, a tympanostomy tube (also called a pressure equalization tube [PE]) is inserted into the incision to keep it from healing right away. The tube, which usually works its way out of the eardrum in 6 to 18 months, allows air to enter the middle ear while the Eustachian tube isn't functioning. If Eustachian tube function doesn't improve over time, tubes sometimes need to be reinserted (this is less common among adults). Ear tubes must remain open to be effective, but they sometimes become clogged with debris (mucus, dried blood, wax). An audiologist can do a test (tympanometry; see Chapter 4) to determine whether the ear tubes are functioning properly.

Barotrauma

The air pressure inside the middle ear should be the same as the air pressure in the ear canal and outside world. This balance is maintained by the Eustachian tube. For example, as an airplane takes off, the air pressure inside the cabin becomes less than the air pressure on the ground, meaning that the air pressure in the ear canal is less than the air pressure inside the middle ear. This causes the air inside the middle ear to expand and the eardrum to bulge outward. Normally, when we swallow, yawn, or chew, the Eustachian tube opens and air escapes from the middle ear, making the pressure on both sides of the eardrum equal. Even when the Eustachian tube isn't working well, it's relatively easy for air to get *out* of the middle ear through the Eustachian tube. During the plane's descent, the air pressure in the ear canal becomes greater than the air pressure inside the middle ear, causing the eardrum to bulge inward. When the Eustachian tube isn't working well (and can't be opened by swallowing, etc.), it's much more difficult for air to get *into* the middle ear to equalize pressure. When the Eustachian tube can't equalize pressure during dramatic altitude changes (during airplane travel and especially during underwater diving), the condition is known as *barotrauma*.

Barotrauma can cause an uncomfortable, plugged sensation or severe pain; in extreme cases, it can draw fluid into the middle ear space, cause bleeding, rupture the eardrum, or even dislocate the ossicles. It's most likely to occur when the Eustachian tube isn't functioning well, and therefore it's best to avoid extreme pressure changes when you have a cold or allergy symptoms. If such situations can't be avoided, check with your doctor first. She might advise you to take a decongestant beforehand. Avoid problems during a flight by sucking on candy, chewing gum, or swallowing sips of water during ascent and descent. Try not to fall asleep, because you'll swallow less often. If your ears feel plugged, try unblocking them by closing your mouth, pinching your nostrils shut, and *gently* forcing air into the back of your nose (as if you were trying to blow your fingers off your nose). Most patients with barotrauma get better quickly without complications. If problems persist, a myringotomy might be necessary.

Conductive Hearing Loss Caused by Head Trauma

A blow to the head, particularly the side of the head, can cause a skull fracture (specifically a temporal bone fracture) that runs through the ear canal, eardrum, and middle ear. The skin of the ear canal can be torn, the eardrum can be perforated, and the ossicles can be broken apart. The damage can generally be repaired, and normal hearing can usually be restored.

Ossicular Chain Disruption

The ossicular chain can be broken, partially broken, or broken and healed with a fibrous (soft tissue) connection. Depending on the degree of damage, conductive hearing loss can reach the maximum (a severe hearing loss). Damage is usually the result of trauma or disease. In the case of trauma, a blow to the head can fracture or dislocate the ossicles, or they can be injured when an object (such as a cotton-tipped swab) is pushed through the eardrum. In the case of disease, the ossicles can become eroded or destroyed by a cholesteatoma (see previous discussion), or broken during surgery to treat chronic middle ear infection. Reconstructive surgery can often reestablish the connection.

Glomus Tumors

Glomus tumors are the most common benign (noncancerous) tumors of the middle ear. Glomera are tiny, neural clusters that can be found at various sites in the body. They're thought to be chemoreceptors that regulate the physical and chemical composition of blood. Tumors that grow on glomera are called *glomus tumors*. They can cause hearing loss when they arise in the middle ear or grow into the middle ear from the area surrounding the jugular vein (which is located just below the middle ear). When the tumor mass prevents the ossicles from moving, a conductive hearing loss results. Occasionally, the tumor grows into the cochlea or CN VIII, causing a mixed hearing loss. Typically, only one ear is affected.

Glomus tumors are slow growing and rarely spread (metastasize) to other parts of the body; however, they can affect the function of nearby cranial nerves, especially those responsible for facial movement, swallowing, voice quality, and movement of the tongue. In extreme cases, they can invade the brainstem or brain. Women are more likely to have glomus tumors, and they appear to be to be inherited in at least some cases.

Because these tumors have a rich blood supply, the first symptom is sometimes tinnitus that's synchronized with the patient's heartbeat (called *pulsatile tinnitus*). When the ear is examined with an otoscope, a reddish mass behind the eardrum that appears to pulsate with the patient's heartbeat can often be seen. Other symptoms may include pain and a feeling of fullness in the affected ear. Treatment typically involves surgery.

Causes of Sensory Hearing Loss

As discussed, problems that affect the cochlea or CN VIII cause *sensorineural* hearing loss. More specifically, problems that affect the cochlea cause *sensory* hearing loss, and those that affect CN VIII cause *neural* hearing loss. However, because sensory and neural hearing losses can't be differentiated without special tests, they're usually grouped together and labeled *sensorineural*. The problems that are described first primarily affect the cochlea. In most cases, these losses are permanent.

Hereditary (Genetic) Hearing Loss

This book focuses on hearing loss that begins in adulthood. We usually think of hereditary hearing loss as being congenital (present at birth); however, some cases don't become apparent until later in life. Mutations that can lead to hearing loss have already been discovered in more than fifty different genes; scientists predict they will identify many more. Although researchers have identified many of the genes responsible for childhood deafness, those responsible for hearing loss that develops later in life are not as well understood.

Approximately 30,000 genes determine our personal characteristics by providing a blueprint for the way we develop and function throughout life. Genes occur in pairs—one member of each pair is inherited from each parent. Genetic hearing loss can involve a single pair of genes (and the particular pair may differ from one person to the next), an interaction among multiple gene pairs, or interactions between genetic and environmental factors (for example, exposure to aminoglycoside antibiotics appears to trigger a particular type of genetic hearing loss). In fact, the degree to which factors such as aging, noise exposure, ototoxic drugs, or some combination of those factors will affect your hearing probably depends on your genetic make-up. This means that you and a friend could be exposed to the same noise (or the same drug) for the same length of time, but only one of you will develop a hearing loss. One of you is more susceptible to damage than the other, and that difference is probably genetic.

The two genes that form a pair may give the same instructions or different instructions. For example, let's say that eye color is determined by a single pair of genes. Both genes in the eye color pair may give the same instructions—like brown and brown. Alternatively, the two genes might give different instructions—like brown and blue. A gene is *dominant* if its effect shows up even when the other gene in the pair gives different instructions (for example, the brown-eye effect might dominate the blue-eye effect).

In the case of dominantly inherited hearing loss, a gene for hearing loss dominates a gene for normal hearing; hearing loss will appear even though the instructions from the other gene in a pair are for normal hearing. In most cases, a person with this type of hearing loss has a parent with a similar hearing loss. In other words, there are no *carriers* or parents who don't have hearing loss themselves but pass it on. Because the affected parent has one dominant gene for hearing loss and one gene for normal hearing, with each conception there's a 50–50 chance that he or she will contribute the gene for hearing loss. This gene will dominate the gene for normal hearing contributed by the normally hearing parent, meaning that with each pregnancy there's a 50 percent chance the child will have a hearing loss. This type of inheritance accounts for approximately 15 to 20 percent of all genetic hearing losses.

Another 70 to 80 percent of genetic hearing losses are recessively inherited (the few remaining cases are due to all other forms of genetic inheritance combined). With recessive inheritance, an effect appears only when both genes in a pair give the same instructions (for example, blue eyes and blue eyes). The affected person's parents typically have normal hearing. Each parent *carries* a gene for hearing loss, but it's dominated by the paired gene for normal hearing. Hearing loss occurs only when two carriers mate and each contributes the gene for hearing loss to their child. Thus, a person with recessively inherited hearing loss ends up with *two* genes for hearing loss in a gene pair. When normally-hearing parents carry the *same* recessive gene, each pregnancy carries a 25 percent risk that the child will inherit a hearing loss (and a 50 percent risk that the child will be a carrier).

Most of us carry some faulty genes, but (luckily) the normal genes with which they're paired dominate. For example, many people carry a recessive gene for hearing loss, but relatively few people actually produce children with hearing problems. This is because the probability of mating with someone who carries the *same* gene for hearing loss is low (remember, mutations in many different genes can cause hearing loss). This is true even among parents who are deaf. In many marriages between deaf people, all of the children are hearing—often because the parents carry different recessive genes for deafness.[2]

Age-related Hearing Loss (Presbycusis)

The word *presbycusis* comes from the Greek language and roughly translated means "old man hearing." Although this gender specificity makes the term politically incorrect, it's not totally inappropriate, because men tend to suffer from earlier and slightly more severe age-related hearing loss than women. Large numbers of people are affected by age-related hearing loss. In this country, approximately one third of all people between the ages of 65 and 75 years and one half of all people over the age of 75 years have hearing loss. Along with arthritis and high blood pressure, hearing loss is one of the three most common chronic conditions affecting older adults.

Eventually, nearly everyone who lives long enough develops some degree of hearing loss, but some of us develop it sooner (and with greater severity) than others. In part, this is determined by our genetic make-up. However, it's also determined by the things to which we expose ourselves over the course of a lifetime, especially noise. We know that people who spend their lives in remote, undeveloped places don't show the same decline in hearing with age. For example, in 1960, the hearing of 500 members of a tribe living near the convergence of the Blue and Red Nile Rivers in Sudan was studied.[3] At that time, the Mabaans had spent their entire lives in the absence of loud, unnatural sounds. Although elderly tribe members had some age-related hearing loss, it was significantly less than that typically observed in people of the same age who lived in developed societies. Moreover, scientists now believe that exposure to "subhazardous" noise (noise that's not dangerously loud) can accumulate and make an ear more vulnerable to aging. In addition to noise, there are other factors that probably contribute to age-related hearing loss. These factors are likely to include smoking, poor diet, exposure to pollutants, bacterial and viral infections, high fever, exposure to ototoxic medications and chemicals, allergies, head trauma, and other health conditions (for example, diabetes, high blood pressure, and heart disease). Fortunately, some of these causes are preventable.

The age at which presbycusis becomes apparent varies. Typically, a bilateral hearing loss develops very gradually, beginning at the high frequencies. In fact, we begin losing high-frequency hearing at a relatively young age. Some teenagers have found a way to capitalize on the superior high-frequency hearing enjoyed only by the young. Some high school students in the United Kingdom and now in the United States are using a ring tone with a frequency of approximately 17,000 Hz for their cell phones. Because most adults over the age of 30 years can't hear the tone, teenagers can be alerted to the arrival of text messages without the knowledge of their parents and teachers. The idea is based on the same principle as an antiteen loitering device known as *the Mosquito* (because it's small and annoying). The Mosquito creates a loud, piercing sound that's painful, but only to the young ears that can hear it. The device was designed for British shopkeepers who wanted to prevent teenagers from loitering around their businesses and driving other customers away.

Age-related hearing loss tends to worsen gradually over time. The hearing loss may be accompanied by tinnitus, sensitivity to loud sounds, and reduced ability to understand speech. In general, the maximal speech perception scores (see Chapter 4) of older adults are poorer than those of younger adults with the same degree of hearing loss. In addition, poor listening conditions cause greater difficulty for older listeners than for younger listeners. In part, this may be due to deterioration in the ascending pathways of the central auditory system (see Chapter 3) or to more general changes related to aging (for example, reduced short-term memory, lengthened reaction time, difficulty maintaining attention in distracting environments, etc.).

The diagnosis of presbycusis should be one of exclusion; treatable conditions should be ruled out first. Presbycusis can't be treated medically or surgically. Nonmedical treatment options include hearing aids, assistive listening devices, and hearing rehabilitation therapy.

Noise-induced Hearing Loss

After aging, noise exposure is the most common cause of sensorineural hearing loss in this country. The increasing noisiness of our society is largely responsible for the sharp increase in hearing loss over the last 30 to 40 years. During that time, the number of Americans with hearing loss has more than doubled. Loud noise affects our hearing, our physical health, and our sense of well-being. Much more information about the threats posed by noise can be found in Chapter 11.

There are two different types of noise-induced hearing loss. Acoustic trauma results from a single, brief, intense exposure to impulse noise at close range (for example, the noise produced by a gunshot, explosion, or firecracker). In this case, the physical limits of structures within the ear are exceeded. In the middle ear, the eardrum can rupture, and the ossicular chain can be dislocated. In the cochlea, hair cells can be partially or completely destroyed. In extreme cases, CN VIII fibers can be stretched or torn. The hearing loss is immediate.

In contrast, repeated exposure to less extreme levels of hazardous noise (for example, occupational or recreational noise) results in metabolic exhaustion of hair cells. In other words, repeated exposure gradually wears hair cells out. Imagine a healthy lawn; individual blades of grass will recover if you walk across them once or twice. However, if people use the same path over and over, individual blades of grass eventually fail to recover, and permanent damage results. When enough hair cells have been destroyed (25–30 percent), we begin to experience hearing loss.

Initially, exposure to hazardous noise causes a hearing loss that goes away after several hours. This is known as *temporary threshold shift* (TTS). Hearing recovers because there are enough healthy hair cells left to allow normal hearing. If exposure to loud noise continues and more hair cells are destroyed, however, a permanent hearing loss develops. See Chapter 11 for information about how to prevent this from happening.

The hearing loss associated with noise exposure typically has a distinctive notched configuration on an audiogram. In addition to a reduction in loudness, the loss is usually accompanied by reduced speech perception ability, tinnitus, and an abnormal sensitivity to loudness (resulting in a reduced dynamic range; see Chapter 4). This is definitely a loss to be avoided, and it's almost entirely preventable. The first line of defense is to avoid exposure to harmful noise. When it can't be avoided, give your ears a break as often as possible (at least every hour), and by all means use hearing protection (see Chapter 11).

Ototoxicity

Taken literally, *ototoxicity* means ear poisoning. Certain medications can damage the cochlea, the vestibular apparatus, or both portions of the inner ear. Ototoxicity can cause hearing loss, tinnitus, and vestibular problems (vertigo, dizziness, or a sense of imbalance) that can be temporary or permanent. More than 200 medications are known to be potentially ototoxic. Among the most infamous are a group of antibiotics commonly known as the aminoglycosides. These drugs are widely used to treat serious or life-threatening conditions because they're highly effective and have a low incidence of resistance. Their relatively low cost makes their use especially common in other parts of the world (according to some sources, aminoglycoside ototoxicity is the leading cause of acquired severe sensorineural hearing loss in China). As resistance to other antibiotics increases, physicians may find it necessary to use aminoglycosides more often.

Aminoglycosides aren't the only ototoxic drugs. Taken in high enough doses, even aspirin can cause temporary tinnitus and hearing loss. Other drugs known to cause temporary hearing loss include powerful diuretics administered intravenously in high doses to patients with problems like congestive heart failure, renal failure, cirrhosis, and hypertension. Drugs used to treat malaria (for example, quinine, chloroquine, and quinidine) can also cause temporary hearing loss. Antimalarial drugs are sometimes used to treat nighttime leg cramps, but the doses used for that purpose typically don't affect hearing.

Of far greater concern are the anticancer drugs that cause permanent hearing loss, sometimes after just one dose. Cisplatin is the most ototoxic drug in common clinical use. A hearing loss can occur after the first treatment, or it can occur months after the last dose. Hearing sometimes continues to worsen over a long period of time, even after treatment has ended.

Ototoxicity is dose related; that is, the risk is related to *how* a drug is given (intravenous administration is most dangerous), *how long* it's given (the longer it's taken, the more dangerous it becomes), and *how much* is given (higher doses carry greater risk). There are no safe limits, because susceptibility differs from one person to the next. Susceptibility is based in part on a person's genetic make-up, but additional risk factors include poor liver or kidney function (the liver is the body's major detoxification system, and the kidneys are responsible for ridding the body of toxins); poor general health; very young or very old age; prior use of ototoxic drugs; preexisting sensorineural hearing loss (especially if it resulted from ototoxicity); concurrent noise exposure; concurrent radiation treatment; and concurrent use of another ototoxic drug. The effects of exposure to noise or taking a second potentially ototoxic drug during treatment can be synergistic (that is, greater than the effects of the two factors simply added together). Patients should avoid exposure to loud noise during and after cisplatin treatment.

Prevention of ototoxicity involves careful dose calculations, close monitoring of kidney function (some ototoxic drugs can also damage kidney function), and measuring drug levels in the blood. Prevention should also involve measuring hearing thresholds before, during, and *after* drug use (see Chapter 11). Because some drugs can remain in the cochlear fluids long after they've been discontinued, hearing loss or balance problems can begin months later. When a change in hearing is detected during treatment, it's sometimes possible to reduce the dose or discontinue the drug before hearing is damaged further. When hearing loss can't be prevented, it tends to affect both ears equally, and tinnitus is common.

Examples of Drugs That Can Harm Hearing

- Cisplatin, carboplatin, nitrogen mustard, and vincristine are chemotherapy agents used to fight cancer. Drugs that kill cancer cells can also kill cochlear hair cells. Damage to hearing is often permanent. Toxicity is enhanced when these drugs are taken with other ototoxic medications, like aminoglycoside antibiotics or loop diuretics. These drugs might also increase susceptibility to noise-induced hearing loss.
- Certain antibiotics can be ototoxic (for example, amikacin, gentamycin, kanamycin, erythromycin, neomycin, netilmicin, streptomycin, tobramycin, and vancomycin can cause permanent inner ear damage). Some are primarily vestibulotoxic (they damage the vestibular system more than the cochlea), some are primarily cochleotoxic (they damage the cochlea more than the vestibular system), and some are both cochleo- and vestibulotoxic.[4]
- Aspirin and aspirin-containing products taken in high doses (6–8 or more tablets a day) can cause tinnitus and hearing loss that typically goes away when the medication is discontinued.
- Nonsteroidal antiinflammatory drugs (for example, ibuprofen [Advil, Aleve, Motrin]) taken in high doses (6–8 pills or more a day) can cause temporary tinnitus and hearing loss.
- Quinine is contained in several medications as well as tonic water. It can be ototoxic in very high doses, but the effects are usually temporary.

- Loop diuretics can cause hearing loss when given intravenously or in very high doses. Damage is more likely to be permanent if a loop diuretic is taken along with another ototoxic drug (like a chemotherapy agent).

Remember, never discontinue a drug without consulting your physician first.

Ménière's Disease

This disease of the inner ear is characterized by episodes of vertigo (a sensation of spinning), sensorineural hearing loss, tinnitus, and a feeling of fullness or pressure in the affected ear. The attacks of vertigo, which are often accompanied by nausea and vomiting, can range from mild to debilitating and can last minutes, hours, or days. They can occur often or once every few years. The hearing loss, tinnitus, and fullness tend to increase before and during episodes, sometimes providing an aura that warns of an impending attack. The patient is likely to feel unsteady for days afterward. In the early stages of the disease, symptoms can improve (or even go away) between attacks, but eventually they become more constant.

Hearing tends to become worse over time—sometimes quickly, sometimes slowly. Some people lose all usable hearing in the affected ear. Both ears are affected in only about 15 percent of patients. The hearing loss is somewhat distinctive in that it's unilateral, and the low frequencies are affected first. In contrast, most sensorineural hearing losses are bilateral, and the high frequencies are affected first. Eventually, all frequencies can be affected. Along with a loss of hearing sensitivity, speech perception can become extremely poor, and loud sounds are likely to be uncomfortable. Some people experience extreme pressure in the affected ear, whereas others experience little or no pressure at all. Tinnitus can be an unpleasant roar.

Ménière's disease is caused by overproduction or underabsorption of endolymph, the fluid that fills the middle chamber of the cochlea (the scala media) and surrounds the hair cells (see Figure 3.6 in Chapter 3). Too much endolymph causes the membranes that form the chamber to stretch until they rupture. This allows endolymph to mix with perilymph, the fluid that fills the other chambers of the cochlea. The cause for this is unknown at this time.

Initial treatment is aimed at providing relief from symptoms; this often involves the use of antivertigo, antinausea, and other medications. The patient's physician may also attempt to reduce endolymph volume by prescribing a diuretic ("water pill") and encouraging the patient to reduce his salt intake. Patients might also be instructed to reduce their intake of substances such as alcohol, nicotine, caffeine, and chocolate. Habits consistent with a healthy lifestyle are encouraged: eating well, getting plenty of sleep, exercising regularly, and avoiding stress. Patients who continue to experience disabling vertigo are sometimes candidates for other therapies.

My Dad

My dad began experiencing symptoms that suggested Ménière's disease about 25 years ago. Fortunately, his symptoms didn't progress much until recently. For the first 20 years, he experienced some unsteadiness and a mild sensorineural hearing loss in his left ear. He functioned quite well. But a few years ago, he began to have full-blown episodes of vertigo and nausea, the hearing in his left ear began to deteriorate, and he experienced a roaring tinnitus that was difficult to bear. The disease has since "burned itself out," but the hearing loss in his left ear is considerable, and he has lost all speech perception ability in that ear. How my dad found relief from his tinnitus is explained in Chapter 6, his hearing aid arrangements are discussed in Chapter 7, and his use of hearing assistance technology is discussed in Chapter 9.

Sensorineural Hearing Loss Caused by Head Trauma

A severe blow to the head, particularly from the front or back, can fracture the part of the temporal bone that contains the inner ear. If the fracture line goes through the cochlea or the bony tube that carries CN VIII and CN VII to the brainstem, hearing, balance, or facial nerve function can be damaged on the injured side. Depending on the nature of the injury, hearing may change (fluctuate) for as long as 6 months following the traumatic event. Hearing can become better, worse, or stay the same; in extreme cases, the loss of hearing is complete and permanent. Balance problems are likely to improve spontaneously, and facial nerve function that doesn't improve on its own can sometimes be improved with medical treatment.

Perilymphatic Fistula

Trauma can also cause the delicate membranes covering the round and oval windows to rupture, allowing perilymph (the fluid that fills two chambers of the cochlea; see Figure 3.6 in Chapter 3) to leak into the middle ear. The leak is called a *perilymphatic fistula*. Ruptures can also be caused by straining, lifting, coughing, sneezing, barotrauma (discussed earlier), or a virulent infection in the middle ear (see previous discussion). Some even occur spontaneously. A sudden hearing loss accompanied by vertigo, nausea, and tinnitus—especially after recent trauma, rapid pressure change, straining, sneezing, or violent coughing—could suggest a perilymphatic fistula. When a fistula is suspected, a period of bed rest with the head elevated approximately 30 degrees may be recommended. The patient may be instructed to avoid sudden head movements, straining, or forceful nose blowing, and stool softeners may be recommended. If no improvement occurs, surgical exploration of the middle ear with possible patching of the fistula may be undertaken. Successful patching can keep the hearing loss from getting worse.

Labyrinthitis (Inflammation of the Inner Ear)

Labyrinthitis is an inflammation of the inner ear "labyrinth" that affects both hearing and balance. The cause is unknown, but it often follows a viral or bacterial infection (for example, a cold, the flu, or a middle ear infection). Symptoms can include vertigo, dizziness, or unsteadiness; nausea and vomiting; hearing loss; and tinnitus. Although the inflammation usually resolves spontaneously over several weeks, it's best to see a doctor who can treat the symptoms. In most cases, hearing returns to normal.

Sudden Idiopathic Sensorineural Hearing Loss

Each year, more than 4,000 people in this country experience a sudden hearing loss in one ear. Although this disturbing event can occur at any age, it happens most often to young and middle-aged adults.

The term *sudden idiopathic hearing loss* is used to describe an abrupt sensorineural hearing loss with no known cause (no known cause makes it "idiopathic"). The operational definition is a hearing loss of 30 dB or greater at three adjacent frequencies (see Chapter 4) that develops over a period of 3 days or less. Most often, the change is noticed upon waking in the morning. The loss can occur instantly or develop over minutes, hours, or days (minutes or hours is most common). About half the time, the hearing loss is preceded, accompanied, or followed by feelings of unsteadiness. Tinnitus is reported by most patients, and some also report a sensation of fullness in the affected ear. Occasionally, patients remember hearing a popping sound when the loss occurred. Sudden idiopathic hearing loss is nearly always unilateral, but in a few cases (about 2 percent) the other ear is affected months or years later.

Many conditions can cause sudden hearing loss (for example, impacted earwax, Eustachian tube dysfunction, labyrinthitis, Ménière's disease, acoustic tumor, head trauma, acoustic trauma, ototoxicity, multiple sclerosis, etc.), and these conditions must be ruled out before a sudden hearing loss is labeled idiopathic. When no cause can be determined, possible explanations include viral infection, problems involving blood flow to the inner ear, and unknown factors. Sudden hearing loss is always considered a medical emergency that requires immediate attention.

Hearing can be unstable for several weeks after the loss begins. During that time, it might improve, become worse, or stabilize. In many cases (30–60 percent), hearing returns to normal without treatment within about two weeks. This outcome is more likely when the audiogram doesn't show a sloping configuration, the hearing loss is not severe, there are no balance problems, and the patient is not elderly. The presence of otoacoustic emissions (see Chapter 4) is another hopeful sign.

Because there's probably more than one cause of sudden idiopathic hearing loss, no single treatment is effective with all patients; however, the sooner that treatment is initiated, the better. The most common treatment is a course of steroids. In the past, these had to be given orally, which often resulted in unpleasant side effects. Today, steroids can be placed inside the middle ear (where they can be absorbed into the cochlea) by injecting them through the eardrum. This approach reduces side effects and allows the medication to be concentrated where it's actually needed. In some cases, the patient is also asked to limit her physical activity; noise exposure; and use of salt, alcohol, tobacco, and caffeine.

Autoimmune Inner Ear Disease

The immune system is designed to detect and fight off infection throughout the body. In autoimmune disease, a malfunctioning immune system attacks the body's own healthy tissues. The cause appears to be genetic. Autoimmune disease can affect the entire body (for example, lupus) or any part of the body: the pancreas is affected in diabetes, the thyroid is affected in Graves' disease, joints are affected in rheumatoid arthritis, the skin is affected in psoriasis, and the brain is affected in multiple sclerosis. In autoimmune inner ear disease (AIED), the immune system mistakes normal cells in the inner ear for harmful cells and attacks them. This produces an inflammatory reaction that can result in a bilateral sensorineural hearing loss that becomes worse rapidly. Left untreated, the condition can lead to total deafness. AIED was thought to be a relatively rare condition (accounting for approximately 1 percent of all hearing losses); however, recent research suggests that immune mechanisms may play a role in some cases of Ménière's disease and sudden idiopathic sensorineural hearing loss, especially those that are bilateral.

Diagnosis of AIED is based on patient history, physical examination, blood work, and the results of hearing and vestibular tests. Signs that point to a diagnosis of AIED are the presence of another autoimmune disorder and improvement in hearing with steroid treatment. Because prompt initiation of treatment is critical, it's important to recognize the symptoms of AIED: sudden, progressive sensorineural hearing loss that's bilateral or begins in one ear and progresses rapidly to the other, fullness in the ear(s), vertigo, and tinnitus.

Powerful antiinflammatory steroids can stabilize or even improve hearing and speech perception ability, making AIED one of the few causes of sensorineural hearing loss that responds to medical treatment. Unfortunately, steroids can produce side effects that can limit their long-term use.

When medical treatment is unsuccessful, hearing aids can be helpful. Patients who progress to profound sensorineural hearing loss often do very well with cochlear implants (see Chapter 8).

Causes of Neural Hearing Loss

Problems that affect the cochlea or CN VIII cause sensorineural hearing loss. Those that affect the cochlea cause sensory hearing loss and those that affect CN VIII cause neural hearing loss. The problems in this section primarily affect CN VIII.

Auditory Neuropathy/Auditory Dys-synchrony

Auditory neuropathy/auditory dys-synchrony (AN/AD) is a condition in which sound energy enters the cochlea but is unable to reach the brain without being degraded. In other words, the neural connection between the cochlea and the brain is bad. The cause is unknown; in fact, there are probably multiple causes. Many patients with AN/AD also have other neuropathies (neurological problems) outside the auditory system. There appears to be a genetic component to the disorder, as some families have more than one member with AN/AD.

The hearing loss associated with AN/AD can fluctuate (change), be asymmetric (different between ears), and worsen over time. Most important, speech perception is often poorer than would be expected given the severity of the hearing loss, particularly in background noise. Some people are unable to understand speech at all in difficult listening conditions. Hearing aids may or may not be useful, but assistive listening devices that improve the signal-to-noise relationship are of value (see Chapter 9). Learning to sign and use finger spelling can also be helpful. Alternatively, when CN VIII function is adequate, patients with AN/AD can be successful with cochlear implants.

This condition is diagnosed when otoacoustic emissions (see Chapter 4), which assess outer hair cell function, are normal but the auditory brainstem response (ABR) and acoustic reflexes, which assess CN VIII function, are abnormal. This pattern of findings suggests that the problem lies beyond the outer hair cells.

Acoustic Tumors of CN VIII

Tumors on CN VIII are slow growing, noncancerous (meaning they don't spread to other parts of the body), and typically affect only one ear. The first symptom might be a unilateral hearing loss, often affecting the high frequencies. The onset can be gradual or sudden, and speech perception can be surprisingly poor given the degree of hearing loss. In some cases, hearing remains within the normal range, but the patient perceives a change in the quality of hearing, and speech perception is degraded. Other complaints can include tinnitus; a feeling of fullness in the affected ear; and vertigo, dizziness, or unsteadiness. Less often, the patient experiences weakness of the facial muscles on the affected side. ABR testing may be used to assess CN VIII function, but enhanced magnetic resonance imaging (MRI) is necessary to make the definitive diagnosis.

Acoustic tumors tend to originate in the bony canal through which CN VIII and CN VII (the Facial Nerve, which is responsible for movement of the facial muscles) pass as they make their way to the brainstem. The tumor is likely to grow beyond the bony canal into a space at the base of the brainstem known as the cerebellopontine angle (CPA).

Most acoustic tumors are surgically removed. In some cases, radio-surgical treatment (the *gamma knife*) is used. When the patient is not a surgical candidate (because of age, health, or preference) and the tumor is small, it's sometimes monitored and left untreated. There are advantages and disadvantages (risks) associated with each treatment choice.

Causes of Mixed Hearing Loss

Any of the conditions that cause conductive hearing loss can coexist with any of the conditions that cause sensory or neural hearing loss. When conductive and sensorineural pathologies exist in the same ear, the result is a mixed hearing loss. Often, the conductive component of the hearing loss can be corrected, improving hearing but not restoring it to normal. In this case, hearing is improved only to the level of the permanent sensorineural hearing loss (see Chapter 4).

Causes of Central Auditory Dysfunction

The incredibly intricate duplication and overlap of pathways and functions within the central auditory system make it possible for the brain to reorganize itself in the face of injury or disease. This means the brain can often find alternative ways to hear and understand *simple* sounds like pure tones and words spoken in quiet. More complex problems might not be revealed by conventional testing. Instead, these sorts of problems (for example, problems determining where sounds are coming from or problems separating a conversation of interest from other conversations) are revealed through case history information and special auditory tests. Conditions that affect central auditory function include brain tumors, vascular events (that is, strokes), infections such as meningitis or encephalitis, degenerative diseases such as Parkinson's or multiple sclerosis, brain damage caused by trauma, and asphyxia.

Auditory Processing Disorder

Auditory processing disorder (APD) can be defined as difficulty understanding information that comes through the hearing channel, particularly when listening conditions are difficult (when a talker speaks rapidly, the talker has a foreign accent, or there's background noise). This difficulty is not caused by any of the medical conditions listed previously, nor is it the result of peripheral hearing loss as shown on the audiogram (although it can *coexist* with medical conditions or peripheral hearing loss). Instead, the problem seems to involve neural "wiring."

Because the central auditory system is vast and complex, there are different types of auditory processing disorders. For example, in a small number of people, the brain has difficulty coordinating information coming from the two ears. Signals are "out of synch," which is distracting. When this is the case, listeners may find it more beneficial to wear one hearing aid rather than two; however, this is the exception rather than the rule (see Chapter 7).

Because understanding speech in the presence of background noise is a common problem in APD, hearing rehabilitation strategies can be very helpful (see Chapter 10). Some adults with APD (or very poor speech perception) do better when assistive listening devices are used to supplement hearing aids in certain situations (see Chapter 9). Such devices can increase the speech signal over background noise, improving speech understanding in difficult listening conditions.

Dizziness

The inner ear houses structures for two different sensory systems: the auditory system (hearing) and the vestibular system (balance). Structures within the vestibular system tell the brain about the position of the head, whether the head is moving, in which direction it's moving, and whether the movement is speeding up or slowing down. The brain combines this information with the visual picture coming from the eyes and information coming from muscles, joints, and tendons throughout the body. A balance disorder involving the inner ear can cause a person to experience dizziness (lightheadedness or unsteadiness) or vertigo (a special type of dizziness in which there's a sensation of movement).

Dizziness is a symptom rather than a disease. In fact, it's the third most common reason people over 65 years of age visit their doctor. Doctors are able to determine the cause of dizziness in about 75 percent of cases. Even when no cause can be found, however, the symptoms can be treated.

CHAPTER 6

Tinnitus: "To Ring Like a Bell"

Oh! dreadful is the check—intense the agony—
When the ear begins to hear . . .
The Prisoner, Emily Brontë

The word *tinnitus* comes from a Latin word meaning "to ring like a bell." Whether you say "TIN-a-tus" or "tin-EYE-tus" (both are correct), *tinnitus* refers to the perception of sound within the ears or head that has no external source. It's most often perceived as high-pitched ringing, but it's also described as roaring, whooshing, humming, buzzing, hissing, chirping, clicking, popping, crackling, boiling, pulsing, or whistling. It can be heard in one ear, both ears, or somewhere in the head. Tinnitus is never perceived as words (hearing voices is another matter entirely) and only rarely described as having a melody.

Nearly everyone experiences tinnitus from time to time, but for some people it's constant and frightfully annoying. According to the American Tinnitus Association, 50 million Americans experience tinnitus more than occasionally; of those, 12 million are bothered enough to seek medical treatment. There are 2 million people for whom tinnitus is debilitating, causing problems like sleep deprivation, poor concentration, depression, and thoughts of suicide. For them, tinnitus affects the ability to function on a daily basis.

ORIGINS OF TINNITUS

The physiologic mechanisms that underlie tinnitus remain a mystery. At this point, no one knows what *causes* tinnitus. For some, tinnitus may originate in the *peripheral* auditory system, most often the cochlea and less often the Cranial Nerve (CN) VIII (see Chapter 3). In many cases, however, tinnitus originates in the brain. Based on what we know about brain plasticity, pathologic changes in the inner ear cause central pathways and structures to adapt (see Chapter 10). In other words, when the brain receives diminished or altered input from the ears, it adapts to accommodate that input. Unfortunately, these accommodations can result in the perception of tinnitus. Support for the central origin of tinnitus includes the observation that, for some patients, severing CN VIII (and therefore disconnecting the ear from the brain) doesn't bring relief from tinnitus.

Most people who have tinnitus also have hearing loss. Almost any condition that can cause hearing loss can also be associated with the onset of tinnitus (for example, impacted wax in the ear canal, middle ear infection, Eustachian tube dysfunction, mastoiditis, otosclerosis, rupture of the oval or round windows, Ménière's disease, ear trauma, CN VIII tumors, or auditory neuropathy/dys-synchrony; see Chapter 5 for a review of pathologic conditions that affect the ear). However, the most common trigger is exposure to loud noise. Many people with tinnitus have some form of hearing damage resulting from noise exposure; in fact, some can link the onset of their tinnitus to a specific event. A one-time exposure to hazardous noise (like a loud concert or a leaf blower) can be just as dangerous as exposure that occurs over time, such as in the workplace. Either type of exposure can lead to a lifetime of tinnitus.

Exposure to certain medications is another common trigger. More than 300 medications list tinnitus as a potential side effect, and this doesn't take possible drug interactions into account. In rare cases, tinnitus originates outside the auditory system. Nonauditory factors that are occasionally associated with tinnitus include head and neck injuries, vascular and cerebrovascular disorders (for example, strokes, aneurysms, and blood clots), heart disease, systemic conditions (for example, diabetes or high blood pressure), infectious diseases, thyroid disease, autoimmune disorders, and TMJ syndrome. In a large number of cases, however, the trigger is simply normal aging.

Drugs That Can Trigger Tinnitus[1]

- Aminoglycoside antibiotics
- Antidepressants
- Aspirin and other salicylates
- Beta-blockers (for example, Inderal)
- Chemotherapy agents such as cisplatin and carboplatin
- Heavy metals (for example, those used to treat parasitic infections)
- Furosemide (Lasix) and other loop diuretics
- Marijuana

- Nonsteroidal antiinflammatory drugs (NSAIDS) used to reduce pain, fever, and inflammation (for example, ibuprofen and naproxen); these drugs are used in many over-the-counter pain relievers
- Oral contraceptives
- Quinine

It's important to understand that tinnitus does not *cause* hearing loss, nor does it make hearing loss worse. In fact, tinnitus usually has no meaning at all. Tinnitus has been compared to the phantom pain sometimes experienced by amputees. Whereas amputees perceive pain in a limb that doesn't actually exist, tinnitus sufferers perceive sound that doesn't actually exist. Tinnitus and pain are thought by some researchers to share common mechanisms.

It bears repeating—most cases of tinnitus are triggered by exposure to loud noise, and exposure to loud noise is something that's almost always preventable. Avoid loud noise when you can; when you can't, limit your exposure time and wear hearing protection. To some extent, exposure to medications that cause tinnitus may be preventable as well. If you begin to experience tinnitus while taking medicine, tell your doctor immediately; it may be possible to adjust the dosage or substitute another medication. If you already have tinnitus, warn your doctor so medications that could make the tinnitus worse can be avoided.

It's Always There...

My friend, Jim, has been exposed to lots of noise as a dairy farmer and avid hunter, but he never had tinnitus until he was treated for cancer a few years ago. Nowadays, he wears earplugs to protect his hearing from the potentially harmful noise produced by farm equipment (the noise produced by a tractor without a "soundproof" cab can exceed 100 dB). The earplugs he uses block 29 dB under the best circumstances (see Chapter 11). Even in all that noise—with or without earplugs—Jim still hears his tinnitus loud and clear.

Substances to Avoid if You Have Tinnitus

Some people find that the following substances make tinnitus worse:

- Alcohol
- Aspirin
- Cheese
- Chocolate
- Coffee

- Cola
- Diuretics
- Foods high in sugar
- Marijuana and other recreational drugs
- Monosodium glutamate (MSG)
- Red wine
- Salt
- Tea
- Tobacco
- Tonic water (which contains quinine, a drug that can cause tinnitus)

To isolate possible triggers, try eliminating one item at a time for a period of 2 weeks and keep a record of any changes in your tinnitus. After 2 weeks, isolate a different item, and so on.

CONVENTIONAL TREATMENTS

The first step in dealing with tinnitus is to consult your doctor. She can determine whether your tinnitus is caused by a medical condition that can be treated. Treatment of the medical condition might cause the tinnitus to diminish or disappear. In other cases, relief can be as simple as discontinuing a certain medication that's causing the tinnitus (but do this only in consultation with your doctor).

Most often, however, tinnitus is *not* caused by a medical condition that can be treated. In this case, there's no cure, but nonmedical treatments can bring relief. Most of the treatments described here have not been evaluated in large, well-designed clinical trials; however, they've all been shown to provide relief for some people. In consultation with your audiologist or physician, you probably will need to try several approaches before discovering what works best for you. And take heart—for many people, tinnitus becomes less noticeable over time *without* treatment. In general, people tend to get better rather than worse.

Hearing Aids

Most people who suffer from tinnitus also have hearing loss, and nearly all of them can benefit from hearing aids. Hearing aids make the sounds around us louder, enabling those with hearing loss to hear them. And the better we're able to hear the sounds *outside* our heads, the less we're aware of the sounds *inside* our heads. In other words, hearing aids "inhibit" the perception of tinnitus. Some people even experience residual inhibition, meaning that the tinnitus isn't noticeable for a period of several minutes to several hours after the hearing aids have been removed (often providing enough time to fall asleep). The use of hearing aids is a simple solution that "kills two birds with one stone" and works well for many people.

My Dad

As a result of Ménière's disease, my dad began suffering from hearing loss, unsteadiness, and tinnitus about 25 years ago. I never heard him complain. About 5 years ago, however, he began having really dreadful episodes in which he experienced severe vertigo, nausea, hearing loss, and tinnitus. Each episode left his hearing and tinnitus worse. Following one particularly bad episode, his tinnitus became almost unbearable. He said that it sounded like a train roaring through his head. He told me that he wasn't sure how much longer he could take it, and asked if I thought it would ever go away. My advice was to try wearing hearing aids. Perhaps it was just coincidence, but it worked. If you were to ask my dad today if he still has tinnitus, he would stop, listen, and tell you that it's still there but that it no longer bothers him. This is because he's become habituated to it (see below). He also experiences residual inhibition; he's very lucky on that score. The hearing aids do not help him hear or understand speech perfectly, but they've helped to solve the tinnitus problem.

Cochlear Implants

Cochlear implants can have the same effect as hearing aids; that is, when the sounds outside our heads are louder, the sounds inside our heads are less noticeable. In addition, it's possible that the electrical stimulation supplied by the implant might suppress tinnitus in some cases. In fact, external electrical stimulation of the ear is being explored as a possible treatment for tinnitus. In a handful of cases, however, cochlear implants have reportedly triggered tinnitus.

Tinnitus Maskers

One day in 1973, Jack Vernon, an audiologist and pioneer in tinnitus research, was walking with a physician who had traveled some distance to consult with him about his very severe tinnitus. As they passed an outdoor fountain, the physician came to an abrupt halt and reported that his tinnitus had disappeared. It was the first relief he'd found since the tinnitus had begun 2 years earlier. The sound of the fountain was replicated in the laboratory, and the idea of a wearable masking device for tinnitus relief was born. The physician's experience also became the basis for the *faucet test*, a simple experiment used to determine whether someone is likely to benefit from tinnitus masking. If your tinnitus is diminished when you stand near a faucet running full force (or in the shower), your tinnitus might be "maskable."

Wearable maskers are small electronic instruments that look like behind-the-ear (BTE) hearing aids. They produce low-level static that drowns out (masks) the tinnitus. Although the wearer still hears noise (from the masker), it's noise over which he has some control. This makes it more acceptable and easier to ignore than the tinnitus. Nonetheless, when the masking is turned off, the tinnitus is still there, although some people do experience residual inhibition.

For tinnitus sufferers with normal or near-normal hearing, for whom hearing aids and cochlear implants are not options, wearable maskers may be a good choice. When the listener does have a hearing loss, tinnitus maskers and hearing aids can be combined in the same instrument.

Today, wearable music players (for example, iPods and other MP3 players) are everywhere and can be worn in almost any setting. They may be preferable to tinnitus maskers, which typically present static to one ear. MP3 players can play different types of sounds (music, nature sounds, talk radio) in both ears for hundreds of hours. They're also used to play sounds created specifically for tinnitus relief.

Bedtime Masking

Because quiet surroundings bring tinnitus into sharper focus (a single candle looks brighter in a dark room than it does when the lights are turned on), many people find tinnitus most bothersome at night. If you have difficulty sleeping, it may help to have a noise source in your bedroom. Some people use indoor waterfalls, fish tanks, or fans; others prefer listening to recorded music or nature sounds. Even playing low-volume static on a radio that's been set between stations can be helpful. Special products that produce masking noises are available online, through catalogs, and in specialty stores (refer to the Resources section at the end of this book). Bedside maskers (with or without timers) can be used with tabletop speakers, headphones, or "sound pillows" in which miniature speakers are embedded. Some sound pillows can be connected to a radio, CD player, home stereo system, television, or other sound source.

Masking gives people a way to exert control over tinnitus, rather than allowing the tinnitus to control them. Listeners can decide what they want to hear, when and where they want to hear it, and at what volume.

Tinnitus Retraining Therapy

In the 1980s, Pawel Jastreboff developed what's called the "neurophysiological model" of tinnitus. The model was based on the observation that a patient's description of his tinnitus (for example, its loudness, pitch, and quality) bore no relationship to its perceived severity. In other words, two people might describe their tinnitus in exactly the same way, but their reactions to it might be quite different. One person might have difficulty working, falling asleep, and enjoying life, whereas the other might not be bothered by it. According to Jastreboff, the difference has more to do with the body's reaction to tinnitus than with the tinnitus itself. According to his model, the body's reaction to tinnitus comes from two parts of the brain: (1) the limbic system, the part of the brain involved in emotion; and (2) the autonomic nervous system, the part of the brain that controls bodily functions and triggers the "flight-or-fight" response to danger. Tinnitus might be triggered by damage in the cochlea, but the body's response to it comes from the brain—and the response is based on beliefs and fears inappropriately linked to the tinnitus.

The goal of tinnitus retraining therapy (TRT) is to train the brain to react to tinnitus as it reacts to the sound of the refrigerator running in the kitchen—we're unaware of it most of the time, but when we do hear it, it's not bothersome. This reaction is referred to as *habituation*. Habituating to a sound is different than ignoring it. Ignoring something requires effort; habituation is passive. A few seconds after the refrigerator "kicks on," we're no longer aware of it. The sound disappears from our conscious awareness because it has no importance. It doesn't evoke an emotional response from the limbic system, nor does it evoke a flight-or-fight response from the autonomic nervous system. According to Jastreboff, habituation occurs naturally for approximately 75 percent of people with tinnitus; in other words, most people who have tinnitus are not bothered by it.

Recall that your brain uses hearing to monitor your environment around the clock (see Chapter 2). Most of what you "hear" never reaches conscious awareness. Only sounds that could signal something important (like danger) are pushed into consciousness. Understandably, some people fear that tinnitus indicates danger; they worry that something is wrong with their hearing, their mind, or their brain. As a result, the body makes tinnitus a priority that demands attention. The situation can be made worse by well-intentioned health care professionals who suggest that tinnitus is a psychiatric condition, or that a brain tumor must be ruled out. Other patients feel desperate or panic stricken when they hear that "nothing can be done about tinnitus" and they must "learn to live with it." The goal of TRT is to prevent reactions from the limbic and autonomic nervous systems, thus keeping tinnitus from reaching the level of consciousness.

TRT always consists of two components: intensive one-to-one directive counseling and sound therapy. The process can take 12 to 18 months. Directive counseling demystifies tinnitus and makes it nonthreatening. Sound therapy requires that the patient be surrounded by low-level sound 24 hours a day. For most people, this means wearing ear-level instruments that generate noise. Unlike tinnitus *masking*, however, this noise is not loud enough to cover up the tinnitus. The intent is not to mask tinnitus completely because it's impossible to habituate to a sound that can't be detected. Other forms of "sound enrichment" must be used when the noise generators aren't being worn, for example, at bedtime and during sleep. Bedside maskers or sound pillows are recommended. In time, the listener naturally habituates to the low-level, external sounds, and the tinnitus is habituated along with it.

Audiologists and physicians require special training to provide TRT. If you're interested in this type of therapy, look for a clinician with the appropriate training and expertise. Contact the American Tinnitus Association for help (see the Resources section at the end of the book).

Neuromonics Tinnitus Treatment

This relatively new treatment has been cleared by the U.S. Food and Drug Administration (FDA) for the treatment of tinnitus. Along with a counseling program that involves education, support, and monitoring, the user receives a customized "neural" stimulus for 2 to 4 hours each day over a period of 6 to 8 months. In the initial phase, the stimulus is mixed with relaxing music, which completely masks the tinnitus and provides immediate relief. The stimulus and music are delivered to high-fidelity earphones by the Neuromonics Oasis, a digital device about the size and weight of a cell phone. In the second phase, the stimulus is removed, and the patient continues to listen to customized music. The dynamic nature of the music allows the patient to be exposed to her tinnitus intermittently. This repeated, momentary exposure to the tinnitus in the context of a relaxing and pleasant listening experience facilitates the desensitization process.[2] In other words, even though the patient occasionally hears the tinnitus, she learns to dismiss it.

Cognitive Behavioral Therapy

Cognitive behavioral therapy (CBT) is a type of counseling designed to help a person change his negative thinking about tinnitus. Tinnitus becomes a problem when a patient develops inaccurate beliefs about its cause or meaning.[3] Changing a patient's beliefs can lead to changes in her reaction to tinnitus, and the tinnitus becomes less intrusive. The patient learns not to feel threatened or victimized and to react more realistically.

Biofeedback

Stress makes tinnitus worse. Biofeedback techniques can teach a person how to control his body's reaction to stress. Some techniques involve the use of instruments that measure and display physical functions that usually are unconscious, such as muscle tension, skin temperature, heart rate, blood pressure, and pulse. The patient varies her emotions and observes changes on the display. Using this "biofeedback," the person learns to bring these functions under conscious control, even during times of stress. With practice, it becomes possible to accomplish this without instruments. Less stress often means less tinnitus.

Relaxation Therapy

Because stress makes tinnitus worse, learning to relax can be therapeutic. A common relaxation technique combines an awareness of muscle tension with slow, deep breathing; instructional materials (CDs, DVDs) are available for home use. Other relaxation techniques include hypnosis, meditation, therapeutic massage, and yoga. Many people find listening to music relaxing. Physical exercise can reduce tension, stimulate endorphins, and promote better sleep.

Personal Adjustment Counseling

People who suffer from tinnitus may feel helpless, depressed, angry, or alienated. These emotions may cause them to focus on their tinnitus, which only makes it worse. Working through these feelings with a professional counselor can be very helpful. This type of counseling is sometimes combined with the use of medication.

Medication

Scientists are actively searching for drugs that are effective in the treatment of tinnitus (for example, drugs that would reduce blood flow or neural activity in areas of the brain responsible for tinnitus). At present, medications used to treat anxiety, depression, and sleep disturbance are sometimes prescribed, because these problems can both result from tinnitus and make it worse. The use of these medications is usually combined with personal adjustment counseling. Although no drugs have received FDA approval for the treatment of tinnitus, a few have been reported to reduce its severity in *some* patients (for example, selective serotonin reuptake inhibitors [SSRIs]). Many drugs have side effects, however, and some can even make tinnitus worse.

Tinnitus Support Groups

Self-help groups can be a tremendous source of information and support. A national network of such groups is available through the American Tinnitus Association (ATA; see the Resources section for contact information). The ATA maintains a website; publishes the quarterly magazine, *Tinnitus Today*; supports public policies that positively impact hearing-related issues; funds tinnitus research; and facilitates more than 50 self-help groups. In addition, the ATA offers a Tinnitus Help Network of volunteers who serve as supportive contacts able to answer questions about everything from relaxation techniques to bedtime masking devices. Help network volunteers can be a valuable resource for someone who is without a self-help group nearby. The ATA also provides contact information for physicians, audiologists, hearing aid specialists, and other health care professionals who have an active interest in treating tinnitus.

Suggestions for Managing Tinnitus

- Consult your doctor to eliminate medical causes.
- Avoid exposure to loud noise. When you absolutely can't avoid it, limit your exposure time and wear hearing protection.
- Carry hearing protectors with you at all times. Choose earplugs that are easy to insert and allow you to hear clearly (like musician's earplugs; see Chapter 11).
- Avoid quiet. Because quiet environments tend to make tinnitus worse, use a masker in quiet places (for example, at your bedside). Experiment to learn which sounds and devices are most helpful in each problem situation.
- Keep your ears active; iPods and other MP3 players can be worn in almost any environment. Music provides an auditory background and takes attention away from the tinnitus, but keep the volume low!
- Avoid medications that could make tinnitus worse.
- Exercise daily to reduce stress and improve circulation.
- Get plenty of rest and avoid fatigue (fatigue tends to make tinnitus worse).
- Eat a healthy diet that's low in salt (avoid high blood pressure).
- If your blood pressure is high, do what's necessary to control it (high blood pressure can cause tinnitus).
- Get your mind off tinnitus and spend more time doing things that you enjoy!

ALTERNATIVE TREATMENTS

Many alternative therapies are used to treat tinnitus. For some, the primary benefit is their ability to promote relaxation and reduce stress. Although none has undergone rigorous scientific evaluation, all are reported to have helped someone with tinnitus (this is called *anecdotal evidence*). There's no guarantee that any of these techniques will provide relief from *your* tinnitus; therefore be aware that you could be spending money for something that does not help you. And, of course, always check with your doctor before trying something new. Such treatments include (but are not limited to) acupressure, acupuncture, the Alexander technique, aromatherapy, chiropractic care, craniosacral therapy, ear canal magnets, electrical or electromagnetic stimulation, homeopathy, hyperbaric oxygen, hypnotherapy, low-power laser therapy, magnets and magnetic stimulation, massage, meditation, melatonin, osteopathy, reflexology, Reiki, Shiatsu, Tai Chi, TMJ treatment, ultrasound, and vibrational therapy. In addition, some people have had success with B vitamins, herbal preparations (such as ginkgo biloba), and minerals (such as magnesium and zinc). Again, always check with your doctor before initiating any alternative treatment.

Tinnitus and Military Service

Between 2001 and 2005, the number of veterans receiving service-related disability benefits for tinnitus and hearing loss increased by 275 percent.[4] Tinnitus has always been one of the top five service-connected disabilities, even during peacetime; however, among veterans who began receiving compensation in 2005, it was *the* most frequent service-related disability (hearing loss was second).[5] In 2006, tinnitus disability payments to veterans topped $539 million. If this trend continues, payments are expected to top $1.1 billion by 2011.[6]

Hyperacusis

The term *hyperacusis* describes an extreme sensitivity to sound experienced by some people with normal hearing (often children). Everyday sounds that other people don't find bothersome can be painful or frightening to people with hyperacusis. The cause is unknown, but the condition is often associated with tinnitus. TRT and CBT can be helpful in gradually increasing tolerance to sound.

PART II

Learning about the Solutions

CHAPTER 7

Hearing Aids

All the sounds of the earth are like music.
Oscar Hammerstein II

If you have a permanent hearing loss, using hearing aids is the single most important thing you can do to minimize its negative effects. Very few people with hearing loss cannot benefit from hearing aids. Hearing aids can't make you hear normally, but they can dramatically *improve* your hearing. They can make communication less stressful, less tiring, and more enjoyable for you *and* your loved ones. They can allow you to participate more fully in all aspects of your life and make you feel less isolated, more confident, and more independent.

Only 5 to 10 percent of the hearing losses experienced by adults can be treated with medication or surgery (see Chapters 4 and 5). The remaining 90 to 95 percent can be treated *nonmedically* with hearing aids and other forms of hearing rehabilitation. Amplification (which includes cochlear implants and assistive listening technology as well as hearing aids) is the only nonmedical treatment that addresses hearing loss directly by increasing what a listener hears. Unfortunately, of the more than 31 million people with hearing loss, only about 6 million (20 percent) use hearing aids. Here are a few of the reasons.

Some people are unable (or unwilling) to admit that they have a hearing loss; others admit it to themselves but hope to conceal it from others. Unlike impaired vision, a stigma has been attached to hearing loss (see Chapter 2). Many people fear that wearing hearing aids will make them look old, incompetent, or unattractive. This perception is apt to change as younger people, already comfortable wearing high-tech equipment in and on their ears, begin to experience hearing loss (often prematurely as a result of increased exposure to noise). Other people are reluctant to seek help because they believe their hearing loss isn't "bad enough" to require it. Most people develop hearing loss gradually, so they're unaware of how much they're missing. In other cases, people resist hearing aids because they believe they don't work and therefore aren't worth the money. They may have tried hearing aids in the past or they have friends or family members who were dissatisfied. Sadly, hearing aids suffer from a bad reputation among many people. Today's hearing aids, however, are *not* your father's hearing aids (unless, of course, your father has new hearing aids). To say that today's hearing aids are better than hearing aids of the past is an understatement. The cost of hearing aids is another significant barrier to seeking help; some people can't afford them and for others they're not a spending priority. Unfortunately, Medicare doesn't pay for hearing aids (at this time), nor do most insurance companies. Given the reputation of hearing aids, many people are unwilling to risk thousands of dollars on something that they fear may not work. Finally, in addition to the obstacles of denial, vanity, fear, and cost, most consumers are uneducated about hearing aids. They're confused by advertising claims and about whom to consult. Reading this chapter can make you a better-educated consumer. At the very least, it can prepare you to ask good questions and make informed choices.

DECIDING WHICH HEARING AIDS ARE RIGHT FOR YOU

Despite claims to the contrary, there is no best hearing aid—no best brand, no best model, no set of features that works best for everyone. Hearing loss is an individual experience. Certainly the characteristics of a hearing loss help to determine which hearing aids may be suitable (see Chapter 4), but that's only part of the picture. The biology behind each hearing loss is unique, and so is the way in which each brain processes sensory information. This means that people who have similar thresholds (audiograms) may interact differently with different hearing aids. An individual's success with a particular hearing aid also depends on his unique preferences, expectations, and abilities. Lifestyle is another critical consideration—in what types of situations is it important that you be able to hear well? In other words, the fact that someone you know has been successful or unsuccessful with a particular hearing aid doesn't mean the same will be true for you (and vice versa).

There are dozens of hearing aid manufacturers (hearing aid "brands"), but just a handful make most of the hearing aids sold around the world (these include Oticon, Phonak, Resound, Siemens, Sonic Innovations, Starkey, and Widex). Each major manufacturer offers a line of models, so there are hundreds of models on the market. Each model offers a different combination of features; no single hearing aid includes all available features. Like automobiles, models range from premium (with all the latest features) to entry level (with fewer features and features that were innovative last year). The differences between models are complex, making it difficult to compare them directly. You need an audiologist's help to determine what's most appropriate for you. In fact, given the choices in style, features, and price, it's unlikely that there's only one "best" hearing aid for you. If you consult five audiologists, you might get five excellent (but different) recommendations.

When most people think about choosing hearing aids, they think about choosing a hearing aid *style*. Style has to do with how the hearing aid appears and the way it's worn in or on the ear (more about this later). Hearing aids now come in an array of styles, sizes, shapes, and colors, and most are quite discrete. The choice about style is ultimately yours; however, factors in addition to the way a hearing aid looks should be considered. An example is the severity and configuration of your hearing loss. Not every hearing aid style is able to accommodate every loss. Another example is the anatomy of your ear. Some ear canals are just too small to accommodate hearing aids that fit deep inside.

Your audiologist needs your input to make important decisions about what goes inside your hearing aids, regardless of their style. He needs to know about the aspects of your life that are affected by your hearing loss. Are there activities that you no longer enjoy? Are there situations that you avoid? Which listening environments do you find most troublesome? Are some people particularly difficult to hear? Are there occasions when hearing exceptionally well is important to you, even if only for a short time? Let your audiologist know if music is an important part of your life. The acoustics of music are quite different from the acoustics of speech and require different signal processing capabilities. Tell your audiologist if you're an avid "birder," you enjoy talking on the telephone, or you often participate in meetings with colleagues seated around a conference table. Learning about your needs can help her to choose the features that will maximize your hearing in all situations.

Your audiologist also needs to know if you have physical limitations that might affect hearing aid use. For example, do you have poor eyesight or difficulty handling tiny objects? Very tiny hearing aids with very tiny batteries require adequate eyesight and nimble hands (or assistance from someone else). Unfortunately, sometimes size *does* matter. If your hands don't work as well as you'd like, your audiologist may be able to choose hearing aids with features that adjust themselves automatically or can be adjusted using a remote control.

What are you able to afford? Hearing aids are available at a wide range of prices that vary depending on the style (smaller hearing aids cost more than larger hearing aids; see later discussion), type of circuitry (digital technology costs more than analog; see later discussion), and combination of features inside (premium hearing aids cost more than entry-level aids; see later discussion). The good news is that more features are becoming available in entry-level aids, and not everyone needs a premium aid. Although everyone needs a clear, undistorted signal that's comfortable (that is, loud enough to hear but never uncomfortably loud), not everyone needs all the bells and whistles offered by top-of-the-line models.

People come with a variety of needs, preferences, budgets, and expectations. Think carefully about yours. Answer your audiologist's questions thoughtfully and honestly. Your chances of success are greatest if you work together as partners. Be specific about the problems your hearing loss creates so that your audiologist can address them in the hearing aid fitting. Identifying specific problems also makes it easier to evaluate the benefit that your hearing aids provide. After considering your needs and priorities, your audiologist will make a recommendation and explain it to you. The final decision, of course, is yours, but be open to her suggestions. Many people begin the process with a preconceived notion about what they want—and usually it has more to do with appearance than performance. Your audiologist has experience with different brands and models of hearing aids: their performance, their service and repair records, their warranties, and other attributes. Remember, part of what you're paying for is your audiologist's expertise.

What Makes for a Satisfied Hearing Aid User?
- Improved hearing ability in multiple listening situations
- The ability to hear soft sounds without uncomfortable loudness
- Natural sound quality
- Comfortable fit
- Reliable performance
- Good service

HEARING AID STYLES

Style refers to the way that a hearing aid's circuitry is packaged: the way it looks and the way that it's worn (on the ear, in the ear, in the canal). There is no best hearing aid style; it's a matter of choosing the one that's right for you.

A hearing aid's style affects its function as well as its looks. In general, as the size of a hearing aid decreases, its power decreases, its battery life decreases, and its cost increases. Larger hearing aids have room for more powerful amplifiers, allowing them to accommodate more severe hearing losses. They also have room for more features and a larger battery, which lasts longer. Larger hearing aids also tend to be more durable and easier to manage if eyesight or manual dexterity are limited. In contrast, tiny models

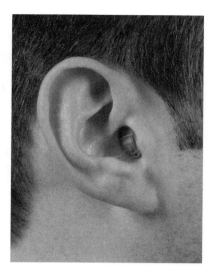

Figure 7.1. Example of a CIC Hearing Aid. (Courtesy of Phonak.)

worn deep in the ear canal (closer to the eardrum) can provide more natural sound quality. Your audiologist considers your hearing needs and preferences in making a recommendation; the final decision is yours.

There are several basic hearing aid styles, and they are discussed here in turn.

Completely-in-the-Canal Hearing Aids

Completely-in-the-canal (CIC) hearing aids are the smallest hearing aids available, and they fit deep within the ear canal. They're virtually invisible when worn, which is something that almost everyone finds appealing. Because they're difficult to reach with one's fingers, a thin, plastic pull cord attaches to the hearing aid and sticks out of the ear canal; the listener pulls on the cord to remove the hearing aid. The "shell" containing the hearing aid's circuitry is custom made from an impression (cast) of the user's ear made by the audiologist (more about this later).

Wearing a hearing aid deep inside the ear canal has several advantages (in addition to being virtually invisible). Placement of the microphone deep in the canal—rather than outside the ear—makes the most of the outer ear's natural ability to collect sounds from the environment and improves the ability to localize the source of sounds. Deep microphone placement provides more natural sound quality and minimizes annoying wind noise. CICs also cause less feedback when using the telephone or headphones (discussed later).

CICs have some important limitations, however. For example, they tend not to be powerful enough to accommodate severe and profound hearing losses; instead, they work best with mild and moderate losses. Also, because the entire hearing aid fits into the ear canal, people with very small or irregularly shaped canals sometimes cannot use them. And they *can* be uncomfortable; some people just can't tolerate wearing a hearing aid deep in the canal. Other people find them difficult to insert. Their size and placement also make some highly desirable features impossible; for example, directional microphones, which have been found to improve speech understanding in noise, are not an option (more about those later). There's also too little space for more conventional user features like a manual volume control or telecoil (more about those later in this discussion). The batteries used in CICs are very small, which makes them more difficult to handle, and they must be replaced more often. CICs are also more susceptible to damage from wax than other hearing aid styles, and for that reason, they have a higher rate of repairs. Because of the need to miniaturize sophisticated technology (and its power source), these aids are also more expensive.

In-the-Canal Hearing Aids

In-the-canal (ITC) instruments are slightly larger than CICs. They fit into the canal but not as deeply as CICs, generally extending a bit into the bowl-shaped depression of the outer ear. They're more visible but still discreet. Like CICs, ITC circuitry is housed in a shell that's custom made to fit the wearer's ear. ITCs are easier to manipulate than CICs, but they're still quite small. They can accommodate mild and moderate (and sometimes moderate-to-severe) hearing losses. As with CICs, microphone placement in the ear canal gives sound a more natural quality. ITCs have more room for features than CICs (for example, multiple programs for different listening environments or manual volume controls) but less room than larger hearing aids. ITC batteries are larger than CIC batteries, meaning they have longer battery life. ITCs are usually less expensive than CICs but more expensive than larger models.

In-the-Ear Hearing Aids

In-the-ear (ITE) aids fill most of the bowl-shaped depression of the outer ear; therefore, they are visible. Like CICs and ITCs, ITE circuitry is housed in a shell that's custom made to fit the wearer's ear. ITEs can accommodate mild, moderate, and severe hearing losses. Because they're larger, they have more space for features like directional microphones and telecoils. Their size also makes them easier to handle. However, they're also more likely to pick up wind noise than CICs and ITCs (although special features can help with that; see later discussion).

A *half shell ITE* is an ITE with a lower profile (that is, it doesn't stick out of the ear canal as far). It's slightly larger than an ITC and slightly smaller

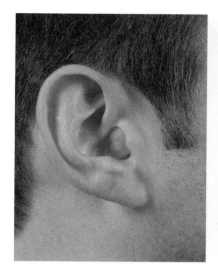 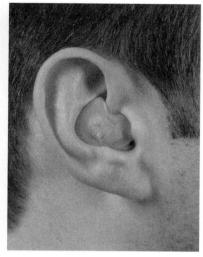

Figure 7.2. Example of an ITC Hearing Aid. (Courtesy of Phonak.)

Figure 7.3. Example of an ITE Hearing Aid. (Courtesy of Phonak.)

than an ITE. Half shell ITEs are usually large enough to accommodate a limited number of features, and like full ITEs, they're suitable for hearing losses that range from mild to severe.

Behind-the-Ear Hearing Aids

The circuitry of a traditional behind-the-ear (BTE) hearing aid is housed in a small case that hooks over the wearer's ear and rests behind it. A clear tube attaches the hearing aid to an earmold, which is usually made of clear plastic. With a BTE, it's the earmold (rather than the hearing aid shell) that's custom made to fit the wearer's ear (CICs, ITCs, and ITEs are known as "custom hearing aids"). The earmold sits in the bowl of the ear and anchors the hearing aid. It also channels sound (from the hearing aid) into the ear canal. BTEs can house larger amplifiers, which means that they can accommodate severe and profound hearing losses. BTEs also have room for more technical features, including those that make hearing aids compatible with assistive listening technology (more about this topic later).

Because of its power and ability to incorporate a wider array of features, the BTE is the most versatile hearing aid style. BTEs are used to accommodate listeners of all ages (infants and children are usually fit with BTEs) and with all degrees of hearing loss. They are the easiest to manipulate, the most durable, and they have the fewest repairs (some are even water resistant). They have room for a larger battery, which means longer battery life. Because the microphone and receiver are separated by a greater distance, the chance of feedback is reduced. Finally, matched for technology

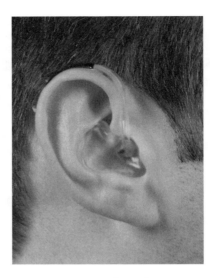

Figure 7.4. Example of a BTE Hearing Aid and Earmold. The ear-mold sits in the ear; the hearing aid hooks over the ear and rests behind it. (Courtesy of Phonak).

and features, BTEs are less expensive than other styles. For these reasons, and because of the recent availability of open canal fittings and mini-BTEs (see later discussion), this style is experiencing a resurgence in popularity. About 50 percent of the hearing aids sold in the United States are BTEs, up from 25 percent just a few years ago.

On the negative side, traditional BTEs have been perceived as big, bulky, and beige—something many people find cosmetically unappealing; however, many new BTEs are small, sleek, and available in high-tech shapes and colors. Some contemporary BTEs can't be distinguished from the high-tech wireless headsets that are used with cell phones. Other limitations include a greater likelihood of wind noise and the need to maintain two pieces of equipment instead of one (the hearing aid plus the earmold).

Open Canal Fittings

Some hearing aid wearers are troubled by something known as the *occlusion effect*. Filling (or occluding) the outer portion of the ear canal with an earmold or custom hearing aid can create an uncomfortable, plugged-up feeling. It can also make the wearer's own voice sound unnatural—like talking in a barrel or a tunnel. Other self-generated sounds (breathing, chewing, coughing, swallowing, throat-clearing) can seem too loud. To experience the occlusion effect, plug your ears by gently pressing your fingers over your ear canals and hum. Continue humming while you plug and unplug your ears. If you hear your voice get louder when your ears are plugged, you're experiencing the occlusion effect.

What Causes the Occlusion Effect?

Sounds made within our heads (including our voices) are transmitted to the ear canal by the bones of the skull (this is called *bone conduction hearing*; see Chapter 4). Although we're unaware of it, the low-frequency components of self-generated sounds typically escape out the ear canal. Plugging the ear prevents these sounds from escaping; instead, they pass through the auditory system, which makes them audible. This is especially troublesome for listeners with good or relatively good low-frequency hearing. Low-frequency energy that becomes trapped in the ear canal causes the hollow voice quality that bothers many hearing aid users.

Have you ever been surprised by the sound of your voice on a recording? Most people think, "Is *that* what I sound like?" Normally, we hear our own voices through a combination of air conduction and bone conduction hearing (see Chapter 4). When we listen to a recording, we hear ourselves by air conduction only. Most people notice the difference.

Another disadvantage of using an earmold or hearing aid that fills the entrance to the ear canal is that sounds are prevented from entering and being heard naturally (without being amplified by the hearing aid). This is especially important for the many people who have normal (or nearly normal) hearing at some frequencies (usually the low frequencies).

One solution to both problems is venting, or putting a hole through the earmold or custom hearing aid shell. A vent allows air into the ear canal, which increases comfort, reduces the likelihood of infection, and allows natural hearing at frequencies for which hearing is reasonably good. Furthermore, it allows self-generated sounds (including the voice) to escape, thereby decreasing the occlusion effect. The larger the vent, the more effective it is at increasing comfort, allowing natural hearing, and reducing the occlusion effect. As the size of the vent increases, however, sound that's already been amplified by the hearing aid escapes from the ear canal. Escaping sounds are picked up by the hearing aid microphone and reamplified again and again, resulting in the annoying squeal known as *acoustic feedback*. Until recently, the solution to feedback has been to decrease the hearing aid's volume, which also decreases the benefit of the hearing aid.

Open canal fittings work like enormous vents. Digital technology has made a new generation of open fittings possible by minimizing the problem

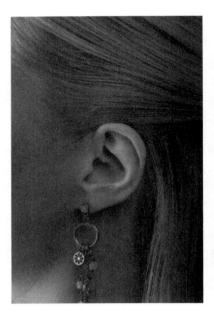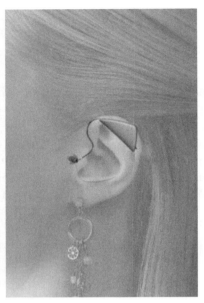

Figure 7.5. Example of an Open Canal Fitting with a Mini- or Micro-BTE Hearing Aid. *Left,* the hearing aid as worn. *Right,* the hearing aid as worn but with the outer ear made translucent. (Courtesy of Oticon Inc.)

of feedback (see later discussion). Here's how modern open fittings work: the BTE hearing aid (often a mini- or micro-BTE) sends amplified sound through a slim, clear, nonreflective tube that follows the contours of the ear into the ear canal (with no BTE earhook and no earmold). Inside the ear canal, a small eartip holds the tube in place but does not touch the ear canal itself. There can also be a clear, flexible *positioner* or *ear grip* that conforms to the contours of the ear, helping to hold the tube in place. The entire arrangement is virtually invisible. Because the ear canal is open, physical comfort is increased, natural hearing is maximized, and the occlusion effect is eliminated. All major manufacturers now offer open canal fitting options.

In addition, manufacturers are now offering open canal models in which the receiver (or loudspeaker, which turns electrical signals back into sound) is located in the ear canal rather than inside the hearing aid. This allows the BTE worn on the ear to be even smaller. The receiver is attached to the hearing aid by a thin, flexible, insulated, nonreflective wire. This arrangement improves sound quality and allows greater amplification or volume. Like other open fittings, receiver-in-the-ear (RITE) fittings are virtually invisible.

Open fittings combine the comfort of an open ear canal with cosmetic appeal. And without the need to make an earmold impression that must be sent away to a laboratory (see later discussion), the initial fitting can

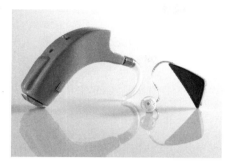

Figure 7.6. *Left,* example of a Conventional BTE Hearing Aid. The earhook on the right end of the aid attaches to an earmold that fits in the ear (not shown). *Right,* example of a Mini- or Micro-BTE. The receiver is in a "dome" that sits inside the ear canal without touching it. The dome is attached to the hearing aid by a thin, flexible wire. (Courtesy of Oticon, Inc.)

be accomplished in just one visit. This means that the user can leave the audiologist's office knowing exactly how her new hearing aids will sound and feel. For all these reasons, digital BTEs with open canal fittings have become very popular in a relatively short time. However, this type of fitting is not suitable for all degrees and configurations of hearing loss, although the range of losses that can be accommodated continues to expand.

Mini-BTEs

Mini- or micro-BTEs have been created to go with the new open canal fittings. These tiny hearing aids often have nontraditional high-tech shapes and colors. Mini-BTEs are usually too small to accommodate some of the user controls discussed later; however, such controls are less important for mini-BTE users who tend to have milder hearing losses and less need to make adjustments to their hearing aids.

My Dad

My dad recently got a new mini-BTE with an open canal fitting. He absolutely *loves* the comfort that it provides. He's always had problems with earmolds not fitting properly and being uncomfortable. This aid is so comfortable that he almost forgets to take it off at night.

Factors to Consider When Choosing a Hearing Aid Style[1]

- If your outer ear is small or deformed, you may be unable to wear a BTE.
- If your ear canal is small or deformed, you may be unable to wear a CIC or an ITC.
- If the "bowl" of your outer ear is shallow, you may be unable to wear a full shell ITE.
- If your vision or manual dexterity are limited, you may have trouble wearing a CIC or an ITC (tiny hearing aids and tiny batteries require adequate vision and nimble fingers—or assistance from someone else).
- If your ears produce an unusual amount of wax, you may be unable to wear a CIC or ITC.
- If you have a draining ear, you may need a large vent or a BTE with an open canal fitting (so that air can enter your ear canal).
- If you have a high-frequency hearing loss and normal or nearly normal low-frequency hearing, you may be most comfortable with a large vent or a BTE with an open canal fitting (this should allow you to hear low-frequency sounds naturally and reduce or prevent the occlusion effect).
- If you have a severe or profound hearing loss, you may need the power available only in a BTE; however, an open canal fitting may be impossible because of feedback.
- If you need technical features that increase comfort and improve understanding in noisy situations, you may need a larger hearing aid (BTE or ITE).
- If you're making a decision on the basis of how the aids look, you may find that an open canal fitting with a mini-BTE is less conspicuous than other styles—take a look!

SPECIAL TYPES OF HEARING AIDS

Wireless CROS or BICROS

The acronym *CROS* stands for contralateral routing of the signal, which is a special hearing aid arrangement sometimes used by listeners who have very poor hearing (or very poor speech perception ability; see Chapter 4) in one ear and normal hearing in the other. Sometimes hearing or speech perception is *so* poor that it's unusable, even with a hearing aid. With a CROS system, a microphone worn on the bad ear (in what looks like a conventional hearing aid) picks up sounds and transmits them (by FM radio waves—no wires are necessary) to a receiver worn on the good ear (in what also looks like a conventional hearing aid). This allows the listener to hear sounds on her bad side that would otherwise be missed. Having a microphone on the "dead ear" also can improve the listener's ability to localize the source of sounds.

A BICROS system (bilateral CROS) is similar, but it's used when the hearing in one ear is unusable and the hearing in the other ear is not normal. This is actually the more common arrangement. A microphone worn on the bad ear picks up sounds and transmits them to the better ear. The hearing aid on the better ear amplifies sounds coming from both sides and delivers them to the better ear. Traditionally, wireless CROS and BICROS systems have been housed in BTEs. They're now available in ITEs as well. A variety of digital signal processing features (see later discussion) can be incorporated.

My Dad

My dad has suffered from Ménière's disease for about 25 years (see Chapter 5). A few years ago, the hearing and tinnitus in his left ear became worse. Because I thought wearing hearing aids might bring relief from the tinnitus (see Chapter 6), and because he seemed to be having so much difficulty hearing (his right ear also had some hearing loss, probably because of age; see Chapter 5), I encouraged him to try hearing aids. The hearing in his right ear was still fairly good at that time; therefore his audiologist recommended a hearing aid for the left ear only. Not long after he bought the aid, he had a particularly bad episode (of Ménière's disease) and lost virtually all ability to understand speech in the left ear. A hearing aid was no longer useful in that ear. Fortunately, because it was a digital aid, his audiologist was able to reprogram it for use in his right ear (on which he now had to depend).

Later, I suggested that my dad try using a BICROS hearing aid arrangement. He wore what appeared to be a conventional BTE hearing aid containing a microphone and transmitter on his left ear. Sounds picked up on his left side were transmitted (wirelessly) to the hearing aid on his right ear. On his right ear, he wore a conventional BTE hearing aid that picked up sounds from his right side and also received the signals transmitted from his left side. It amplified signals from both sides and delivered them to the right ear, allowing him to pick up sounds on his left side that he would otherwise have missed and giving him a better sense of where sounds were coming from. He wore this arrangement for several years and thought that it was helpful in some situations but not so helpful in others.

Disposable, Deep-fitting, Extended-wear Devices

In the future, disposable, extended-wear devices that fit deep within the ear canal could become more widely available. The disposable device is placed extremely close to the eardrum by an ENT physician and worn continually for about 120 days, or until the battery ceases to function. The device is completely invisible and said to offer improved sound quality. With its initial release, patients paid about $1,450 to $2,000 per ear, per year.

Middle Ear Implants

A middle ear implant may be an option for a person who is unable to tolerate conventional hearing aids and has too much hearing to be a candidate for a cochlear implant (see Chapter 8). With this type of hearing device, a tiny electromagnetic coil is surgically attached to one of the bones within the middle ear (the incus), and a receiver is implanted under the skin behind the outer ear. An external processor containing a microphone, amplifier, and battery is held over the implanted receiver by a magnet. The external processor picks up sounds from the environment and transmits a representation of them across the skin to the implanted receiver. The receiver sends the signals through a conductor to the electromagnet implanted on the incus. Signals sent to the incus cause the ossicular chain to move, and movement of the ossicular chain transmits energy to the cochlea in the natural manner (see Chapter 3).

Candidates for middle ear implants usually have a sensorineural hearing loss, a normally functioning middle ear, and an unsuccessful history with conventional hearing aids. Using a middle ear implant eliminates the need to wear a hearing aid or earmold in the ear canal, which in turn eliminates problems such as discomfort, the occlusion effect, allergic skin reactions, feedback, and wax damage to the hearing aid. However, surgery is more expensive than buying conventional hearing aids and carries more risks. In the future, it's possible that middle ear implants could be totally implantable and therefore invisible (with the microphone implanted in the ear canal).

Bone Conduction Devices

If you've had a hearing evaluation, the audiologist may have tested your hearing by bone conduction (see Chapter 4). This is done by placing a small box against the bony bump behind your ear (the box would have been attached to a metal band that stretched across your head). A traditional bone conduction hearing aid is similar to that device—awkward and cumbersome to wear all the time. A *bone-anchored* hearing aid is an implantable device that allows the listener to hear by bone conduction without the inconvenience of a traditional bone conduction hearing aid. It's more comfortable, and the sound quality is better, partly because the device stays in place.

Unlike a middle ear implant, which requires a normally functioning middle ear, this type of hearing aid is typically used by listeners who have conductive or mixed hearing loss. Bone conduction hearing aids have traditionally been used by people born without ear canals or with small, misshapen ears that can't support conventional hearing aids, or by people who have chronic middle ear disease that's aggravated by wearing a hearing aid or earmold in the ear canal (for example, people with draining ears).

With a bone-anchored hearing aid, a titanium post is implanted in the bone behind the outer ear, and the post becomes integrated into the bone as it heals. When healing is complete, a hearing aid is attached to the post with an abutment. Sounds processed by the hearing aid cause the implanted post

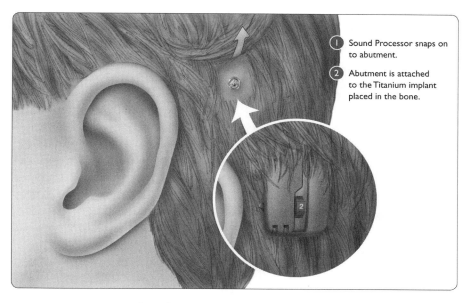

① Sound Processor snaps on to abutment.

② Abutment is attached to the Titanium implant placed in the bone.

Figure 7.7. A Bone-anchored Hearing Aid. (Courtesy of Cochlear Americas.)

to (imperceptibly) vibrate the bones of the skull, stimulating both cochleae by bone conduction (see Chapter 4). The ear canal and middle ear (where the problem lies) are bypassed. As with a middle ear implant, the ear canal remains completely open.

The bone-anchored hearing aid also works for people who have *single-sided deafness* or one ear that can't be aided (in this case, it would be an alternative to a CROS hearing aid system). When hearing is stimulated by bone conduction, the bones of the skull vibrate, and the fluids inside *both* cochleae are stimulated (see Chapter 4). That means sounds picked up by a microphone on the listener's "bad" side reach both cochleae (including the one with better hearing) by bone conduction.

My Dad
A bone-anchored hearing aid might be a good solution for my dad, but he won't consider the surgery.

Other nontraditional bone conduction options are available for people who have single-sided deafness. In one case, a microphone worn on the nonhearing ear converts sounds picked up on the bad side into electrical signals. However, instead of amplifying them and converting them back into sound (like a conventional hearing aid), the electrical signals drive a small "vibrator" that sits in the canal of the nonhearing ear where it makes contact with the bones of the ear canal. When it vibrates, sounds are transferred by the bones of the skull to both cochleae (including the one with better hearing). Because the device is not implanted, surgery is unnecessary.

HEARING AID TECHNOLOGY (CIRCUITRY)

Until recently, the goal of hearing aids was simple: to make all sounds louder. Today, the goals also include making soft sounds sufficiently loud while preventing others from becoming uncomfortably loud and emphasizing sounds that are meaningful while deemphasizing those that are not.

As mentioned, hearing aid style refers to how a hearing aid looks and how it's worn in or on the ear. Hearing aid circuitry refers to the technology inside. At present, existing hearing aids use three types of technology: conventional analog, programmable analog, and digital. With a few exceptions, any type of circuitry can be placed in any hearing aid style. In other words, style has nothing to do with the sophistication of the circuitry inside. The type of technology determines the extent to which a hearing aid can selectively process incoming sounds and the degree to which the aid can be customized to meet individual needs.

Conventional Analog Technology

Until recently, all hearing aids used analog technology to process incoming sounds. For the most part, analog hearing aids simply make all sounds louder. The hearing aid's microphone collects sound waves traveling through air and changes them into electrical signals. The electronic copy of an incoming sound—the sound's "analog"—is amplified (made bigger) and sent to the hearing aid's receiver, which changes it back into sound. The signal that a listener hears is louder than the original (with some distortion thrown in). It may be possible to emphasize some frequencies (for example, the high frequencies) over others; however, this type of selective amplification is crude. The audiologist makes all adjustments manually (on the hearing aid) using a tiny screwdriver. Conventional analog hearing aids are the least flexible in terms of meeting individual needs. Available features generally are limited to telecoils and manual volume controls (see later discussion). However, they are also the least expensive. Although this technology is becoming obsolete, it might be perfectly adequate for people who usually communicate in quiet situations (like people who live alone and don't go out often). It's less effective in difficult listening environments because signal processing features can't be integrated into the circuitry.

Programmable Analog Technology

With a computer microchip inside, programmable analog hearing aids are a step up from conventional analog hearing aids. They still rely on analog circuitry to process incoming sounds, but digital technology (a microchip) is used to program them. An audiologist attaches the hearing aid to a personal computer and uses special software to program the aid for the listener's hearing loss. This is quite an improvement over using a screwdriver to make crude adjustments on an analog hearing aid. The hearing aid can also be reprogrammed to accommodate changes in the hearing loss. With many programmable aids, multiple programs can be created for different listening environments and held in the microchip's memory. The listener selects the appropriate program (for a quiet room, a noisy room, telephone use, listening to music, etc.) by pressing a button on the hearing aid or using a remote control. Programmable analog aids can accommodate more features than conventional analog aids (for example, multiple listening programs, compression circuitry, directional microphones, and telecoils—all described later), but far fewer than digital aids. They're more flexible than conventional analogs in terms of meeting individual needs but less flexible than digitals. As you might expect, they're also more expensive than conventional analogs but less expensive than digitals.

Digital Technology

Fully digital hearing aids represent a giant leap forward in hearing aid technology. In addition to being programmed digitally (like programmable analog aids), they use digital technology to process incoming sounds. As recently as 2002, fewer than one half of the hearing aids sold in the United States were digital, while in 2006, more than 90 percent were digital. In fact, some manufacturers are phasing out conventional analog and programmable analog hearing aids and turning their full attention to more affordable entry-level digitals.

Digital hearing aids use the most advanced technology available today. They offer cleaner, crisper sound quality than do analog hearing aids (similar to the difference between a CD and an audio cassette). A computer (microchip) is housed within the hearing aid and controls all of its operations. The audiologist uses a personal computer and special software to program the hearing aid to fit an individual listener's hearing loss, typical listening environments, and listening preferences. This can be done with far greater precision than is possible with nondigital hearing aids, although maximizing performance often requires fine tuning over several visits.

Digital technology makes it possible to incorporate a variety of sophisticated signal processing features designed to improve speech understanding and maximize listener comfort (more about those features later in this chapter). Not surprisingly, digital technology is more expensive than analog technology; however, the product lines of all major manufacturers now include high-end, mid-level, and economy digital models. Mid- and lower-priced digitals offer more features all the time. Although these aids are still expensive, manufacturers *are* making better technology available at more affordable prices.

How a Digital Hearing Aid Works

A microphone picks up sounds traveling through air and converts them into a stream of electrical signals. In an analog hearing aid, the electrical signals are amplified, and then converted back into sounds by the hearing aid's receiver. In a digital hearing aid, however, an analog-to-digital (A/D) converter changes the electrical signals into a computer code (millions of zeros and ones). The computer then applies complicated algorithms (mathematical formulas) to the incoming streams of numbers to analyze sounds in the environment (are they noise, speech, music, feedback?) and decide how they should be processed. Based on those decisions, different features perform complex actions on the signal. Millions of adjustments are made, theoretically providing the clearest, most natural sound quality possible. Reducing sounds to numbers allows them to be processed in an infinite number of ways, very quickly, and without distortion. After adjustments have been made, the streams of numbers are converted back into electrical signals by a digital-to-analog (D/A) converter. The hearing aid's receiver then changes the electrical signals back into sounds that get sent into the ear canal. And all of this happens in an instant!

HEARING AID FEATURES: DIGITAL SIGNAL PROCESSING

Different hearing aid models incorporate different features or combinations of features. These features have been designed to solve the problems long associated with hearing aid use (for example, understanding speech in noisy situations, acoustic feedback, and uncomfortable loudness). Conventional analog aids offer virtually no signal processing features, and programmable analog aids offer very few. Larger hearing aids (BTEs and ITEs) can accommodate more features than can smaller aids (ITCs and CICs). And, of course, more features cost more money.

In many cases, digital signal processing means greater listening comfort and improved speech understanding in difficult listening conditions. However, no hearing aid—no matter how advanced—can block out all background noise, nor can any hearing aid eliminate the distortion that can be caused by sensorineural hearing loss. Having realistic expectations increases your probability of success with hearing aids.

The research and development teams employed by hearing aid manufacturers continually search for new ways to solve old problems. The strategies that manufacturers develop are often proprietary (patented) and called by different names. This makes comparing hearing aids like comparing apples and oranges (and dozens of other fruits). Manufacturers routinely claim that their particular strategy or feature is "the first," "the only," or "the best" solution to a particular problem. Your audiologist can help you to sort through advertising claims and set priorities.

Some examples of the features available in hearing aids today are included here. The intent is not to showcase any particular processing strategy or any particular manufacturer's features; rather, the intent is simply to give you a sense of what's available. Dozens of features exist, and they are continuously evolving. By the time you read this, new ones will have been developed. These examples, described in simplistic terms, are meant to be representative only.

Adaptive and Automatic Sound Processing

Digital technology made it possible for hearing aids to offer sophisticated signal processing features, but the features were sometimes cumbersome to operate. Sometimes it was difficult for users to know *when* to use advanced features. Other times, it was difficult for users to make adjustments in ever-changing listening environments. And as more processing features became available, adjustments to one feature had the potential to interact with adjustments to another. It seemed that listeners might not be able to take advantage of the features they had. Today, *intelligent* or *smart* hearing aids have features that work adaptively and automatically. The hearing aid continually analyzes the listening environment by performing millions of calculations (per second), and then adapts to it *automatically*. The hearing aid makes internal adjustments so that the user doesn't have to make *manual* adjustments; the aid is essentially on "auto-pilot." In contrast, when aids are not automatic, the user considers the listening environment and makes adjustments manually by touching a button on the hearing aid or using a remote control (for example, the listener can adjust the volume manually or change listening programs to suit the environment). Many listeners appreciate never having to adjust their hearing aids, but others prefer to be able to make adjustments themselves. Some hearing aids are fully adaptive and automatic, yet allow the user to manually override some of the computer's decisions by using controls on the hearing aid or a remote.

Manufacturers of fully adaptive and automatic hearing aids claim that they provide the best combination of sound quality, speech understanding, and comfort in all listening situations. The computer finds the optimal combination of settings and provides the best amplification scheme for any environment. The good news: all this happens in a heartbeat and is imperceptible to the listener. The bad news: there are still situations in which listening is difficult.

Data Logging

Some hearing aids analyze and store information about the amount of time a listener spends in different listening environments and how the hearing aid's features are adjusted (manually or automatically) to accommodate those environments. That is, the hearing aid keeps track of its own performance and builds a profile of the listener's needs and preferences. The audiologist can access the stored information and use it (along with the listener's feedback) to further fine tune the hearing aid's features. In some cases, the hearing aid's computer can even make suggestions about how settings can be improved.

Some hearing aids are trainable. This technology is based on the observation that individual listeners have consistent preferences about how they like to hear in different environments. For example, as a listener adjusts the volume control to his preferred setting in a variety of listening environments, the trainable hearing aid remembers and learns. Soon, the hearing aid automatically adjusts volume to levels that match that listener's preferences. A possible future development is an *experience monitor* that periodically signals the listener (through the hearing aid) that a test is about to take place. A paired comparison of two different feature settings would be presented, and the listener would "vote" her preference by pressing a button on the hearing aid. Over time, the hearing aid would learn the listener's preferences in various environments, and the monitor would become unnecessary.

Multichannel Processing

Most digital hearing aids (entry level to premium) divide incoming sounds into different frequency "channels." In the very simplest example, there would be a high-frequency channel and a low-frequency channel. Sound processing is controlled independently in each channel; for example, high-frequency sounds might be amplified more than low-frequency sounds. The way in which signal processing features are programmed in one frequency region (channel) doesn't affect the way they're programmed in other regions. Theoretically, processing sounds in smaller "slices" is more precise; the greater the number of channels, the greater the ability to tailor a hearing aid's performance to meet an individual listener's needs.

Loudness Compression

Listeners with sensorineural hearing loss (more specifically, listeners with damage to the cochlea) are likely to find loud sounds uncomfortable. In fact, "too much loudness" has long been a complaint among hearing aid users. In an effort to solve this problem, several loudness *compression* strategies have been developed. All of them share the same basic goals: to ensure that soft sounds are amplified enough for the listener to hear them but to prevent other sounds from becoming uncomfortably loud. In other words, the normal range of loudness is compressed to fit within the listener's abnormally small comfort range (also called his dynamic range; see Chapter 4). This feature is now basic to most digital hearing aids, including those in the entry-level category.

Without compression, all sounds (whether they're soft, medium, or loud) are amplified by the same amount until the hearing aid's output limits are reached, and the sounds become distorted (as well as unpleasantly loud). With compression, softer sounds receive *more* amplification (but are still perceived as relatively softer), and louder sounds receive *less* amplification (but are still perceived as relatively louder). In hearing aids with multiple channels (see previous discussion), compression settings can be adjusted independently in different frequency regions. This allows more compression in some frequency channels (perhaps the high-frequency channels where hearing loss and the need for compression are greatest) with less in others.

Digital Feedback Reduction

Feedback is the annoying (and often embarrassing) high-pitched squeal that a hearing aid sometimes makes. It happens when sound that's been amplified leaks out of the ear canal and passes through the hearing aid again. It's more likely to happen when sound is trapped close to the ear—as when a listener cups her hand around the hearing aid, wears a hat over the hearing aid, gets a hug, or uses the phone. Feedback also occurs when the earmold or hearing aid shell is poorly fitted or inserted into the ear improperly, or when the aid's volume is turned up too high. Occasionally, it means the hearing aid is malfunctioning.

Before the availability of digital signal processing, feedback was controlled by turning down the volume on the hearing aid. This reduced the feedback, but it also reduced the benefit provided by the hearing aid. With digital signal processing, most (but not all) feedback can be controlled by the hearing aid's computer. When feedback occurs, the hearing aid detects it and introduces an internal signal that's exactly the same but 180 degrees out of phase. Signals that are the same but opposite in phase cancel one another. Digital feedback management has made the new generation of open canal fittings possible. Without it, sound would leak out of the open ear canal and cause constant (or nearly constant) feedback. This is another basic feature now found in most digital hearing aids (entry level to premium).

Directional Microphones

Difficulty hearing in noisy conditions is the most common complaint among hearing aid users. The directional microphone is a feature that's been shown to improve speech understanding in noisy environments. In fact, this is one of the two best technologies available today for improving speech understanding in noise (read on for the other one). Traditionally, hearing aids have had one *omnidirectional* microphone that picks up sounds from all directions. Omnidirectional microphones most closely represent the way we typically hear—from all around us. They give listeners a sense of where sounds are coming from and the most natural connection to the rest of the world. Today, most digital hearing aids (entry level to premium) also have a second microphone, called a *directional microphone*. In the simplest example, a directional microphone emphasizes sounds coming from one direction (usually the front), while deemphasizing sounds coming from other directions. This means that in a noisy situation, the directional microphone targets conversation (which is usually in front of the listener) and reduces (but does not eliminate) distracting sounds coming from the sides and rear. This works best when the user is close to the sound that she wishes to hear and the noise is coming from another direction.

Depending on the hearing aid, switching between microphones may be done manually (by pressing a button on the hearing aid or a remote control) or automatically (the hearing aid's computer analyzes the listening environment and selects the most appropriate microphone arrangement). Directional microphones work best with BTEs; they're also available in ITEs and, less often, in ITCs. Directional microphone technology isn't possible with CIC hearing aids because of their small size and position deep within the ear canal.

Digital Noise Reduction

Many digital hearing aids (entry level to premium) have sophisticated features designed to reduce noise and enhance speech. Each manufacturer has developed its own approach. In general, a hearing aid with a noise reduction feature performs millions of calculations (per second) to determine whether incoming sounds are speech or noise (or some combination of the two). In a simple example, the hearing aid recognizes speech sounds as short and constantly changing and noise as steady and continuous (for example, fan noise, appliance noise, or traffic noise). In this case, the solution is to reduce amplification in the channels containing continuous sounds while preserving the amplification of speech sounds in all other channels.

Noise reduction systems do a reasonably good job of analyzing the sounds coming into a hearing aid; that is, determining whether they're speech or noise. They're not as good at treating the two signals differently. The speech signal is made up of a broad range of frequencies; therefore every frequency channel contains some of the speech signal. When amplification is reduced in a channel containing noise, the speech sounds in that channel are reduced as well, and that makes speech harder to understand.

Hearing aids amplify all sounds, not just those we want to hear. To some extent, a person's success with hearing aids depends on his ability to tolerate background noise. Many hearing aids are capable of *emphasizing* some sounds over others, but no hearing aid can completely separate unwanted sounds from those that are of interest. Clinical tests generally fail to show an improvement in speech understanding as a result of digital noise reduction. Nonetheless, users often report that noise reduction makes listening in noisy environments more comfortable, less stressful, and less tiring. And many users think that's worthwhile.

Wind Noise Reduction

This is a special type of noise reduction. Some hearing aids can be programmed to recognize wind noise and suppress it, while preserving the speech signal to the extent possible. In extremely windy conditions, some hearing aids can momentarily reduce all amplification to prevent discomfort.

Multiple Listening Programs

Most digital hearing aids (entry level to premium) can store several preset programs in their memories. The audiologist creates different programs for different listening situations—it's like having several different hearing aids all in one. For example, a listener might have different programs for listening in quiet, in noise, or on the telephone. Another listener might have a program for comfortable listening and a different program for critical listening when it's important to be able to hear very well for a brief period of time. Yet another listener might have a program for bird watching. Some listeners have a program especially designed for appreciating music. The listener can change programs by pressing a button on the hearing aid or using a remote control. Many digital hearing aids change programs automatically. Without multiple programs in memory, the same internal hearing aid settings are used for all listening environments.

My Dad

The right hearing aid in my dad's BICROS hearing aid arrangement (see earlier description) had three preset programs. Program 1 (signaled by one beep) was used for quiet conditions; it used the omnidirectional microphones on the right and left ears. Program 2 (signaled by two beeps) was used for noisy conditions; it used the directional microphone on the right hearing aid and the omnidirectional microphone on the left ear. Program 3 (signaled by three beeps) was also used for noisy conditions; it used the directional microphone on the right hearing aid and deactivated the microphone on the left ear. Deactivating the microphone on the left side reduced noise coming from anywhere but the front (where the directional mic on the right ear was pointed). My dad changed programs manually by pressing a button on his right hearing aid. My dad's programs were simple. In many cases, switching among programs means more than switching microphones on and off.

My dad's new hearing aid is fully adaptive and automatic (that is, it analyzes the listening environment and then automatically makes adjustments that adapt to it). However, I also wanted him to have a program switch that would allow him to override the automatic adjustments. Program 1 is for quiet listening conditions (omnidirectional microphone), Program 2 is for noisy conditions (directional microphone), and Program 3 is for critical listening situations (in which he needs extra volume). He also has a program for the telecoil setting (see later discussion and Chapter 9).

HEARING AID FEATURES: COMPATIBILITY WITH ASSISTIVE LISTENING TECHNOLOGIES

Hearing aids, especially those with features like those just discussed, can improve speech understanding in noise. The only thing more effective is combining hearing aids with assistive listening technology (this is *the* best way to improve speech understanding in difficult listening conditions). Although these technologies are discussed in detail in Chapter 9, the features that make them compatible with hearing aids are included here. Basically, these features allow a hearing aid to receive input directly from an external source (for example, a microphone worn by another person), without passing through the microphone on the hearing aid. In this case, the speech signal is louder and clearer than the background noise. If you're interested in using assistive listening technology (and you probably should be), choose a hearing aid that can support it (like a BTE or ITE).

Ear-level FM

To understand speech clearly, people with sensorineural hearing loss need better listening conditions than do people with normal hearing. More specifically, they need a better signal-to-noise relationship (SNR); for them, speech must be louder than the background noise by approximately 20 dB. Because sound is measured on a logarithmic scale, this means speech must be ten times louder than the noise (see Chapter 3). In many situations, this SNR cannot be achieved with hearing aids alone. One way to improve the SNR is to move the talker closer to the listener. Ideally, the talker's mouth would be 8 to 12 inches from the listener's ear at all times, but, of course, that's unrealistic. A better solution is to use *remote microphone technology* in which the microphone is "remote" to the user's hearing aid. In other words, we put a microphone close the talker's mouth and transmit the signal by FM radio waves to a receiver worn on the listener's ear. It's like a tiny FM radio station with a single transmitter and receiver—no wires or cables are involved. When the microphone/transmitter is worn by the talker, the effects of distance are eliminated because sound is transmitted directly from the talker's mouth (which is close to the microphone) to the listener's ear. It's as if the talker is speaking into the ear of the listener. The effects of noise and reverberation are reduced because the signal from the talker's mouth is closer to the microphone and therefore louder than the background. The SNR can also be improved, to a slightly lesser degree, by placing the microphone near the talker or holding the microphone and aiming at the talker.

The signal from the talker's microphone bypasses the hearing aid's microphone. It can be the only signal that the listener hears or the microphone on the hearing aid can also be active, making it possible for the listener to communicate with others nearby. Using both microphones can make the

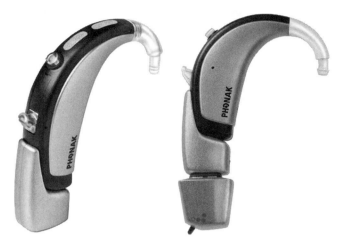

Figure 7.8. Examples of Ear-level FM Receivers and Adapters. *Left*, an FM receiver *integrated* into a "boot" adapter (*bottom*) that attaches to the end of a compatible BTE. *Right*, an FM receiver (*bottom*) that plugs into to a universal boot adapter (*center*) that slides onto the end of almost any BTE (*top*). (Courtesy of Phonak.)

SNR less favorable, so amplification of the two inputs must be properly balanced by the audiologist. The remote microphone/transmitter can also be connected to an external source such as a television, radio, telephone, CD player, or personal computer. In this case, the hearing aid's microphone is turned off, and the listener hears only the input from the external source.

To receive an FM signal, the listener must wear an FM receiver. Traditionally, the receiver has been worn like a pager (see Chapter 9), but several ear-level options are also available. Some BTE hearing aids have an FM receiver built inside (not shown in Figure 7.8). Others are compatible with a special *boot* or *audio shoe* adapter that contains an FM receiver. The boot attaches to the bottom of a compatible BTE hearing aid (see Figure 7.8 left). In other cases, an FM receiver plugs into a *universal* boot adapter that connects to the bottom of almost any BTE (see Figure 7.8 right). Switching to the FM mode can be done by pushing a button on the hearing aid or using a remote control. With many digital hearing aids, the FM receiver automatically activates when it senses the presence of a signal from an FM transmitter.

Telecoils

A *telecoil* is an optional hearing aid feature originally intended to make listening over the telephone easier. Telecoils have been around for a long time (they're one of the few features available on analog and programmable analog hearing aids); however, their versatility has sparked renewed interest. For example, in addition to their use with telephones, they can conveniently double as receivers for the assistive listening systems used in public places (see Chapter 9).

To use a telecoil with the telephone, the hearing aid is switched to the telecoil setting, and the telephone handset is placed over the hearing aid. The telecoil picks up electromagnetic energy produced by the telephone. This energy is amplified and converted back into sound by the hearing aid's receiver. The hearing aid's microphone is turned off, dramatically reducing the interference of room noise and eliminating the feedback that normally occurs when the handset is held over the hearing aid's microphone.

Telecoils are tiny; ten or more could fit on the surface of a dime. They fit in BTEs, ITEs, and some ITCs. CIC hearing aids are too small to accommodate them. In hearing aids with multiple programs, the telecoil setting can be one of the programs held in the hearing aid's memory. A telecoil can be manually activated by touching a switch or a button on the hearing aid or by using a remote control. Some digital hearing aids switch into and out of the telecoil mode automatically when a telephone is moved toward or away from the hearing aid. This is particularly helpful for listeners with poor manual dexterity.

Direct Audio Input

Direct audio input (DAI) is an optional feature that allows an external sound source (for example, a telephone, television, stereo, radio, computer, external microphone, CD player, or assistive listening device) to be plugged into a hearing aid with a patch card. The direct connection is made by a DAI jack (available on a limited number of hearing aids) or a universal DAI boot that slips over the end of almost any BTE hearing aid. Like all assistive listening devices, direct audio input bypasses the hearing aid's microphone.

Compared with the telecoil, DAI has at least two advantages: DAI is subject to less electromagnetic interference than a telecoil (interference from computers, florescent lights, and other electronics can cause buzzing in a telecoil), and signal strength is unaffected by head position or orientation (which can cause "dead" spots with a telecoil). On the other hand, a telecoil is wireless, and DAI is not. FM technology eliminates all of these problems, but it's more expensive.

HEARING AID FEATURES: LISTENER CONVENIENCE AND COMFORT

Delayed Start-up

Some hearing aids can be set (by the audiologist) to turn on several seconds after the battery compartment door has been closed. This gives the listener a few seconds to place the hearing aid in or on the ear without the annoying feedback that usually occurs when a hearing aid is being handled.

Audio Signals

Some hearing aids use beeps or tones to let the listener know the status of his hearing aid (which listening program or volume setting has been selected, when the battery is low, and so forth). For listeners who have difficulty remembering the significance of tones, voice indicators are also available (in several languages). Some aids can even be programmed to provide voice reminders about maintenance and follow-up visits.

Diagnostic Tools

Some hearing aids have internal diagnostic capabilities and can provide the user with a performance report on the hearing aid's circuitry, receiver, and microphone.

Wind Noise Protector

Some hearing aids are equipped with a microphone hood that helps to reduce wind noise. Wind noise that does enter the microphone can be further reduced digitally by some hearing aids.

Remote Control

Some digital (and programmable analog) hearing aids have features that can be operated by remote control (such as volume, program selection, and activation of FM receivers). Using a remote control allows changes to be made without having to touch the hearing aid, and some users feel that's more discreet. In addition, using a remote device is easier for listeners who have dexterity problems. Remote controls sometimes allow features to be incorporated into ITC or CIC hearing aids, which are too small for buttons, switches, and wheels. More sophisticated remote devices also display a hearing aid's settings and battery status. For listeners who wear two hearing aids, one remote can be used to control both. Remote control devices come in a variety of styles that range from the traditional television-type to watches, key chains, necklaces, and belt clips.

Manual Volume Control

In the past, virtually all hearing aids had manual volume controls. As hearing aids become smaller and more models have features that are adaptive and automatic, however, fewer have them. Nonetheless, many listeners prefer to have a manual volume control. They may be accustomed to having one, they may find the automatic volume control feature doesn't meet their needs in all listening situations, or they may simply feel that they want more control over their hearing aids. As stated previously, it's very important to discuss *your* needs and preferences with your audiologist.

HEARING AID BATTERIES

All the work that a hearing aid does is powered by one tiny battery. Today, most hearing aid batteries are the zinc air type (see Appendix A), although a few hearing aids are now available with rechargeable batteries.

TWO EARS (OR HEARING AIDS) ARE NEARLY ALWAYS BETTER THAN ONE

People are meant to have two ears that hear equally well; that's the normal listening condition. Two ears working together provide the brain with a complete "picture" of the surrounding sound environment. Our brains are wired to receive input from both ears, and remember, we hear with our brains, not with our ears. For these reasons, people who have hearing loss in both ears are usually advised to wear two hearing aids (often referred to as *binaural hearing aids* or *bilateral hearing aids*).

Binaural hearing or hearing in stereo has several important advantages. For one thing, it allows us to know where sounds are coming from. This ability is called *localization*. Imagine yourself with normal hearing in both ears; as you step into the street you hear a siren. In that instant, your brain compares the information that it receives from your right ear to the information that it receives from your left ear. If the siren is on your right side, the sound reaches your right ear slightly ahead of when it reaches your left ear (sound reaching your left ear has to go around your head). It also reaches your right ear with slightly greater loudness. Based on these very slight differences in timing and loudness, your brain determines that the potential hazard is on your right side and directs your attention there. Of course, your brain makes these comparisons in an instant and without making you consciously aware of them. The ability to localize also improves speech understanding in some situations. Imagine that you're in a situation with more than one speaker. As the conversation quickly shifts from one person to the next, you need to be able to identify the current speaker without hesitation. With only one hearing aid, everything sounds like it's coming from your aided side. You must search for the talker with your eyes (whose lips are moving?). By the time you identify her, you may have missed an important part of the message, making it difficult to catch up—or the conversation may have already moved on to someone else. Hearing with two ears allows us to localize sounds almost instantly.

Hearing without Stereo

I recently had an experience that gave me a sense of what it's like to hear with only one ear or one hearing aid. I was attending a meeting of my county's Planning Commission. Seven men were seated at a ∩-shaped table on a platform at the front of the room. Each spoke into a microphone, so it was easy for me to hear. Because there was only one loudspeaker, however, all the voices (as I heard them) came from the same place. The men were unfamiliar to me, so I couldn't immediately recognize their voices. Each time the conversation moved to a new talker, I had to search all the faces to see whose mouth was moving. Had it *also* been difficult for me to hear, I surely would have missed part of the message while I was searching for the talker.

There are other important advantages to binaural hearing. Everyone realizes that it's harder to hear when there's background noise. Imagine yourself at a party. You're having a conversation with someone (or at least trying to), but a dozen other conversations are going on in the room at the same time. People with two equally hearing ears have some ability to separate the conversation they want to hear from those that they don't. The brain compares the input coming from each ear and uses the differences to separate the signal of interest (the foreground) from the background. Binaural hearing allows the brain to "squelch" the background noise to some extent. Wearing two hearing aids at a party also means that you're less likely to ignore (or appear to ignore) someone who's speaking to you on your unaided side.

There are other advantages to wearing binaural hearing aids. People who wear two hearing aids need less amplification (that is, hearing aid volume need not be turned up as high) because of *binaural summation*. Less amplification means background noise and loud sounds are less annoying and less stressful. Less amplification also means less feedback. In addition, being able to listen twice (once at each ear) to the same sounds provides an advantage. Sounds are more easily distinguished when heard by both ears. This is known as *binaural redundancy*.

Recent research has brought yet another advantage to light. When hearing is impaired in both ears, but a hearing aid is worn in only one ear, the aided ear does all the work. Over time, the brain's ability to process information coming from the unaided ear deteriorates because of a lack of stimulation (this is termed *late-onset auditory deprivation*). It's a classic case of "use it or lose it." Whether the deterioration can be reversed by adding a second hearing aid at a later date is unclear at this point. If too much time goes by, it's possible that the advantages of binaural hearing could be lost forever.

Finally, hearing with two ears is just more natural, more balanced, and more comfortable. Hearing in stereo (like listening to music in stereo) improves sound quality, giving it greater richness, clarity, and depth. With only one ear, sounds can be shallow and flat.

Because of the many benefits of binaural hearing, two hearing aids are usually recommended for listeners who have hearing loss in both ears, even if the hearing loss is different in each ear. About 80 percent of all hearing aid fittings in this country are binaural. In most cases, there's a helpful synthesis of information (*binaural integration*) when sounds are presented to the two ears. This means that binaural aided performance is better than the aided performance of either ear alone. However, there are a few people for whom binaural hearing aids are not the best choice. Occasionally, and especially if the listener is elderly, wearing two hearing aids can cause *binaural interference*. In rare cases, information coming from the two ears is out-of-synch and distracting. This is an auditory processing disorder (APD) that results from a problem within the central auditory pathways that are responsible for transferring information from one side (hemisphere) of the brain to the other (see Chapter 5). If you're not getting good benefit from binaural hearing aids, you should discuss this with your audiologist. She might advise you to try wearing both aids at the same time, then wearing an aid only on your right ear, and then wearing an aid only on your left ear. Be sure to try each arrangement for the same period of time (perhaps 2 weeks) and in comparable listening conditions. If you find that wearing one hearing aid is more helpful than wearing two, report it to your audiologist. Remember, however, that for the vast majority of people with bilateral hearing loss, two hearing aids really *are* better than one.

Until recently, wearing binaural hearing aids meant wearing two aids that worked independently. Today, some digital hearing aids can be programmed to communicate with one another and operate as a unit. Like many other digital hearing aids, these aids continuously analyze incoming sounds and make adjustments to fit the listener's needs. In this case, however, information about sounds coming into the two aids is shared, and adjustments are automatically made to both aids. If the listener uses manual controls (for changing volume or switching programs, for example), making adjustments to one hearing aid changes both simultaneously. The program button might be located on one aid and the volume control on the other, allowing the aids to be smaller and making the controls easier to find. Alternatively, both aids can be controlled with a single remote device. Coordination between hearing aids is intended to make the listener's experience more like true binaural hearing (with potentially improved localization and better speech understanding in noise).

BUYING HEARING AIDS

Where to Buy Hearing Aids

Hearing aids are complicated devices—far more complicated than eyeglasses. Part of what you're paying for when you buy them is the expertise and guidance of an audiologist. Your audiologist will evaluate the nature of your hearing loss, choose hearing aids to satisfy your needs and preferences, make impressions of your ears so the hearing aids (or earmolds) fit comfortably, teach you how to operate and care for your new hearing aids, fine tune the hearing aids as you become accustomed to wearing them, and counsel you (and your family) about your hearing loss and adjustment to hearing aids. You wouldn't buy eyeglasses through the mail, over the Internet, or from someone who shows up at your door; instead, you'd see a competent optometrist or ophthalmologist. It's important to do the same with hearing aids. In fact, several of the largest, most reputable hearing aid manufacturers have recently developed policies that prohibit the sale of their products through the mail or over the Internet. Oticon, for example, has stated, "People with hearing loss deserve to make the best choices possible. . . . We believe this is best accomplished through a personal relationship with a dispensing professional in a face-to-face setting."[2] Oticon refuses to accept new orders from distributors who provide hearing aids without direct contact. In other words, it's important to see an audiologist who's experienced in hearing aid fitting.

Choosing an Audiologist

Choosing your audiologist is probably the most important decision that you make when it comes to purchasing hearing aids. The audiologist's skill in assessing your needs, providing information and support, and choosing the right combination of technical features is more important than the particular hearing aid brand or model that you buy. If you live in an area where a number of audiologists practice (see Chapter 4 for information about how to locate audiologists), consider scheduling brief appointments to meet several. While you're there, ask some questions of the receptionist or business staff (although be sensitive to the fact that they will be busy with other work).

Issues to Consider When Choosing an Audiologist

- Is the audiologist a member of the American Academy of Audiology (AAA) or the American Speech-Language-Hearing Association (ASHA)?
- How does he stay current with changes in hearing aid technology?
- How many hearing aids does she fit in an average month? (A 2006 survey of hearing aid dispensers reported an average of 15 per month.)
- Does he fit a variety of different hearing aid styles (CICs, ITCs, ITEs, BTEs, and mini-BTEs)?
- Does she offer hearing aids from a variety of different manufacturers?
- Is there a trial period of 30 days or longer?

- If the hearing aids are returned at the end of the trial period, which charges are nonrefundable? (For example, costs related to testing and making custom earmolds or hearing aid shells are nonrefundable.)
- How are hearing aids priced? Can charges be itemized?
- Will there be follow-up visits to discuss progress and fine tune the hearing aids? Are those visits included in the price of the hearing aids? If so, how many visits are included?
- Is financing available?
- Does a written warranty come with the hearing aids? Is the warranty honored by the manufacturer, the audiologist, or both?
- Are repair services offered? How long do repairs usually take? How are repair charges determined? Are repairs guaranteed for some set period? Is a loaner hearing aid available if your hearing aid must be sent away for repair?
- How are hearing aid emergencies handled? Can you drop in with problems, or do you need an appointment? If an appointment is necessary, how long will you wait to get one?
- Is insurance against loss or damage available?
- Are rehabilitation services are offered? Is information provided informally during individual counseling sessions, or is a more structured program available? If a structured program is in place, how many sessions does it include? What do the sessions cover? Is the program intended for groups, individual clients, or a combination of the two? Does the program include family counseling about hearing-related issues? (For more information about rehabilitation services, see Chapter 10.)
- How much do rehabilitation services cost? Are they included in the price of the hearing aids, or is there a separate charge? If a structured program is available, do you pay by the session or for the entire program?
- Does the audiologist sell a variety of hearing assistance technology? (For more information, see Chapter 9.) Is there an opportunity to try an assistive device before buying it?
- Is a written contract or purchase agreement provided? What does it cover? (For example, does it include an itemized price for the hearing aids, the warranty terms, the length of the trial period, any nonrefundable costs associated with the trial period, payment terms, repair policy and repair costs, loaner hearing aid policy, insurance options, and specifics about follow-up visits and hearing rehabilitation services?)
- How will the audiologist measure the benefits provided by the hearing aids that you try or buy? Does he use standardized tools to document improved communication and satisfaction over time?

Hearing Assessment

Before the audiologist can make recommendations about hearing aids, she must thoroughly evaluate your hearing. Hearing assessment is described in considerable detail in Chapter 4.

Medical Clearance

Before you buy hearing aids, the Food and Drug Administration (FDA) requires that your ears be examined by a physician (the examination can be within the previous 6 months). The FDA regulation is designed to protect consumers who might have a hearing-related condition that could be treated medically. Your physician should give you something in writing that says you are a candidate for hearing aids. This is typically referred to as medical clearance. Alternatively, the FDA allows you (as an adult) to sign a waiver stating that you have been advised to see a physician, but you do not wish to do so.

Ear Impressions

Once you've decided to go forward with a hearing aid trial, your audiologist needs to make impressions of your ears (except with open canal fittings, in which case impressions are unnecessary). An impression is used to create a custom earmold (for a BTE) or the shell for a custom hearing aid (ITE, ITC, and CIC). After examining your ear with an otoscope, the audiologist will insert an otoblock (a little piece of cotton or foam tied to a string) that prevents the impression material from going too far into your ear canal. He then pushes soft, putty-like material into the ear canal and outer ear. After a few minutes, the material firms up to form a cast of your ear and ear canal. The impression is gently removed from your ear and sent away to the hearing aid manufacturer or earmold laboratory. Nothing about the process is painful, and it takes only a few minutes; however, the finished hearing aid or earmold may not be ready for a couple of weeks.

Some earmolds and hearing aid shells are now being manufactured digitally. Manufacturers use sophisticated imaging technology to turn the impression into a three-dimensional computer model. Specifications requested by the audiologist can then be added to the model. The ultimate fit should be more accurate and more comfortable. Some companies offer technology that allows audiologists to scan the impression right at their desks and transmit the information to the company electronically. This eliminates the problems that can cause impressions to deteriorate as they travel to the laboratory. In the future, it may be possible to scan the ear directly with no need to make an impression at all.

Hearing Aid Fitting

When your custom earmolds or hearing aids are ready, you can return to the audiologist for the initial hearing aid fitting. This visit is often called a hearing aid orientation. The performance of your new aids is tested in various ways (some tests will probably occur before your appointment). The audiologist uses a computer to customize the new aids to fit your hearing loss and listening preferences. You'll be given an opportunity to listen to different sounds and voices (including your own) and to evaluate how the aids sound to you. The audiologist might do some behavioral testing while you're wearing the hearing aids (for example, you might be asked to repeat sentences in noise). She might also place a small microphone inside each of your ear canals, present sounds, and make measurements with and without the hearing aids in place. These *real ear* (or *probe microphone*) measurements provide an excellent starting point for programming and fine tuning your hearing aids.

You'll also learn what to expect from your hearing aids, how to operate them, and how to care for them. Your audiologist will suggest a schedule that can help you to adjust to your new aids without becoming overwhelmed. You might be asked to complete a pre–hearing-aid-fitting questionnaire that will help you and your audiologist to evaluate the benefits provided by the hearing aids. Post–hearing-aid-fitting questionnaires can be completed during later sessions for comparison. You'll receive a large amount of information during this visit; don't hesitate to ask questions!

Hearing Aid Orientation

Most or all of these topics should be addressed during your hearing aid orientation session(s):

- Setting realistic expectations for hearing aid use
- Operating the hearing aids' features (for example, multiple programs, directional microphones, and telecoils)
- Caring for your hearing aids properly
- Adjusting to your hearing aids
- Knowing how and when to change the batteries, the battery that size you need, where to buy batteries, and how to care for batteries safely
- Learning to put the hearing aids in your ears and take them out
- Avoiding feedback
- Using the telephone with your hearing aids
- The hearing aid warranty
- Hearing aid insurance
- Strategies for improving communication and learning to be assertive about the help you need
- Assistive listening technology and its benefits
- Community resources related to hearing loss
- General information about hearing anatomy and physiology, audiogram interpretation, the causes and effects of hearing loss, and so forth
- Helping family members to cope with hearing loss and improve communication

All of these topics are covered in greater detail in Chapter 10.

Hearing Aid Trial Period

Your hearing aid trial period should be no less than 30 days. It's important that you make the very best use of this time. Follow your audiologist's suggestions for adjusting to your new aids (see Chapter 10). Usually, this means gradually increasing the time that you wear the aids each day and the difficulty of the listening environments in which you wear them. Do not be tempted to wear them in challenging listening situations (like a party or noisy restaurant) immediately! That is *not* a good test of how helpful they can be to you. It takes time for your brain to become accustomed to receiving a new sort of auditory input, and you need to get used to hearing sounds that you've forgotten. By the end of the trial period you should be wearing the aids full time in all listening conditions.

As you begin to wear the aids in a wider variety of situations, they probably will need adjustment by your audiologist. The more that you wear your hearing aids, the more feedback you can provide, and the better your audiologist can fine tune them. Having adjustments made *during* the trial period allows you to make a more informed decision about whether to keep the hearing aids at the end of the trial. You should view the trial period as chance to practice, practice, practice. Practice inserting and removing the aids, adjusting the controls, changing the batteries, and keeping the aids clean. Practice wearing them in a variety of different situations. If you have questions or problems, now is the best time to resolve them.

At the end of the trial period, you may choose to keep the hearing aids. Alternatively, if you've given it your best effort but decide that these aids are not for you, you may return them to your audiologist for a refund, minus a service charge. You can also opt to begin a new trial period with different hearing aids. Policies governing trial periods vary; be sure that you fully understand the terms at the outset, including the policies regarding loss or damage during the trial period and the nonrefundable service fee. Service fees vary but should not exceed approximately one tenth of the total cost of the hearing aid(s). It's always a good idea to have all of this information in writing.

Follow-up Visits and Hearing Rehabilitation Services

Hearing aid fitting is an ongoing process rather than a single event. The greatest advantage of digital hearing aids is that they can be programmed to meet your unique needs and preferences. Keep a journal about your progress, questions, and reactions as you become accustomed to wearing your aids. In fact, your hearing aids may use data logging to keep their own journal. Some audiologists use software that creates virtual listening environments (like clattering dishes, blaring sirens, whistling birds) in the office. Various sounds are played through speakers, and adjustments to the hearing aids are made on the spot. A few hearing aids enable users to record samples of their own listening environments so that they can be recreated in the audiologist's office. Your audiologist will use the feedback you (and maybe your hearing aid) provide to make decisions about fine tuning.

It may take several visits over the first few months to be certain that the physical fit is good, the settings are optimal, and you can manage the hearing aids properly. Follow-up visits are often included in the purchase price of the hearing aids; be sure to ask ahead of time. Don't let a potentially successful fitting fail because you don't know how to use the hearing aids or they need further adjustment. A problem that prevents you from getting the most out of your hearing aids could be a simple one that's easily solved.

Once you've become accustomed to your hearing aids, ask your audiologist if you might benefit from assistive listening technology (for example, a device that would make watching television easier, one that would help you hear better on the telephone, or something that would improve communication in the car). More detailed information about hearing assistance technology can be found in Chapter 9. You should also ask your audiologist about the availability of additional hearing rehabilitation services. Chapter 10 covers these services in greater detail.

Finally, your audiologist will want to recheck your hearing and hearing aids at least annually. If your hearing changes, your hearing aids will need reprogramming.

The Cost of Hearing Aids

Everybody wonders why hearing aids cost so much. Hearing aids—especially digital hearing aids—are expensive. Generally speaking, the more technical features a hearing aid has, the more it costs. Miniaturization is also expensive. Generally speaking, the smaller the hearing aid, the more it costs.

A tremendous amount of research has gone into developing a computer (microchip) small enough to fit inside a hearing aid, yet powerful enough to make millions of calculations per second. And this extremely-tiny-but-ever-so-powerful computer doesn't sit on a desk all day in a temperature-controlled room with good ventilation. This computer must be able to work in a hostile environment—in the case of custom hearing aids, an environment that's warm, damp, and often filled with a damaging substance (earwax). Moreover, this computer gets moved about daily as it's pushed in and pulled out of an ear. In addition, the miniature computer needs a very tiny but portable power supply; researchers had to develop a battery small enough to fit inside a hearing aid that could be as small as a fingertip. These technical demands drive up the cost of digital hearing aids. And there's more to it than just research and development. There are also costs related to hearing aid components, the manufacturing process, marketing, and merchandising. Add to that the fact that manufacturers need and deserve to make a profit.

People often wonder why hearing aids don't become less expensive as the technology becomes more widely available. Many variables affect price, but the most important one may be the size of the market. If as many people bought hearing aids as buy cell phones, or iPods, or desktop computers, economies of scale probably *would* drive prices down. In 2006, however, only 2.37 million hearing aids were sold in the United States (plus several million more worldwide) compared with the 800 million cell phones, 40 million iPods, and more than 200 million desktop and notebook computers sold worldwide. Unless the number of people buying hearing aids increases dramatically, it's unlikely that economies of scale will cause hearing aid prices to drop.

Fortunately, not everyone needs the most expensive hearing aids. All major manufacturers offer economy, mid-level, and high-end digital products. Basically, the difference among them is the number and sophistication of the features that they include. Features affect performance in noise, suppression of feedback, the ability to make soft sounds detectable without making louder sounds uncomfortable, and so forth. There are also features that make hearing aid use more comfortable and convenient, and still others that make hearing aids compatible with assistive listening technology. Not everyone needs (or can afford) the newest and most expensive features, however. In many cases, entry-level or mid-level models (which might carry last year's "premium" features) do just fine.[3]

Unfortunately, it's difficult to comparison shop for hearing aids. There are several reasons for this. First, every manufacturer offers a variety of models, and each model has different features or feature combinations. Often, the features are proprietary (patented by the manufacturer), intended to perform different functions, and called by different names. This makes it difficult to compare hearing aids across manufacturers. Second, it's impractical for audiologists to work with all hearing aid brands and models. Realistically, it would be impossible for an audiologist to have in-depth expertise with hundreds of different hearing aids. Most have special training and expertise with the hearing aids made by a few manufacturers. Third, audiologists' preferences for certain hearing aids can affect their pricing structure. Volume discounts from hearing aid manufacturers sometimes allow audiologists to offer the hearing aids that they fit most often at a lower cost (economies of scale *do* apply here). This makes it difficult to compare the price of a particular hearing aid across audiologists. Finally, most audiologists "bundle" the cost of their services into the price of the hearing aid itself; only a few do not. Services that may or may not be bundled into the cost of a hearing aid include the hearing evaluation, ear impressions, batteries, hearing aid fitting and orientation, follow-up appointments, hearing rehabilitation services, the hearing aid warranty, and insurance coverage.

The cost of a particular hearing aid is determined by its style and technological sophistication. According to an annual survey conducted

Table 7.1. Average Prices of Hearing Aids Sold in the United States in 2007

Hearing Aid Type	Average Cost of One Hearing Aid
Analog (all styles)	$857
Digital	
Low-end	
BTE (behind-the-ear)	1,149
mini-BTE	1,318
ITE (in-the-ear)	1,204
ITC (in-the-canal)	1,309
CIC (completely-in-the-canal)	1,364
Mid-level	
BTE	1,843
mini-BTE	1,861
ITE	1,840
ITC	2,147
CIC	2,023
High-end	
BTE	2,609
mini-BTE	2,672
ITE	2,686
ITC	2,744
CIC	2,860

by *The Hearing Journal* and *Audiology Online*,[4] the *average* price of *all* hearing aids sold in the United States in 2007 was $1,986. Table 7.1 shows the *average* price of hearing aids sold in 2007 by level of sophistication (low-end, mid-level, and high-end), type of signal processing (analog or digital), and style (BTE, mini-BTE, ITE, ITC, and CIC). These prices include all of the services provided by the dispensing audiologist. Remember, the prices shown are merely averages; a single hearing aid can cost anywhere from a few hundred dollars to a few thousand dollars.

In 2007, on average, audiologists charged $375 for the professional services they provided to their hearing aid clients. Usually (87 percent of the time, according to the annual survey) these service charges were bundled into the cost of hearing aids. Only 13 percent of audiologists charged separately for their services related to hearing aids.

Are an audiologist's services too expensive? No. An audiologist must take a history, perform a hearing evaluation, make medical referrals as necessary, discuss listening needs and preferences, take ear impressions, select and fit hearing aids, reprogram the aids when necessary, provide counseling and instruction over several follow-up appointments, and handle repair problems as they occur. It's estimated that an audiologist spends at least five contact hours with each new hearing aid user *plus* some noncontact time. Compare this with the amount you'd be charged if you spent more than 5 hours with your dentist or lawyer. It might help to consider that audiologists have the same amount of education as other professionals such as dentists, lawyers, veterinarians, podiatrists, and optometrists.

The *average* lifespan of a hearing aid is 5 to 7 years, depending on its style (BTEs are most durable; CICs are least durable), how well it's cared for, the amount of earwax the wearer produces, and other issues. Assuming a cost of $3,972 for two hearing aids (realizing that buying two hearing aids might not actually double the cost) and a 5-year lifespan, the cost per day would be about $2.18. Compare that figure to the daily out-of-pocket cost of some common drugs (using the average co-pay charged by the five largest Medicare Part D insurers). In 2006, the cost of celecoxib (Celebrex, a drug prescribed to relieve the pain, inflammation, and stiffness of arthritis) was $2.83 per day. The cost of alendronate sodium (Fosamax, a drug prescribed to prevent bone fractures due to osteoporosis) was $2.21 per day. The cost of lansoprazole (Prevacid, a drug prescribed to relieve the heartburn caused by acid reflux disease) was $4.24 per day. None of these drugs is used to treat a life-threatening condition, but each improves the user's quality of life. Most users consider the money well spent. Similarly, the cost of hearing aids is a quality-of-life investment. Insurance generally doesn't cover hearing aids (more about that later), but the daily cost of hearing aids *without* insurance is more affordable than the insurance co-pay for many commonly used drugs.

Paying for Hearing Aids

Unfortunately, most health insurance plans, including Medicare, don't cover the cost of hearing aids, although they may cover the cost of a hearing evaluation. However, some health insurance plans *do* cover part or all of the cost, so it's worth checking with your provider. You should also check to see if your employer participates in a hearing benefit/discount plan such as HearPO, the National Ear Care Plan, or the Universal Hearing Benefits Plan. In addition, some prescription discount plans allow hearing aids to be purchased at a reduced price, as long as the user works with a participating provider. You might also check with your employer about a flexible spending account that would enable hearing aids to be purchased on a pretax basis.

When insurance doesn't cover the cost, there are some state and federal sources of financial assistance. For example, some veterans are eligible for hearing aids and hearing-related services through the Department of Veterans Affairs (to learn more, visit the Department of Veterans Affairs website at www.va.gov or call the Health Benefits Center toll-free at 877-222-8387). If you need hearing aids or assistive technology to become employed or continue performing your job, contact your state's vocational rehabilitation office (to obtain contact information for the agency in your state, visit www.disabilityinfo.gov and click on Vocational Rehabilitation). The Technical Assistance Project, funded by the U.S. Department of Education Rehabilitation Services Administration, supports state agencies that provide assistive technologies to persons in need. Some of these agencies lend equipment, make loans for the purchase of equipment, offer demonstrations centers, and provide referral information. Visit http://69.89.27.238/~resnaorg/taproject/RESNA.html (click on State AT Programs, and then on State Contact List) to find contact information for the assistive technology office in your state. In addition, each state has a commission or agency that serves citizens who are deaf or hard of hearing. The names of these agencies differ from state to state; to find the agency in your state, visit your state's web page and look for a directory of agencies and commissions. Finally, Medicaid is a medical assistance program for people with low income. Eligibility criteria can be found at www.cms.hhs.gov/MedicaidEligibility/. Hearing aid coverage through Medicaid varies from state to state. This information, with contact information for each state, can be found at www.hearingloss.org/advocacy/medicaid_by_state1.asp. Finally, you might check with your local/state Departments of Social Services and Public Health (check the government listings in the phone book).

The Seattle-based Northwest Lions Foundation for Sight and Hearing (NLFSH) has formed a nonprofit alliance of hearing professionals, hearing aid and earmold suppliers, and other related groups called AUDIENT (see the Resources section). The goal is to provide quality hearing care and hearing aids at a reduced cost to people who couldn't otherwise afford them. To qualify, the patient's household income cannot exceed 2.5 times the federal poverty guideline; therefore, income qualifications change as federal poverty guidelines change (federal poverty guidelines can be found at http://aspe.hhs.gov/poverty). At the 2007 federal poverty level, an individual would qualify with an annual income less than $24,500. The income limit is higher if there are more people in the household ($33,000 for a two-person household; $41,500 for a three-person household—for each additional person, add $8,500). The hearing aids provided are high-quality, fully digital BTEs. In 2007, the cost to the patient ranged from $760 to $1,400 for one hearing aid and $1,290 to $2,400 for two. In addition to the hearing aids, this price included a 30-day trial period, custom earmolds, the hearing aid fitting, three follow-up visits during the first year, and a 1- or 2-year limited manufacturer's warranty. The price did not include the cost of the hearing evaluation. Participating providers receive minimal reimbursement for their services.

More recently, the Lions Clubs International Foundation (LCIF) launched the Affordable Hearing Aid Project (AHAP). LCIF has partnered with Rexton, a hearing aid manufacturer, to make low-cost, high-quality hearing aids available to low-income people. Participating Lions Clubs are responsible for determining the financial eligibility of local applicants. Eligibility is usually based on federal poverty guidelines with the local economy taken into account. Eligible applicants are referred to local hearing aid dispensers who've been recruited by the club to work as partners in AHAP. The hearing aids are ordered from Rexton through AHAP and shipped to the local dispenser. The hearing aid price covered by AHAP does not include shipping costs, the services of the dispenser, earmolds, transportation, and so forth; however, these costs might be covered by the local Lions Club or shared by the Club and third parties.

There are at least two national foundations that give assistance to people who are unable to afford hearing aids: Hear Now (the Starkey Hearing Foundation) and the Travelers Protective Association Scholarship Trust for the Deaf and Near-Deaf (see the Resources section for contact information). In addition, fraternal and charitable organizations sometimes offer reconditioned hearing aids or provide financial assistance for the purchase of new aids. Try contacting local chapters of the following organizations (and others like them) to see if they can provide help on an individual basis: AgrAbility Project, Benevolent and Protective Order (BPO) of Elks of the USA, Civitan International, Knights of Columbus, Kiwanis International, Lions Clubs International, National Easter Seals Society, National Grange, Quota International, Rotary International, Ruritan National, Sertoma International, and United Way. Finally, local speech and hearing centers, often funded by the United Way, sometimes offer hearing aids at reduced rates to their low-income clients.

A few companies offer financing to cover health care expenses, including hearing aids. These companies allow people to buy hearing aids and pay for them over time in monthly installments. Examples include General Electric's CareCredit health care credit card, Citibank's Health Card, and the Helpcard. Generally, patients complete a short application in their audiologist's office (enrollment is free), and the audiologist submits the application online, by fax, or over the telephone. Notice of approval usually arrives within minutes. The terms vary, but a typical arrangement allows the patient to select a no-interest payment plan for 3, 6, 12, or 18 months, or choose a 24-, 36-, or 48-month plan with interest. Occasionally, audiologists offer their own financing plans.

Some audiologists offer leasing plans. A lease agreement usually includes a down payment, a security deposit, monthly payments, and an option to buy the aids at a predetermined price at the end of the leasing period. Leasing allows the user to upgrade his hearing aid every 3 years, which means less need for repairs and a chance to take advantage of ever-improving technology. However, leasing is more expensive than paying for hearing aids all at once.

Finally, the news from Washington is hopeful. Legislation that would provide a tax credit for hearing aids has been introduced (several times) in the U.S. House of Representatives. If passed, the Hearing Aid Assistance Tax Credit Act would provide a tax credit of up to $500 per hearing aid once every 5 years for persons 55 years of age and older (the credit would also be available to parents purchasing hearing aids for a dependent child). Another bill, the Help America Hear Act of 2007, would require certain insurance companies to cover two hearing aids every 3 years (capped at $2,500 per covered person). Finally, the Medicare Enhancement and Auditory Rehabilitation (HEAR) Act of 2007 would provide Medicare coverage for hearing aids and auditory rehabilitation services for seniors with hearing loss. Encourage your elected representatives to support these bills and others like them!

When you spend money for hearing aids, remember that you're doing more than simply buying hearing equipment. Better hearing means a better quality of life for you and the people you love. Buying hearing aids should be viewed as an investment that allows you to participate more fully in your relationships, your work, and the activities you enjoy. And what could be important than that?

Hearing Aid Warranty

New hearing aids come with a 1- or 2-year warranty from the manufacturer. Specific provisions vary, however, so it's important to understand exactly what is (and is not) included in your warranty and for how long. Be sure to ask questions and get important information in writing. In addition to the manufacturer's warranty, there are consumer-direct companies that offer special warranty plans for hearing aids. Examples are Discovery Hearing Aid Warranties and SoundAid Hearing Aid Warranties (see the Resources section). The warranty options offered by these companies pick up where the manufacturer's warranty leaves off, covering loss, damage, and component failure. These companies claim that the cost of a 1-year service warranty is less than the cost of a single repair.

Questions to Ask about Your Hearing Aid Warranty[5]
- When does the warranty period begin and expire? Most hearing aids come with a standard 1- or 2-year warranty from the manufacturer, although some offer an additional year of coverage.
- Can I get additional coverage after the initial warranty period has ended? Extended warranties that go beyond the initial warranty period can usually be purchased from the manufacturer, your audiologist, a general insurance company, or companies that have special warranty plans for hearing aids.
- Which parts of the hearing aid are covered? If the aid must be repaired, is the labor charge covered? Warranties typically cover the internal parts of the hearing aid and any manufacturing defects in the hearing aid case or shell. Coverage for labor charges varies.
- What if I lose the hearing aid or it becomes damaged? Some warranties offer protection only against defects in workmanship, whereas others also cover loss and damage. If loss and damage are *not* covered, hearing aid insurance can be purchased or the hearing aid can added to a homeowner's policy. If

the aid must be replaced, ask if it will be replaced with an upgrade or the same model.
- Will I be charged for modifications and adjustments to the hearing aid? Most modifications and adjustments can be made by the audiologist, but occasionally an aid needs to be returned to the manufacturer, and sometimes it must be remade entirely. Ask if you will be charged for modifications, adjustments, or remakes during the warranty period.
- Will I be charged for shipping costs or office visits? These may or may not be included under the warranty.
- Are earmolds included? Earmolds often have a more limited warranty (30–90 days) that covers fit and workmanship.

Hearing Aid Insurance

Buying hearing aids is a big investment. You may want to insure them against accidental damage, theft, or loss, unless those things are covered by your manufacturer's warranty. Some insurance carriers provide coverage as part of an existing policy, such as a homeowner's policy. Alternatively, there are companies that provide special policies for hearing aids (see the Resources section for examples). In addition to providing coverage against damage, theft, and loss, some offer repair coverage after the manufacturer's warranty expires. You should discuss this with your audiologist, because some policies must be obtained within 90 days of the hearing aid purchase.

Service and Repairs

The average lifespan of a hearing aid is 5 to 7 years. On average, hearing aids need to be repaired by the manufacturer every 1 to 2 years. Remember, hearing aids are worn in an environment that's hostile to electronics. Most repairs are necessary because earwax and moisture accumulate in the hearing aid. Wax accumulates in microphones and receivers, causing distortion, reduced amplification, and an overall deterioration in performance. Moisture causes corrosion or rust in the battery compartment and shorts in the amplifier. Preventative maintenance can dramatically reduce the need for repairs and prolong the life of your hearing aid. Properly cleaning the hearing aid every time it's removed from your ear is well worth the effort (see Chapter 10 for more information). Storing your hearing aids in a drying kit each night is another good idea (see Appendix B for information about drying kits).

Hearing Aid Complaints

Hearing aid problems can almost always be worked out with your dispensing audiologist. In the rare instance when that does not happen, you can contact the state licensing board in your state, your state attorney general, or a local consumer protection agency. You can find contact information in the government pages of your telephone book. In addition, you should report serious problems to the Better Business Bureau (www.bbb.org).

Tips for Buying a Hearing Aid

- Educate yourself. The more you know about hearing loss and hearing aids, the better your decisions will be.
- Be cautious about aggressive sales tactics. No one should pressure you into buying a hearing aid.
- Don't be misled by exaggerated advertising claims about hearing aids that can eliminate all background noise or amplify only one conversation in the midst of many. Remember, if it sounds too good to be true, it probably is.
- Take a relative or friend with you to your appointments. You'll receive a great deal of information at once. Having another person there to listen (and maybe take notes) is helpful and also makes the visit less stressful.
- Keep all of the follow-up appointments with your audiologist (the cost is probably included in the price of your hearing aids).
- Take advantage of other services that your audiologist offers, including hearing rehabilitation services, literature on hearing loss and amplification, guidance on how to adjust to your hearing aids, and information about hearing aid care and maintenance.
- Keep a journal of your daily listening experiences. This can provide valuable information for your audiologist during follow-up visits.
- Be assertive during your appointments. Jot down questions prior to appointments and take them with you. Write down the answers (or ask your audiologist to provide written information).
- Ask about hearing assistance technology that might help you in challenging listening situations.
- Don't be afraid to try other hearing aid models, features, or styles if the first aids you try do not help you.
- Don't assume that the most high-tech or expensive hearing aids are the best ones for you; what you need depends on the nature of your hearing loss, your lifestyle, and your individual hearing needs.

THE SECRET OF SUCCESS

You probably know people who appreciate their hearing aids, people who do nothing but complain about them, and people who own them but never use them. What accounts for the difference? Are people who buy more expensive hearing aids happier with them? Are people who wear a certain hearing aid style (BTE, mini-BTE, ITE, ITC, or CIC) more satisfied than others? Is there a technical feature or combination of features that makes a hearing aid fitting successful? Many factors affect the outcome of a hearing aid fitting, including the listener's type, severity, and configuration of hearing loss; speech perception ability (in quiet and in noise); and dynamic range. But what's the *real* secret to success with hearing aids? The answer is simple, but it isn't always easy: the real secret to success is wanting to hear as well as you possibly can and being willing to do whatever it takes to make that happen.

Success with hearing aids (and nearly everything else in life) is about motivation. In fact, motivation is the single best predictor of success with hearing aids. For example, research suggests that a listener's willingness to tolerate background noise might be more important to his success with hearing aids than his speech perception ability.[6]

If you really want to hear better, you'll have to work at it. Hearing aids alone are only part of the solution; the rest is up to you. Make an effort to adjust to your hearing aids. Wear two hearing aids if you can manage it financially. Take advantage of any hearing rehabilitation services that are available. Learn to appreciate the improvement your hearing aids provide, even though it's less than perfect. The outcome is in your hands. If you decide (in the absence of special problems or circumstances) that you want to hear as well as you possibly can, and you're willing to really *try*, then you're likely to be successful with hearing aids.

The following comments by a hearing aid user provide a good illustration. Notice that the writer never claims hearing aids are perfect; rather, he's able to accept the imperfections and enjoy the benefits. This acceptance is important because there's nothing you can buy that's as good as the human auditory system. Thus far, no feat of engineering can match it. Given the times in which we live, this reality can be difficult to accept; we've come to believe that a technological solution exists for every problem.

Changing the Muted World
by Peter Whitis, MD

I lost my hearing so gradually I barely noticed it. My wife, whose hearing is so exquisite she can hear the conversation at a table 20 feet away in a noisy restaurant, learned to repeat herself rather frequently in our conversations, now going past 50 years.

I subtly withdrew from most group activities, movies, concerts, parties, as it just got too difficult to understand people. I would nod my head for most of the conversation and then make some inane remark off the subject and see this stunned look. I often had a ten-second delay in processing the conversation while trying to fill in the gaps I couldn't hear. It would be like trying to read this article with parts of the words erased. It was easy for my mind to wander. My work was affected and I decided to retire earlier than I had planned.

My wife wondered if I really heard the music she loved to play. I didn't know if I did or not. How could I know what I didn't hear? I found myself leaving music out of my life too and even began thinking why did so many people think it such an important part of their lives.

People with soft voices, accents, rapid speech, high- or low-pitched tones out of my hearing range were the most difficult to hear. My son and his wife could converse from either end of the dining room table in their normal voices and I, sitting in the middle of the table, could not comprehend them.

My spouse would try to seat me at places in church or concerts where the acoustics were favorable. Friends at lectures would scout out the seats for me nearest the auditorium speakers. In the car, we used an amplifier with a microphone attached to my wife's shoulder seatbelt.

With all these limitations, I was losing contact with people. Increasingly my life was dominated by reading, closed-captioned TV whenever I watched it, solitary pursuits like bird-watching, the Internet, long-distance running, biking. Tennis, my passion, continued to be fun but my partners knew I couldn't hear let calls or had to come to the net to talk to me.

On the whole, at work and home, people were kind, considerate and forgiving of my hearing loss. But I knew it was not easy to have to repeat themselves for my benefit or raise their voice to talk to me.

Then the digital age arrived. I was fitted with a pair of behind-the-ear (BTE) hearing aids to replace my 13-year-old canal aids. Abruptly, my aural world boomed.

It's a noisy world out there.

My bilateral BTE aids are automatically programmed to switch for music listening, phone mode, TV or conversation in noisy environments, have a volume switch and a mute button. By hooking them up to her computer, my audiologist can tell how much volume I have increased in different listening situations, how much time I've spent in voice/noisy or voice/quiet situations. She can reprogram them individually depending on my needs and comfort level.

Now I could hear the furnace turning on and the washing machine spin cycle take off like a jet engine. The dishwasher sloshed through its cycles with impressive violence. Stacking plates and bowls in the cupboard was fearfully noisy with each plate sounding like a pistol shot. I understood now why my wife used to leave the kitchen to make the bed when I began to put away the dishes. I could hear the coffee gurgling and the toaster pop up.

Best of all, I could now talk to people and understand what they were saying better. I still needed to face the person, voices behind me were lost, background noise interfered but less so, fast talkers still had to slow down for me. Playing tennis was a totally new experience. Now I could hear the ball being hit with an exhilarating sound like chopping wood.

. . . I noted that the poetry I had written over the years used singular visual imagery. New aural imagery became possible ("the gate swinging to and fro" could become "a creaky swinging gate".) Being a backyard bird-watcher I longed to hear and identify birdcalls but knew it was impossible to hear them before. With my new aids, I confidently bought a book and tape of common birdcalls.

It's not all peachy. All this ambient noise is stressful at home, in the car, and in social situations. It's understandable why some choose not to use hearing aids. But there is some relief when the TV is too loud at the health club (as it usually is), when I'm trying to read and the washing machine is gaining altitude, when I just need quiet, there is that little mute button. Then I know my hearing loss is no longer just a handicap, but a blessing.

Peter Whitis, MD, is a 73-year-old child/adolescent psychiatrist working part-time in a residential adolescent treatment center in Eau Claire, Wisconsin. Along with an active sports program including strength training, tennis, running, and biking, he loves to read, write, and is active in current affairs. He and his wife Martha have been married 53 years and have four sons and ten grandchildren.

Adapted from the September/October 2006 issue of *Hearing Loss Magazine*, with permission from the Hearing Loss Association of America.

CHAPTER 8

When Hearing Aids Are Not Enough: Cochlear Implants

The renowned poet John Keats wrote,
"Heard melodies are sweet, but those unheard are sweeter,"
but he was wrong.

Ode on a Grecian Urn, John Keats

Hearing aids provide substantial benefit to most users, but for people with severe-to-profound sensorineural hearing loss, they may not be enough. Basically, hearing aids work by making sounds louder, then sending them through a dysfunctional auditory system. In most cases, the dysfunction is caused by damaged or missing hair cells within the cochlea (see Chapters 3 and 4). People with mild, moderate, and sometimes even severe hearing losses have enough working hair cells to transmit the amplified sound energy to Cranial Nerve (CN) VIII and the brain, however imperfectly. When hearing loss is more severe, however, there may not be enough working hair cells to make the connection. In this case, the auditory fibers that form CN VIII are available to carry information to the brain, but there aren't enough hair cells to trigger the neural activity (or the activity that *does* get through is too degraded to be useful). When this is the case, a cochlear implant may be the solution. A cochlear implant converts sounds into patterns of electrical pulses; these electrical pulses bypass most of the auditory system and stimulate CN VIII fibers directly. CN VIII then carries the bioelectrical (neural) information to the brain, which interprets it as sound. Cochlear implants are a true miracle of modern medicine; they're the only medical technology to functionally restore a human sense.

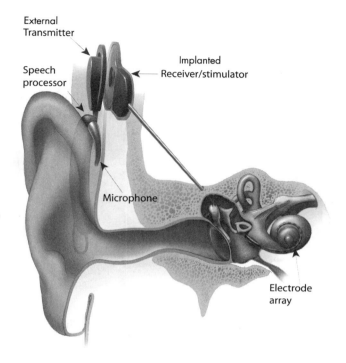

External
Transmitter

Speech
processor

Implanted
Receiver/stimulator

Microphone

Electrode
array

Figure 8.1. External and Internal (Implanted) Components of a Cochlear Implant. (Artwork courtesy of National Institutes of Health [NIH] Medical Arts.)

HOW A COCHLEAR IMPLANT WORKS

A cochlear implant is an electronic device made of several different parts. External components are worn outside the body; internal components are surgically implanted under the skin and within the cochlea. Figure 8.1 shows where the external and internal components are placed. Figure 8.2 shows the components themselves; the numbers in the figure correspond to the numbers in the text.

Similar to a hearing aid, an ear-level microphone (1) picks up sounds from the environment. Sound information is sent to a speech processor (2), which may be worn on the ear like a behind-the-ear (BTE) hearing aid or on the body like a pager (processor controls [3]). The processor contains a tiny computer that digitizes sound information and organizes it into patterns according to a code. The patterned information travels through a cable (4) to a transmitter (5), which is worn on the head behind the ear. The transmitter sends the information to a receiver/stimulator (6) implanted under the skin. The transmitter and receiver, each about the size of a quarter, are held together by magnets. No wires or cables pass through the skin, reducing the chance of infection. The receiver converts

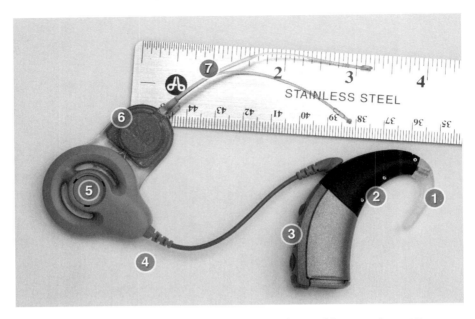

Figure 8.2. External and Internal Components of a Cochlear Implant. (Courtesy of Cochlear Americas.)

digitized information into patterned electrical pulses and sends them through tiny wires to the electrode array (7) that winds through the cochlea. The array has tiny electrodes attached to it (at present, a maximum of 24 electrodes substitute for more than 16,000 hair cells). The electrodes deliver the coded electrical pulses at very high rates to auditory nerve fibers located in different frequency regions of the cochlea (see Figure 3.7 in Chapter 3). The auditory nerve fibers come together as CN VIII and carry the bio-electrical (neural) information to auditory centers in the brain. With practice, the brain learns to interpret the coded electrical pulses as meaningful sound.

COCHLEAR IMPLANT CANDIDACY

Food and Drug Administration (FDA) regulations allow infants 12 months of age and older to receive cochlear implants; however, infants younger than 12 months have been implanted under special conditions. There is no upper age limit, and people in their 90s have been implanted very successfully.

Generally speaking, adult candidates must have a severe-to-profound sensorineural hearing loss in both ears (thresholds of 70 dB or poorer) and receive limited benefit from hearing aids. Limited hearing aid benefit is a criterion because conventional implantation procedures sacrifice residual

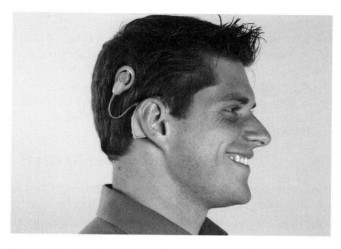

Figure 8.3. Ear-level Speech Processor and Transmitter. (Courtesy of Cochlear Americas.)

(remaining) hearing in the implanted ear. Hearing loss criteria continue to change (always becoming less stringent); therefore if you were told in the past that you had too much hearing, it might be worth checking again. If your audiologist thinks you may derive more benefit from an implant than from hearing aids, he will refer you to a cochlear implant center for extensive evaluation by members of a cochlear implant team. The evaluation might require more than one visit, and it will likely include sessions with the implant team coordinator, a physician, an audiologist, and a psychologist or social worker.

The physician/surgeon will evaluate your overall health and the condition of your ears to be sure that it's physically possible to perform the surgery and implant the device. She will examine images of your cochlea (CT scan or MRI) in search of anatomic variations that could affect insertion of the electrode array into the cochlea. The audiologist will do a comprehensive hearing evaluation, with and without hearing aids. If you don't currently wear state-of-the-art hearing aids, you may be required to try them for 3 to 6 months to evaluate their benefit. The implant audiologist must be convinced that you're likely to receive greater benefit from an implant than from hearing aids or no device at all. Members of the implant team will also want to know about your expectations, motivation, and family support. Team members must determine that you have the personal resources to handle a cochlear implant and keep it working over a lifetime.

Members of the team will discuss all aspects of the process: the hearing evaluation, the medical evaluation, the surgical procedure, surgical risks, postsurgical recovery, activation and programming of the device, and long-term follow-up care. Team members will provide information about the level of success that you can reasonably expect and the limitations that you might face. They will also discuss the relative advantages and disadvantages of the implant devices available to you. They will discuss costs, warranties, and insurance coverage. Armed with this information, you and your family can decide if you want an implant and, if so, which device is best for you.

EXPECTED OUTCOMES FOR COCHLEAR IMPLANT USERS

Chapter 2 suggested that hearing occurs on three levels: primitive, warning, and symbolic. At the *primitive level*, hearing provides a constant auditory background that makes us feel connected to the world around us. The auditory background includes everything from the drone of traffic noise to more enjoyable sounds like birds chirping overhead, leaves crunching underfoot, and children laughing in the distance. In nearly all cases, a cochlear implant can restore the auditory background and reduce feelings of isolation.

An implant also restores hearing at the *warning level*. At this level, sounds provide information about what's happening around us (even in places we can't see, like behind us, through walls, and in the dark). A smoke alarm signals danger. An unexplained noise could signal the presence of an intruder. A scream could signal a need for help. An inability to hear warning sounds creates feelings of anxiety and insecurity. A cochlear implant almost always makes the user feel safer and more independent.

The third level of hearing, the *symbolic level*, is the most important. At this level, hearing is used to understand speech. Success with implants at this level is more variable. With therapy and practice, most users learn to understand speech with considerably less need for speechreading. Many are able to communicate over the telephone, and newer technologies are making it possible for more users to appreciate music. Not all implant users achieve the same level of success, however.

Success depends on many factors. Those that are especially critical include the age at which hearing loss began, the duration of deafness, past use of hearing aids, and age at the time of implantation. Generally speaking, two groups of patients experience remarkable success: children who are implanted at a very young age and adults who lose their hearing later in life (after developing speech and language). In contrast, expectations are somewhat lower for adults who were born deaf (or became deaf before speech and language developed) and have not relied on hearing for communication in the past. In this case, CN VIII and hearing areas in the brain haven't been adequately stimulated, and benefit from an implant might be more limited. Even in this case, however, it's likely that an implant will improve speechreading ability by allowing the user to combine visual cues with the rhythm of speech, which can be heard with an implant.

Factors That Affect Outcome with Cochlear Implants

- The person's age when he became deaf (adults who have been deaf since birth or early childhood tend to benefit less from an implant, especially if they haven't relied on hearing for communication in the past)
- The length of time that the person was deaf before receiving an implant (the shorter the time, the greater the chance of success)
- The person's past use of hearing aids (past use increases the probability of success, because the brain has been receiving sound stimulation)
- The person's age at the time of implantation (very young children do best because their brains are more adaptable or "plastic"; however, adults, even elderly adults, often do remarkably well)
- The physical condition of the cochlea and CN VIII (malformation of or damage to the cochlea or CN VIII reduces the probability of success)
- The listener's auditory skills before the implant (people with more residual hearing and better speech perception tend to do better with implants)
- The presence of other medical conditions (medical conditions can make surgery, postsurgical recovery, and rehabilitation more difficult)
- The person's expectations (an implant doesn't restore normal hearing, and those with that expectation will be disappointed)
- The person's motivation
- Family support
- Participation in a hearing rehabilitation program following surgery

COCHLEAR IMPLANT SURGERY

The surgical procedure, performed under general anesthesia, typically takes 2 to 5 hours. Patients usually go home the same day or the next morning. A "bed" for the receiver is hollowed out of the mastoid bone behind the ear, and an opening is made into the cochlea through the middle ear. The receiver is then anchored in the mastoid bone, and the flexible electrode array is threaded through the spirals of the cochlea. Generally, an audiologist in the operating room tests the electrodes to be sure they're working before the incision is closed. Most people resume normal activity within a week. All surgery involves risks, but those associated with cochlear implant surgery are comparatively small.

DEVICE ACTIVATION AND PROGRAMMING

After the incision has healed, the patient returns to the cochlear implant center to have the implant activated. The audiologist fits the speech processor and transmitter to the user, turns on the device, and speaks. Voilà! Hearing! This is an unforgettable (and often very emotional) moment for the patient and family. The audiologist then connects the processor to a special computer with special software (specific to each implant manufacturer) and programs the device.

Each implant manufacturer offers several processing or coding strategies from which the audiologist can choose. A coding strategy is a set of rules that determine how the processor translates the characteristics of incoming sounds (for example, pitch, loudness, and timing) into patterns of electrical pulses and how the electrodes are stimulated. Implant manufacturers are continually developing new coding strategies and improving existing ones.

Electrodes are activated one by one; the audiologist sets each electrode's minimal and maximal current levels, ensuring that incoming sound information will be loud enough to hear but not loud enough to cause discomfort. Like fine tuning hearing aids, mapping is an ongoing process rather than an event; it can take multiple visits to achieve the best map, although this varies. Some processors allow several programs to be stored in memory so that the user can select the program that best suits the listening environment.

Implant centers provide assistance, information, and support to users and their families long after device activation and programming. Rehabilitation may be provided by professionals at the implant center or arranged closer to home in consultation with implant team members. Learning to listen through a cochlear implant is an adjustment that often takes time, instruction, and practice. Rehabilitation is designed to help the user adjust to a new type of "sound" and learn to use the technical capabilities of the device. The rehabilitation program typically focuses on auditory training, perhaps combined with speechreading practice. The program should also include instruction about assistive listening technology, communication strategies, and maintaining the implant. For some, it might also include personal adjustment counseling as the user makes the transition from being deaf to being hard of hearing. Family counseling is another important component. Finally, the implant center may offer a support group in which implant candidates can meet experienced users and connect with other new users. In addition to implant centers, implant manufacturers offer extensive and personalized support services that can be accessed online or by telephone.

CHOOSING AMONG COCHLEAR IMPLANT DEVICES

Like hearing aids, cochlear implants have become smaller and more technically sophisticated over the years. Initially, all processors were worn on the body (usually in a pocket or clipped to a belt) with a cable connecting the processor to the transmitter on the head. Today, all manufacturers offer ear-level processors that look something like BTE hearing aids. Although ear-level devices are less cumbersome, body-worn processors, with larger controls, may be preferred by people with vision or dexterity problems. Like hearing aids, processors offer increasingly sophisticated technical features that automatically adjust to improve listener comfort and speech understanding in difficult listening situations.

If you become a cochlear implant candidate, you might be asked to choose the device with which you'll be implanted. Three manufacturers have a presence in the United States: Advanced Bionics, Cochlear Americas, and Med-El. Some implant centers work with only one manufacturer's implant, whereas others work with all three devices. Users of each device show a wide range of performance; however, studies have shown that the same level of success is possible with any of them. Cochlear implants are designed to last a lifetime. All three implants have a low failure rate. This is important, because internal device failure generally means a second surgery. All three implants are built to handle future upgrades and enhancements. As new technologies emerge, users are able to take advantage of them without the need for further surgery. All three implants cost about the same. The total cost of evaluation, surgery, the device itself, and rehabilitation ranges from $45,000 and $70,000. Most insurance companies, Medicare, and the Department of Veterans Affairs cover part or all of the cost.

There are important technical differences in the way each device processes and codes incoming sounds; however, a distinction that's probably more apparent to the user is the manner by which each device connects to external sound sources. All three processors can be connected to telephones, FM systems, induction loops, televisions, computer speakers, portable CD/DVD players, and personal listening devices such as iPods. The means for making these connections differs by manufacturer and speech processor style. Another important distinction is the implant's battery supply; implants use considerable power. Devices use rechargeable batteries, disposable batteries, or both.

There's no evidence that one implant is inherently better than the others. Members of your implant team can discuss the relative advantages and disadvantages of the implant devices that are available to you.

Factors to Consider When Choosing an Implant Device

- Device failure rate
- Device durability
- Weight of the external components
- Comfort (try the external components on)
- Appearance of external components
- Ability to see and adjust controls on the processor
- Number of coding strategies available
- Flexibility of programming
- Ability to incorporate future technological improvements
- Availability of technical features designed to improve speech understanding in difficult listening conditions
- Type of batteries used (rechargeable or disposable) and their cost
- Battery life
- Ease of connecting to the telephone and assistive technology

- Customer service
- Warranty

AUDITORY BRAINSTEM IMPLANTS

Most of the problems that cause deafness lie within the cochlea. Damage to the cochlea results in sensory hearing loss. A problem that results in damage to CN VIII can cause neural hearing loss. For example, surgery to remove a tumor on CN VIII might result in permanent and total deafness in one ear. People affected by Neurofibromatosis Type II (NF2) often develop CN VIII tumors on *both* sides, and removal of the tumors can result in total bilateral deafness. Hearing aids and cochlear implants are ineffective because CN VIII is unable to carry sound information to the brain. Auditory brainstem implants are designed to treat this type of deafness. They involve placement of a multichannel electrode on the cochlear nucleus, the site in the lower brainstem where CN VIII normally delivers the sound information it carries. A speech processor worn outside the body collects sounds from the environment and codes them; electrical stimulation of the cochlear nucleus results in the perception of sound. The ability to understand speech with this device is somewhat limited at this time.

CURRENT AND FUTURE TRENDS

When single-channel cochlear implants first became available in the mid-1980s, only people with adult-onset, profound hearing loss and speech perception scores of less than 10 percent were considered candidates. Since then, outcomes have improved, and candidacy criteria have broadened considerably, enabling infants, children, and adults with more hearing and better speech perception to benefit from this technology. It's expected that hearing criteria will continue to expand in the future and that devices will continue to become smaller and more sophisticated. Future devices might be totally implantable, with no need for external components at all.

Bilateral Cochlear Implants

Hearing with two ears has important advantages (see Chapter 7). For example, when hearing is approximately the same in both ears (either naturally or through two hearing aids), slight differences in the timing and loudness of a sound arriving at the two ears allow us to localize its source. Hearing with two ears also enables us to separate the signal of interest from background noise; the brain compares the signals coming from the two ears and filters out much of what is unwanted. Until recently, cochlear implants have been used in only one ear. Because of concerns about the destruction of hearing in the implanted ear and the unknown effects of long-term electrical stimulation, the goal was to save residual hearing in the nonimplanted (better) ear for future advances in hearing science. However, implant outcomes are now excellent for most users, and many implant centers are offering bilateral implants (implants in both ears). Research shows that bilaterally implanted listeners have improved localization ability, better hearing in noise, and a greater sense of well-being. Among other things, candidacy for bilateral implants depends on how much hearing there is in the better ear. Of the 100,000 people who've been implanted thus far, perhaps 15 percent have been implanted bilaterally. Insurance companies are beginning to cover the cost of two implants.

Electro-acoustic Stimulation

Candidacy criteria for cochlear implants are now being broadened to include people who have severe or profound high-frequency hearing loss with mild or moderate low-frequency loss. These listeners often do quite well wearing hearing aids in quiet, but they have difficulty understanding speech in noisy situations because they're missing critical high-frequency information. Hearing aids may be unable to amplify high-frequency sounds because there aren't enough functioning hair cells in high-frequency regions of the cochlea to pass information along to CN VIII (these areas are sometimes referred to as *cochlear dead regions*). In the past, these listeners derived limited benefit from hearing aids, yet didn't qualify for cochlear implants because of their "good" low-frequency hearing. Implant manufacturers are now testing hybrid devices that combine hearing aid and cochlear implant technologies, and there are new surgical techniques that allow low-frequency residual hearing to be preserved (for example, use of a "short" electrode array that doesn't reach all the way to low-frequency regions of the cochlea). The listener wears a device that amplifies the low frequencies *acoustically* and stimulates the middle and high frequencies *electrically*. Research suggests that patients implanted with hybrid devices have better speech understanding in noise and improved music perception. Although there's some indication that it might be more difficult to adjust to electro-acoustic stimulation than to either a hearing aid or cochlear implant alone, this technology appears to represent a major advance in the treatment of high-frequency hearing loss.

Bimodal Fittings

A bimodal fitting is one in which a hearing aid is worn on one side (acoustic hearing) and a cochlear implant (electrical stimulation) is worn on the other. Initially, bimodal fittings were discouraged because of concerns about the brain's ability to integrate two different types of input (which could result in binaural interference). In addition, implant criteria required that there be little hearing in the nonimplanted (better) ear. However, improvements in cochlear implant performance have led to expanded candidacy criteria, meaning that people with considerably more hearing in both ears now receive implants. Researchers have found that the two inputs actually provide complementary information, resulting in better speech perception in noise and improved localization. Listeners report that hearing is more natural and sound quality is better with a hearing aid in the nonimplanted ear. The arrangement also prevents auditory deprivation (over time, speech perception in the nonimplanted ear may deteriorate due to lack of stimulation), and provides the listener with a backup device should one fail. Disadvantages include greater cost (two devices cost more than one) and more maintenance. Adjustment to bimodal hearing takes more time and skill, and a few listeners probably *will* experience binaural interference. In the future, however, bimodal fittings may be recommended for all listeners with unilateral implants who have usable hearing in the nonimplanted ear, even if the loss is severe or profound. For many people, this solution will be more practical and much less expensive than two implants.

Optical Stimulation

Researchers are exploring the use of light, rather than electrical signals, to stimulate CN VIII. In contrast to electrical stimulation, in which a broad spread of current stimulates a broad range of nerve fibers that are responsive to a broad range of frequencies, an optical cochlear implant could stimulate nerve fibers with greater precision. Stimulation that is more frequency specific should result in a more accurate representation of sound being sent to the brain. This in turn should result in clearer hearing, including improved speech perception in background noise. Optical stimulation might also decrease tissue damage, because electrodes wouldn't touch neural tissues to stimulate them.

Auditory Nerve Implants

Researchers are also exploring the possibility of implanting an ultrathin electrode array directly in CN VIII.[1] Conventional electrode arrays are implanted in the cochlea, which is separated from auditory nerve fibers by fluid and bone; according to researchers, the effect is like talking to someone through a closed door. The intraneural implant would eliminate those barriers. This type of implant has the potential to activate nerve fibers associated with specific frequencies more precisely and reduce interference among electrodes when they're stimulated simultaneously, both of which should increase hearing clarity. In addition, it could be better in terms of preserving low-frequency residual hearing. If the initial success with animal studies is borne out, a human auditory nerve implant could be 5 to 10 years away.

Questions to Ask When Considering a Cochlear Implant[2, 3]

- How well should I expect to hear and understand speech with the implant?
- Which ear should be implanted?
- Am I a candidate for two implants?
- What is the surgeon's experience with implant surgery? (How many surgeries has she performed? How many times has she implanted the device that I will receive?)
- What are the surgical risks?
- How long will the surgery take?
- How long will I be in the hospital?
- How will I feel when I wake up after surgery?
- How much work will I miss?
- When can I go back to my exercise routine?
- Do I need a meningitis vaccination?
- How often do I need to return to the implant center after surgery?
- How much time should I plan to devote to postsurgical rehabilitation?
- Which implant is best for me?
- How does the implant connect to the telephone and assistive listening devices?
- What kind of batteries does the device use? How much do the batteries cost?
- Can I use a hearing aid in the other ear?
- Does insurance cover the surgery, the device, and rehabilitation?

CHAPTER 9

Hearing Assistance Technology

Sweet is every sound, sweeter the voice, but every sound is sweet.
                                                        Alfred Lord Tennyson

If your hearing loss can't be corrected medically, obtaining two hearing aids and learning to make the very best use of them should be among the first steps you take. Only a tiny percentage of people with hearing loss can't be helped by hearing aids. Hearing aids can improve your ability to function in nearly all situations; nevertheless, some situations will be difficult even *with* hearing aids, especially if your hearing loss is severe. Hearing assistance technology (HAT) supplements the benefits provided by hearing aids. HAT is designed to improve your ability to function independently and to communicate in difficult listening situations, whether you use hearing aids or not. It can benefit people with *any* degree of hearing loss. Although some technologies are especially helpful to persons with severe and profound hearing loss, others can substitute for hearing aids if the listener's hearing loss is mild. Every person with hearing loss should consider hearing assistance technology.

If you don't wear hearing aids, you can benefit from almost any type of assistive listening technology by wearing headphones or earbuds. If you *do* wear hearing aids, there are a variety of ways to achieve a direct (wired or wireless) connection between your hearing aids and nearly any sound source: a movie, telephone, concert, television, computer, worship service, stereo, lecture, personal music player, or friend wearing a microphone. With hearing aids, it's all about connectivity. The hearing aids that allow the greatest connectivity are behind-the-ear (BTE) hearing aids.

HEARING ASSISTANCE TECHNOLOGY

Hearing assistance technology (HAT) is an umbrella term that's used to cover a broad range of services and technologies designed to help people with hearing loss. HAT can be divided into four general categories: assistive listening devices and assistive listening systems (ALD/S), telephones and telephone accessories, auxiliary aids and services, and alerting devices.

Assistive listening devices (ALDs) and assistive listening systems (ALSs) make up a large and diverse category. ALDs are personal units that allow people to receive sound directly from almost any source, in most cases with a wireless connection. ALSs work in conjunction with the sound systems used in public facilities. While the sound system is broadcasting to normally-hearing patrons through loudspeakers, the ALS is transmitting the same signal directly to receivers worn by patrons who are hard of hearing.

Another large and diverse category includes telephones and telephone accessories. Using the telephone can be very challenging for people with hearing loss (visual cues are unavailable, important frequencies are filtered out, and volume is often inadequate). Dozens of specialty telephones and telephone accessories are available to improve telephone communication with or without hearing aids.

The auxiliary aids and services category represents a blend between services and technology, and includes captioning, computer-assisted real-time transcription (CART), computer-assisted note-taking, interpreter services, and the use of written materials.

The final category includes devices that substitute light or vibration for sounds in the environment; for example, a flashing light or vibration might let a listener know when a smoke alarm goes off, a doorbell rings, or an alarm clock buzzes. For the most part, these technologies are intended for people who have considerable hearing loss.

Unfortunately, assistive services and technologies usually aren't covered by Medicare or private health insurance plans (although one should always check). Depending on the circumstances, they may be provided in conjunction with the Americans with Disabilities Act (ADA; see Chapter 10). State vocational rehabilitation agencies, the Department of Veterans Affairs, and Medicaid can be other sources of funding. Assistive devices are most often purchased through mail order catalogs, over the Internet, and in specialty retail stores (for example, Radio Shack and Best Buy). Some audiologists offer them in their offices, but not often enough, and the selection is usually limited. Because the array of devices is vast, diverse, and ever changing, it's difficult for audiologists to stock, display, and dispense them in their practices.

Hearing assistance technology can be incredibly helpful; however, most consumers are unaware that such technologies exist, or they don't know where to find them. And regrettably, audiologists often fail to provide adequate information about HAT. The Rehabilitation Engineering Research Center (RERC) at Gallaudet University (Washington, DC) is developing a software program that can assist audiologists in analyzing a person's needs and identifying particular assistive technologies to meet those needs. The program highlights specific devices and vendors and suggests other hearing rehabilitation procedures that could be of benefit.[1] In the meantime, you'll probably need to do some research on your own. This overview is intended to give you an idea of the types of products and services that are available and to encourage you to try some of them. Use the information provided in the Resources section to search for the best possible solutions to the problems that *you* experience and to stay current; assistive technologies change constantly as new features and new devices are introduced. The annual convention of the Hearing Loss Association of America (formerly SHHH) is probably the best place to see new technologies and learn about them from company representatives. Always consult with your audiologist before making a purchase, however, so that she can advise you about a device's compatibility with your hearing aids.

Connectivity is an important issue that should be considered when you're fit with hearing aids. Hearing aids with features like telecoils, FM receivers, and direct audio input (DAI) capability (more on this later in the chapter; also see Chapter 7) offer the most flexibility in terms of interfacing with assistive technology. These features are most often found in BTE (and, to a lesser degree, ITE) hearing aids. BTEs offer more options than any other hearing aid style.

ASSISTIVE LISTENING DEVICES AND ASSISTIVE LISTENING SYSTEMS

Situations in which people with hearing loss have the greatest difficulty understanding speech typically are characterized by one or more of these problems:

- Distance separating the listener and speaker (or the listener and another sound source of interest). Loudness decreases quickly over distance, and the weakest sounds (which are most important to speech understanding) are lost first. Furthermore, the range of a hearing aid microphone extends only 6 to 12 feet.
- Background noise that competes with the speaker's voice. Although contemporary hearing aids have features designed to make understanding speech in background noise easier, this remains a challenge (see Chapter 7). Even the most advanced hearing aid can't compete with the human ear when it comes to understanding one conversation in the midst of many. For optimal understanding, speech (the signal) must be considerably louder than the competing noise (this is known as a favorable signal-to-noise relationship [SNR]).

- Reverberation or poor room acoustics. A reverberant room is one with lots of hard surfaces (hard walls, hard floor, hard ceiling, hard furniture) and few sound-absorbing materials (drapes, carpeting, ceiling tile, upholstered furniture). Sounds bounce off the hard surfaces, creating echoes that reach the ear at different times. Overlapping signals blur the original signal, "smearing" it and making it difficult to understand. Classrooms, cafeterias, and gymnasiums tend to be highly reverberant.

Distance, noise, and reverberation are classic "degraders" of speech understanding. They cause difficulty for *all* listeners, even those with normal hearing. For listeners with hearing loss who are already missing cues important to speech intelligibility, however, it takes less distance, less noise, and less reverberation to degrade speech understanding.

What's the solution? It's not turning up the volume on your hearing aids; that increases the signal, but it also increases the noise. Moving closer to the speaker would be a better solution. Putting your ear 8 to 12 inches from the speaker's mouth would be ideal, but it's not very practical. Fortunately, the same thing can be accomplished using remote microphone technology. *Remote microphone technology* increases the loudness of the signal (the *signal* is the sound you want to hear) without increasing the background noise. In other words, remote microphone technology makes the relationship between the signal and the noise more favorable. Technically, the signal-to-noise relationship is called the *signal-to-noise ratio*, or SNR. Improving the SNR is *the* most effective way to improve speech understanding in poor listening conditions.

What is remote microphone technology? Instead of relying on the hearing aid's microphone to pick up the speaker's voice, the speaker uses a remote microphone (remote from your hearing aid), and her voice is sent directly to you (more about *how* it's sent coming up). The ALD/S creates a wireless connection between you and the speaker, bypassing the noise and reverberation in the room. You can increase the loudness of the speaker's voice as much as you like without increasing the loudness of the noise. It makes no difference where you are in the room; your ability to hear the speaker is the same. In fact, all listeners wearing receivers can hear the speaker above the noise.

Let's imagine how this works. Let's say that you're attending a meeting in a large room with 20 people seated around or near a conference table. The presenter is standing at one end of the room; you arrived late, so you're seated at the opposite end. She uses her computer to make a portion of the presentation. For this segment, the lights are dimmed and her back is to you. The other people in the room are listening, but they're also making noise (clearing their throats, moving their chairs and feet, shuffling papers, pouring water/coffee, consuming doughnuts). Because the room is reverberant, noises bounce off hard surfaces and "smear" the presenter's words. The room noise (original and reverberated) is closer to you—and therefore louder—than the soft-spoken presenter. In a situation like this, the SNR is poor and you struggle to hear. How *much* you struggle depends on your hearing loss, the vocal qualities and speech characteristics of the presenter, the size of the room, and room acoustics. The presenter's words, already weakened by distance, can be overwhelmed. To make matters worse, you can't depend on visual cues. Now imagine that you're using a *personal ALD*. You've asked the presenter to clip a tiny microphone to her lapel (there are other microphone options as well). You wear a small receiver of some sort, perhaps it's inside your hearing aids. There are no wires, cords, or cables connecting the two of you. Now the presenter's words go directly to your hearing aids. The distance between you has effectively been eliminated, and her voice doesn't mix with the noise and reverberation in the room. Even when she turns away, the signal stays strong and clear because the microphone is still close to her mouth. The SNR is improved by as much as 20 dB; in other words, her voice is perhaps ten times louder than the noise in the room.

Let's make one more adjustment to this scenario. With the hearing aid microphone turned off, the presenter's voice coming from the remote microphone is the only input to your hearing aid. This gives you the very best SNR. Now, however, you have difficulty hearing your colleagues when they ask questions and make comments. Ideally, your hearing aid microphones can be activated along with the remote microphone. In this case, the remote microphone provides the primary input, and the hearing aid microphones provide secondary input. Although using both microphones at the same time decreases the SNR a bit, the signal from the remote microphone is adjusted to be louder than signals picked up by the hearing aid microphones. Either way, the presenter's voice is louder and clearer than it would have been using hearing aids alone.

Assistive Listening Systems

The Americans with Disabilities Act (ADA) requires public and private facilities that provide sound systems for their patrons to offer an assistive listening system for patrons who are hard of hearing or deaf. This includes theaters, movie houses, concert halls, auditoriums, arenas, stadiums, meeting rooms, lecture halls, performance spaces, courtrooms, and more. Facilities of this type normally amplify sound and broadcast it through loudspeakers to the audience. By adding special equipment to the regular sound system, the same signal can be transmitted directly to people wearing special receivers. Assistive listening systems can make a remarkable difference in the ability to enjoy recreational, social, cultural, educational, political, and civic activities. Although exempt from the law, many places of worship offer assistive listening systems as well.

Imagine that you go to a theater to enjoy a play or movie, or maybe you're attending a service at your place of worship. Unless you're sitting very close to the loudspeaker, it may be difficult for you to understand the words that are spoken. Connecting to the facility's assistive listening system can enable you to hear the words as if they were spoken 8 to 12 inches from your ears. The effects of distance and background noise are effectively eliminated.

The law requires that clearly visible signs be posted at a facility's entrance indicating the availability of an assistive listening system and the location where receivers can be obtained (see Appendix C). Patrons borrow the equipment and return it before leaving the facility. There's no charge, but a driver's license (or another form of identification) may be required as a deposit. At least one employee should be available to instruct patrons about how to use the system.

Unfortunately, some expensive assistive listening systems merely collect dust. There are several possible reasons for this. Often, people are simply uninformed about their right to have this type of accommodation. In addition, facilities sometimes do a poor job of advertising a system's availability, or staff members are unable to instruct patrons about its use. Patrons may be confused about how the system works with their hearing aids or have concerns about hygiene. However, the *most* likely reason is that people fear they will be conspicuous. Unfortunately, when a system gets little use, a facility's staff may be uninformed, and equipment may be poorly maintained (for example, batteries may not get recharged). People need to look (or ask) for accommodations in public places and use them. A little advance scouting can be helpful. When planning to attend an event, drop by the facility ahead of time so that you can learn about the system and how it can meet your needs (if that's not possible, call the facility or visit their website).

Why suffer through an event when it's possible to hear better? Why not *enjoy* the event that you've paid to see? If a facility already has an ALS, teach yourself to use it (don't worry; it's quite simple). Once you've done that, you can educate other patrons and even employees. If you encounter a facility that doesn't have a system, politely ask that one be installed. Be assertive; the ADA says that disabled people have the right to access the same goods, services, and facilities that are available to nondisabled people. If you use a wheelchair, you have the right to a ramp. If you have a hearing loss, you have the right to an assistive listening system.

Assistive Listening Devices

An ALD is a sound system on a smaller scale. Usually, a microphone is worn by a speaker or placed close to a sound source of interest. The listener wears a special receiver (which can be part of a hearing aid). ALDs can improve communication in virtually any situation. They can also relieve the stress and fatigue that difficult situations create.

An ALD can also create a direct connection between an external sound source—like a television—and a listener. People with hearing loss often drive everyone else in the house (or on the block!) crazy when it comes to television volume. In fact, television volume often tops the list of complaints from family members. An ALD transmits sound directly from the TV to a receiver worn by the listener (again, the receiver can be part of the listener's hearing aid). This makes sound from the television louder and clearer because it's not degraded by distance and noise in the room. The user can increase the volume on the hearing aids or the ALD without increasing the volume on the TV itself; the TV can even be muted. The connection between the listener and the television can be wireless or hard wired.

Wireless Signal Transmission

How does the signal travel from the remote microphone to the receiver worn by the listener? There are three different means of wireless transmission: induction loop (IL), frequency modulation (FM), and infrared (IR). All three can provide a high-quality signal and improve the SNR by roughly the same amount. All three can be used with personal ALDs as well as the systems used in public places, and all three can be used with or without hearing aids. Each has advantages and disadvantages that can make it the best choice in a particular situation.

To some extent, all three types of wireless transmission work in a similar fashion. For example, a remote microphone can be worn by a speaker. The job of any microphone is to pick up sound and change it into an electrical signal that can be amplified. The amplified signal is then transmitted (by a transmitter) to a receiver worn by a listener. The job of a receiver is to receive the electrical signal and change it back into sound. The sound then gets delivered to the listener's ears through a headset or the listener's hearing aids. The *difference* between the three wireless technologies is *how* sound is carried from the source to the receiver.

Induction Loop Transmission and Telecoils

With induction loop (IL) technology, sound is picked up by a microphone worn by a speaker, changed into an electrical signal, and sent to the system's amplifier, which makes it stronger. The electrical signal from the amplifier is sent to a wire that loops around a listening area. The electrical signal in the wire creates an electromagnetic field inside the loop that can be picked up by a telecoil inside a hearing aid (H/A). The telecoil, originally designed to improve telephone communication (see Chapter 7), serves as the ALD/S receiver, making a separate receiver and headset unnecessary. When a telecoil is used with an ALD/S, the hearing aid may allow the remote microphone and hearing aid microphone to be active at the same time, making it possible to hear the speaker more clearly while still hearing people nearby. In contrast, when a telecoil is used with a telephone, the hearing aid's microphone is turned off (eliminating room noise), and the telephone provides the only input to the hearing aid.

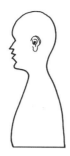

Telecoil in H/A works with IL (*no body-worn receiver necessary*)

Listeners who wear hearing aids *without* telecoils can remove them and wear an IL receiver with headphones or earbuds. However, this means that the signal isn't customized by the settings programmed into the hearing aids. It's sometimes possible to wear headphones over hearing aids, especially if they're completely-in-the-canal (CIC) aids. It may be necessary to turn down the hearing aid volume (to avoid feedback) and turn up the

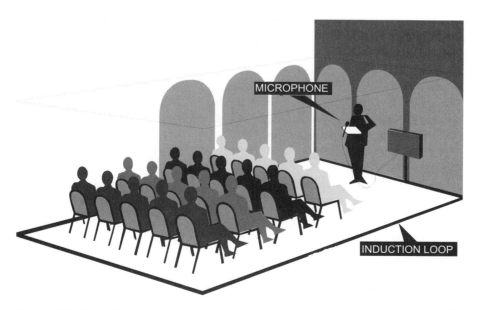

Figure 9.1. Example of an Induction Loop Assistive Listening System. The speaker's voice is picked up by the microphone, amplified, and sent to a wire that loops the room. Within the loop, an electromagnetic signal is picked up by the telecoil inside a listener's hearing aid or by a body-worn IL receiver worn with a headset. (Courtesy of Ampetronic Ltd.)

ALD/S volume to compensate, however. Headphones made of soft materials are less likely to cause feedback. Listeners *without* hearing aids can also use an induction loop by wearing a receiver with headphones or earbuds.

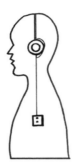

Headphones or earbuds work with FM, IL or IR receiver

The primary disadvantage of induction loop technology is that most hard of hearing people don't wear hearing aids, and among those who do, many don't have telecoils. Despite their versatility and relatively low cost, telecoils are included in only about 60 percent of the hearing aids sold in this country, probably because they don't fit inside smaller hearing aids like CICs. In the United Kingdom, both telecoils and induction loop systems are far more popular. Listeners in the United States have become more aware of telecoils due to the efforts of David Myers, a psychology professor at Hope College in Holland, Michigan. Traveling in Great Britain, Myers, who's severely hard of hearing, discovered the convenience and outstanding sound quality offered by loop systems. He described his experience in an 800-year-old abbey with high stone walls:

> ...noticing a hearing assistance sign...my wife suggested I activate the telecoils that came with my new hearing aids. When I did, the transformation was dramatic. Suddenly the babble of people awaiting the start of the service was replaced by the pure harmonies of the musicians—whom I had not even heard—playing in front of microphones across the abbey. It was like listening to a CD over a headset. When the liturgy began, the leader's words seemed to travel directly from her microphone to the center of my head. Her voice could not have been more distinct.[2]

Myers returned to start the "Let's Loop America" campaign (see the Resources section for contact information). Subscribing to the philosophy of "if you build it, they will come," Myers believes that if communities begin looping listening areas in public places, more people will opt for hearing aids that contain telecoils. Indeed, in Myers's small community, dozens of churches and public facilities have been "looped" within the past several years, and more people are opting for hearing aids with telecoils. Myers believes the public will gradually come to see loop systems as the most convenient and cost-effective assistive listening format. He notes, for example, that areas where it would be impractical to check out and return equipment (such as ticket windows, airport gates, and information desks) could be looped. People would simply switch their hearing aids to the telecoil setting and communicate with someone wearing a small microphone.[3,4]

William and Christine Diles, California audiologists, make residential loop installation a complementary option for anyone who purchases hearing aids with telecoils. They've "looped" more than 1,000 homes, 40 banks, several churches, a pharmacy, and a movie theater. They report that their patients are enthusiastic about using loops and telecoils at home and in facilities around their communities.

Advantages of Induction Loops and Telecoils

- Listeners who have telecoils in their hearing aids don't need to wear special receivers and headsets to use an induction loop system; they simply switch their hearing aids to the telecoil setting (this can be done by touching a button on the hearing aid or a remote control).
- Listeners with telecoils don't need to borrow receivers and headsets to use the ALS at a public facility. They can attend an event confident that their receivers are working properly, rather than relying on receivers maintained by the facility.
- All telecoils work with all induction loops, eliminating compatibility issues between personal receivers (telecoils) and the IL systems used in public places.
- Used with a neckloop or silhouettes (see later discussion), telecoils make hearing aids compatible with other wireless transmission systems (FM and infrared), personal communicators, and external sound sources.
- Listeners with telecoils hear a signal that is customized by the settings programmed into the hearing aids.
- Listeners with two telecoils receive a binaural signal.
- The transmitter of a personal IL unit can be plugged into an external sound source (like a television); within a looped space, sound from the television is picked up by the telecoils inside a listener's hearing aids (the connection between the television and the listener is wireless).
- Many hearing aids allow the telecoil and hearing aid microphones to be active at the same time (allowing listeners to communicate with the people around them); in this case, the telecoil provides the primary input to the hearing aid, and the hearing aid microphones provide secondary input.
- Telecoils and induction loops are less expensive than FM or IR technology.

Disadvantages of Induction Loops and Telecoils

- Most people who are hard of hearing don't wear hearing aids, and among those who do, many don't have telecoils.
- Telecoils fit in all behind-the-ear (BTE) hearing aids and some mini-BTE, in-the-ear (ITE), and in-the-canal (ITC) hearing aids. However, they typically don't fit in CIC aids.

- The signal from an induction loop is not always consistent; occasionally, reception can be affected by head orientation or a listener's position in the room (there can be "dead spots" in the electromagnetic field).
- Telecoils are subject to electromagnetic interference (buzz) produced by computer monitors, computer power supplies, fluorescent lights, dimmer switches, microwaves, power lines, copiers, fax machines, and some appliances.
- The signal from an induction loop can spill over into another room (a potential problem when privacy is a concern, as in a courtroom).
- Personal IL devices don't offer the portability and versatility of personal FM units.

Induction Options

There are three induction options:

Area Loops

- Almost any area can be looped (classrooms, reception windows in offices, lecture halls, car interiors, kitchen tables, information desks, teller windows, family rooms, or favorite chairs).
- The induction loop wire can be permanently installed under a carpet, along the baseboards, on the ceiling, in the basement, or in the attic. Installation is relatively simple; many people do it themselves (when that's not possible, check with a carpet installer or an electrician). After installation, the loop should be relatively maintenance free.
- Temporary loops can be set up for meetings or special events.
- Everyone inside the loop who has telecoils in their hearing aids can pick up the signal.

Neckloops

- A neckloop is worn like a long, loose-fitting necklace by someone who has telecoils inside his hearing aids. The neckloop creates an electromagnetic field around a listener's head similar to the electromagnetic field created by an induction loop that encircles a room. The telecoils inside the hearing aids pick up the signal from the electromagnetic field. The neckloop can be plugged into an FM or infrared (IR) receiver, making any hearing aid with a telecoil compatible with FM and IR wireless transmission.
- A neckloop can be worn under clothing; there are no cords or wires connecting it to the hearing aids.
- A neckloop can be plugged into almost any external sound source (such as a television).

Silhouettes

- A silhouette looks like a very thin, flat BTE case with a cable coming out of the bottom; it hooks over the ear like a BTE.

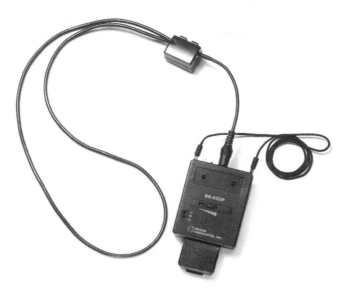

Figure 9.2. Example of a Neckloop Plugged into an IR Receiver. (Courtesy of Sound Associates, Inc.)

- The cable plugs into the receiver of an FM or IR assistive listening device or system, making any hearing aid with a telecoil compatible with FM and IR wireless transmission.
- A silhouette can also be plugged into almost any external sound source (like a television).
- A silhouette is less sensitive to head orientation than are area loops or neckloops.
- A silhouette is worn closer to the telecoil than an area loop or neckloop, which means that a more powerful electromagnetic signal is available for listeners with more severe hearing loss. If the additional power is not needed, the electromagnetic signal can be kept relatively low, making it less susceptible to interference.

FM Transmission

An assistive listening device or system that uses FM transmission is basically a small radio station. With a personal ALD, the signal from a remote microphone (worn by a speaker, for example) is broadcast via FM radio waves to a listener wearing a receiver that's tuned to the same frequency. Similarly, an ALS in a public facility takes the signal from the sound system and broadcasts it via FM radio waves to audience members wearing receivers tuned to the appropriate frequency.

With a personal FM device, the microphone/transmitter can be worn by the speaker, held and aimed at the speaker by the listener, placed on

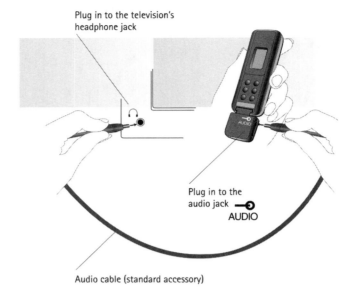

Figure 9.3. Example of an FM Microphone/Transmitter Plugging into the Headphone Jack of a Television. The transmitter will broadcast the signal directly to an FM receiver worn by the listener. The connection to the listener is wireless. (Courtesy of Phonak.)

a podium, or set in the middle of a conference table. Personal FM devices can be used virtually anywhere; they're more portable and more versatile than personal IL or IR units. For example, a couple (or anyone else) could use an FM device in a noisy restaurant, in the car, or while taking a walk or a bicycle ride. Alternatively, an FM transmitter can be plugged into an external sound source (like a television). The connection between the sound source and the listener is wireless.

The FM signal can be delivered to the listener's ears in one of several ways:

- Some BTE hearing aids have FM receivers built inside; therefore there's no need to wear a separate receiver. Some automatically switch to FM mode when they sense an FM signal and switch back to microphone mode when the signal is no

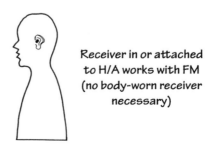

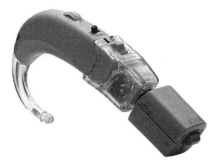

Figure 9.4. Top (*left*) to bottom (*right*), BTE Hearing Aid, Boot (Audio Shoe) Adapter, and FM Receiver. (Courtesy of Oticon, Inc.)

longer present. In other cases, the listener switches to FM mode manually by touching a button on the hearing aid or remote control.

• A tiny receiver can be connected to a boot or audio shoe adapter and snapped onto the bottom of almost any BTE hearing aid; again, this eliminates the need for a separate receiver (Figure 9.4).

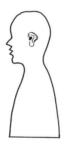

Receiver in or attached to H/A works with FM (no body-worn receiver necessary)

• If the hearing aid has a telecoil, a neckloop (see Figure 9.2) or silhouette can be plugged into the earphone jack of an FM receiver.

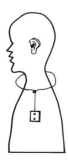

With neckloop, telecoil inside H/A works with FM or IR receiver

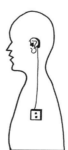

With silhouette, telecoil inside H/A works with FM or IR receiver

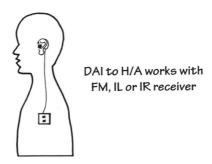

DAI to H/A works with
FM, IL or IR receiver

- A hearing aid with direct audio input (DAI) capability or a DAI boot (see later discussion) can be connected to an FM receiver with a patch cord.
- If the hearing aids don't have integrated FM receivers, telecoils, or DAI (and the hearing loss is not too severe), a listener may be able to remove the aids and use headphones or earbuds connected to an FM receiver. In this case, the signal would not be customized by settings programmed into the hearing aids. Occasionally, listeners can wear headphones over their hearing aids, especially if the aids are CICs. A listener *without* hearing aids can also wear headphones or earbuds connected to an FM receiver.

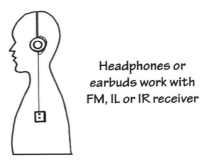

Headphones or
earbuds work with
FM, IL or IR receiver

Advantages of FM Transmission

- Receivers can be incorporated into BTE hearing aids or connected to BTE hearing aids with adapters (see Figures 7.8 and 9.4), eliminating the need for a body-worn receiver and headset. A body-worn receiver is similar to a pager and can be worn under clothing, in a pocket, or clipped to a belt.
- If the signal goes through the hearing aids, it is customized by the settings programmed into them by the audiologist.
- Listeners with two ear-level receivers receive a binaural signal.
- Personal FM units are highly portable and highly versatile; they offer the greatest flexibility of movement.
- A listener can pick up the FM signal throughout the house (no more shouting from room to room).
- FM is the only wireless transmission mode that can easily be used outdoors.

- The transmitter for a personal FM unit can be plugged into an external sound source (like a television). Sound from the television is broadcast directly to a personal FM receiver; the connection to the listener is wireless (see Figure 9.3).
- Many hearing aids allow the FM and hearing aid microphones to be active at the same time (allowing the user to communicate with the people around him).
- No installation is required.
- FM transmission offers more power to accommodate severe and profound hearing losses.

Disadvantages of FM Transmission

- FM transmission is subject to interference from other communication devices operating in close proximity, such as nearby radio stations, pagers, police band radios, emergency vehicles, walkie-talkies, other FM devices/ systems, etc.
- The FM signal can spill over into other rooms (a problem when privacy is a concern).
- Ear-level FM receivers (in or attached to hearing aids) generally require BTE hearings aids. Some people prefer custom hearing aids.
- FM units are relatively expensive.

Wireless Communication for Small Groups

A new system addresses the need to hear multiple talkers in a group setting. Although the transmission technology differs, this system functions like a variation on a personal FM device—with a significant advantage. A conventional FM device has a single microphone/transmitter that broadcasts to one or more receivers (as would be used in a classroom setting, for example); in contrast, this system has a single receiver and up to four microphones/transmitters. This means that one to four companions can wear remote microphones that transmit to a listener wearing a receiver, making it possible for the listener to interact comfortably with more than one person at a time (see figure 9.5). This means, for example, that the user could dine with up to four other people in a noisy restaurant or play cards as part of a foursome. The unit can also be used like a traditional FM device for one-to-one communication.

Infrared Transmission

With infrared transmission, invisible beams of light are used to carry sound from its source to one or more listeners wearing receivers. Infrared receivers have not been built into hearing aids, nor are they available

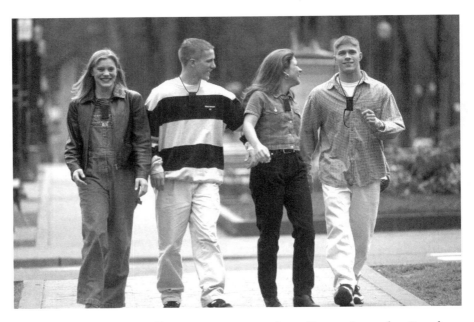

Figure 9.5. Up to Four Talkers Wearing Microphone/Transmitters that Broadcast to a Receiver Worn by the Listener. (Courtesy of Etymotic Research, Inc.)

in adapters that connect to hearing aids. Instead, infrared is used with telecoils in hearing aids, hearing aids that have direct audio input (DAI; discussed later), or, more commonly, headsets that replace hearing aids:

• Listeners with telecoils in their hearing aids can plug a neckloop or silhouettes into the IR receiver.

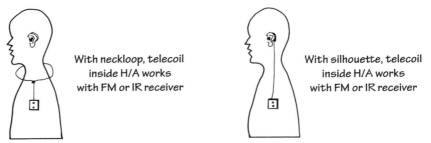

• Listeners with hearing aids that have DAI capability can plug the IR receiver into their hearing aids using patch cords.

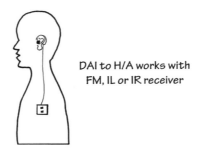

- If the hearing loss is not too severe, the listener can remove the aids and use headphones or earbuds connected to the IR receiver, although in this case the signal isn't customized by the settings programmed into the hearing aids. Occasionally, listeners can wear headphones over their hearing aids, especially if they're CICs. Listeners *without* hearing aids can wear a receiver with headphones or earbuds.

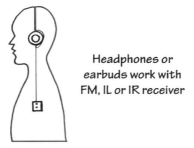

Headphones or earbuds work with FM, IL or IR receiver

A popular IR receiver style looks something like a stethoscope attached to earbuds. The lightweight receiver hangs below the chin. There are also

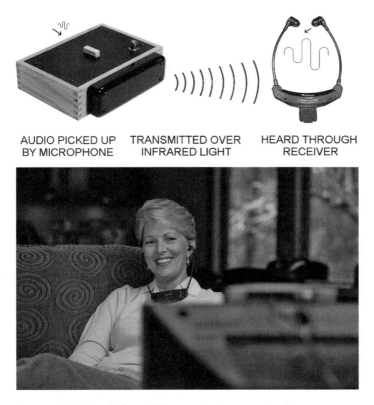

AUDIO PICKED UP   TRANSMITTED OVER   HEARD THROUGH
BY MICROPHONE   INFRARED LIGHT   RECEIVER

Figure 9.6. *Top*, Infrared Transmission to a Stethoscope-type Receiver. *Bottom*, Stethoscope-type Receiver Worn by a Listener Watching Television. (Courtesy of Sound Choice Assistive Listening, Inc. [*top*] and Clarity, a division of Plantronics, Inc. [*bottom*].)

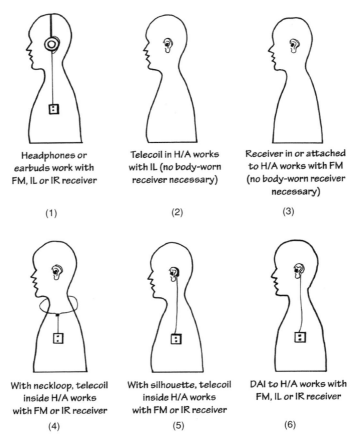

Figure 9.7. Receiver Options for Wireless Technology. *Left to Right:* (1) Listeners *without* hearing aids can wear headphones/earbuds plugged into an FM, IL, or IR receiver. Listeners *with* hearing aids can remove them and wear headphones/earbuds with a receiver. In some cases, listeners can wear headphones over their hearing aids. (2) Listeners with telecoils in their hearing aids simply switch to the telecoil setting to receive an IL signal. (3) Listeners with FM receivers in their hearing aids (or attached to them with boot adapters) don't need a separate receiver to receive an FM signal. (4) Listeners with telecoils in their hearing aids can wear a neckloop plugged into an FM or IR receiver. (5) Listeners with telecoils can wear silhouettes plugged into an FM or IR receiver. (6) Listeners with DAI capability can plug their hearing aids into an FM, IL, or IR receiver with a patch cord. (Adapted from work created by Cynthia Compton-Conley.)

wireless earphones with built-in infrared receivers. Some receivers contain a microphone that enables the listener to hear others in the room while using the IR unit. Personal IR devices are especially popular for television viewing.

Advantages of Infrared Transmission

- Unlike IL and FM transmission, the infrared signal doesn't spill over into other rooms, which is important when privacy is a concern (for example, during courtroom proceedings, business meetings, performances using copyrighted material).
- An unlimited number of individual transmitters can operate simultaneously in the same building, as long as they're in separate rooms.
- An IR transmitter can be plugged into an external sound source (like a television). Sound from the television is broadcast directly to the IR receiver. The connection between the television and listener is wireless.

Disadvantages of Infrared Transmission

- Unlike IL and FM, IR receivers have not been built into hearing aids or adapters that connect to hearing aids; this usually makes wearing a receiver and headset necessary.
- Sometimes IR units can't be used outdoors or in rooms with exceptional natural light because of light interference.
- The receiver must be able to "see" the IR light; this means it can't be worn under clothing.
- Personal IR units don't offer the portability and versatility of personal FM units.

Hard-wired Assistive Listening Devices

Direct Audio Input

Direct audio input (DAI) capability is an optional feature on some BTE hearing aids (see Chapter 7). Some hearing aids have DAI jacks; in other cases, a universal DAI boot adapter slips over the end of almost any BTE hearing aid. Using a special patch cord, it's possible to plug a hearing aid directly into an external sound source (the sound source could be a television, telephone, stereo, radio, computer, personal music player, or something else). A hearing aid with DAI capability can also be plugged into the receiver of an assistive listening device or system. DAI enables sound to be customized by the settings programmed into the listener's hearing aids.

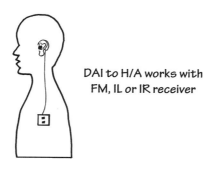

DAI to H/A works with
FM, IL or IR receiver

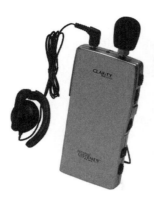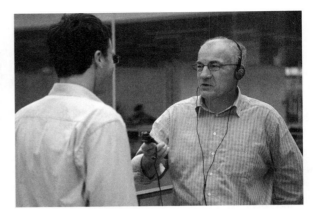

Figure 9.8. Examples of Personal Communication Devices. The device connects to the listener with a cable. (Courtesy of Clarity, a Division of Plantronics, Inc. [*left*] and Phonic Ear [*right*].)

Personal Communication Devices

Personal communication devices, sometimes called *one-to-one commu-nicators* or *personal amplifiers*, are hard-wired devices in which a cable connects the microphone and the listener. The unit is generally about the size of a pager or television remote and contains a microphone, amplifier, and battery; it attaches to headphones or earbuds with a cable. The microphone can be built into the unit or it can be detachable. In some cases, an additional microphone can be ordered. The microphone can be worn by the speaker, held by the speaker, placed close to the speaker, or held by the listener and aimed at the speaker. In any case, the microphone and the listener are connected by cables. Alternatively, the unit can be plugged into a sound source (like a television, telephone, or ALD receiver). Although personal communicators generally aren't worn with hearing aids, hearing aid users with telecoils can plug a neckloop or silhouette into the unit and hear through their hearing aids.

Hard-wired devices are portable, easy to use (no installation is necessary), and considerably less expensive than wireless systems (less than $200). A personal communicator can be a reasonable substitute for hearing aids in certain situations (for example, during a hospital stay when wearing hearing aids isn't possible, when hearing aids are away for repair, or for a homebound listener whose listening needs are minimal). Mobility is limited by the cable connection, however.

My Dad

My dad isn't ready to make a big investment in HAT (like many people, he thinks that he's already made a big enough investment in hearing aids). When he bought his last hearing aid, however, I insisted that he get a telecoil (even though he hears quite well on the phone). Because I also wanted him to have an open canal fitting (which he *loves*), and I hoped that he'd be able to use a mini-BTE, I asked his audiologist to choose a mini-BTE that could accommodate a telecoil.

As a first step (toward using HAT), I bought him a personal communicator and a neckloop. Although this doesn't offer the freedom and convenience of wireless technology, it's a start. At home, he detaches the microphone and mounts it on the TV (a little plastic mount came as part of the package). The microphone plugs into the unit (which looks something like a remote control) with a long cord. He plugs his neckloop into the unit and switches his hearing aid to the telecoil setting. He hears better and watching TV is more relaxing. In the car, he plugs the neckloop into the unit, and my mother attaches the microphone to her lapel. At church, he can plug the neckloop into the receiver for the assistive listening system. If he needs to, he can plug his neckloop into the phone. My next goal is to convince him to try an induction loop in the room where he and my mother watch television. With that, he could just walk into the room and switch his hearing aid to the telecoil setting.

Cochlear Implants and the Use of Hearing Assistance Technology

Virtually all of the information in this chapter applies to cochlear implants as well as to hearing aids. All implants have DAI capability, meaning that they can be plugged into televisions, personal music players, computers, telephones, and other audio sources with special cables. All implants offer telecoil options that allow them to be used with hearing aid–compatible telephones and induction loops. Implants can be connected to FM and IR receivers with special cables; in some cases, FM receivers are built into the speech processor or connect to it with an adapter.

TELEPHONES AND TELEPHONE ACCESSORIES

The ability to communicate by telephone continues to be vitally important in our society. Unfortunately, it can be a formidable challenge for people with hearing loss (visual cues are unavailable, important frequencies are filtered out, volume may be inadequate). Fortunately, dozens of products are available to improve telephone communication. Some are meant to work with hearing aids, some are meant to work without them, and some can be used either way (which can be helpful when the phone rings in the middle of the night or you're just getting out of the shower). Others use a text format that makes the issue of hearing aids irrelevant.

Hearing Aid Compatibility

Holding a telephone handset over a hearing aid usually causes feedback. Telecoils were originally designed to improve telephone communication by minimizing feedback and room noise (the hearing aid microphone is turned off when a telecoil is used with a telephone). Telecoils were developed to take advantage of telephone technology that's now obsolete. Years ago, magnets drove the speakers in telephone handsets, and some of the electromagnetic signal leaked out. The leaking signal could be picked up and amplified by a telecoil. As telephone technology improved, however, magnets were no longer used, and the electromagnetic signal disappeared. Eventually, telephones were no longer compatible with telecoils. The Hearing Aid Compatibility Act of 1988 required manufacturers to begin making landline phones (corded and cordless) that were compatible with hearing aids. As a result, virtually all modern landline telephones are now *hearing aid compatible* (HAC). Landline phones that are HAC contain electronics that generate an electromagnetic signal for telecoil use. Unfortunately, standards don't regulate electromagnetic signal strength; therefore users must be careful to choose a phone that meets their particular needs (portable devices that amplify the electromagnetic signal are also available).

Landline Telephones

Listeners with telecoils achieve a direct connection with HAC telephones by switching their hearing aids to the telecoil setting and placing the handset over the hearing aid. It can take some experimenting to find the right spot for the handset relative to the hearing aid. Without a telecoil, using the telephone with a hearing aid is likely to cause feedback, although this is less likely with CIC hearing aids. It may be easier to remove the hearing aid and use a telephone with amplification. Hard-of-hearing listeners *without* hearing aids can also benefit from telephone amplification. There are several types from which to choose, with many models in each category.

In-Line Amplifiers

In-line amplifiers can be used with virtually all modular, corded telephones. Most telephones today are modular, meaning that the handset can be unplugged from the base. The curled cord attached to the handset plugs into the amplifier, and the amplifier plugs into the telephone's base

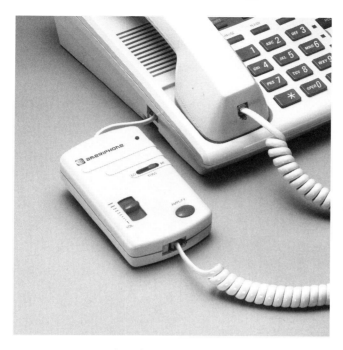

Figure 9.9. Example of an In-line Telephone Amplifier. (Courtesy of Clarity, a division of Plantronics, Inc. and Harris Communications.)

(where the curled cord on the handset would normally plug in). A volume control enables telephone conversations to be amplified by as much as 50 dB (depending on the model). It also enables the volume to be turned down so the telephone can be used by people without hearing loss. Some models have a tone control that gives the high frequencies an extra boost. In-line amplifiers typically can't be used with trimline models in which the dialing mechanism is in the handset.

A telephone mouthpiece normally amplifies our words slightly and sends the amplified signal to the earpiece, allowing us to monitor our own speech; however, any room noise that reaches the mouthpiece is also amplified. If you're using a telephone with amplification, room noise is amplified even more. Some telephone amplifiers have a control that allows the telephone's microphone to be muted while you're listening, which minimizes noise. Alternatively, you can cover the telephone's mouthpiece with your hand while listening.

Replacement Handsets

Another option is to replace the handset on your telephone with one that contains an amplifier and volume control. Again, a volume control allows

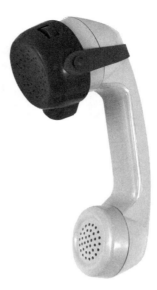

Figure 9.10. Example of a Portable (Strap-on) Telephone Amplifier. (Courtesy of Global Assistive Devices, Inc. and Harris Communications.)

the telephone to be used by people without hearing loss. Replacement handsets work with most modular corded telephones; however, they're not compatible with trimline models in which the dialing mechanism is in the handset.

Portable Amplifiers

A portable amplifier is a small device with a volume control that fastens to the handset of a corded or cordless telephone with a strap. Most have volume controls so that they can be left on telephones used by people without hearing loss. In addition to amplifiers that boost the acoustic signal, there are also portable "induction amplifiers" that boost the electromagnetic signal.

Amplified Ringers

Special ringers are available for use with corded and cordless landline telephones. Most models offer some combination of a very loud ringer (with a volume control); ringer frequency options (the user chooses the frequency that's easiest for her to hear); ringer pattern options (horn, siren, warble); and a flashing light, strobe, or vibrator that can be activated along with the ringer. The device plugs into a telephone outlet on the wall; at the other end, it plugs into a jack on the base of the telephone.

Amplified Telephones

Stand-alone telephones have been designed especially for people with hearing loss. Both corded and cordless models are available, and they're all HAC. These telephones increase the voice signal by as much as 55 dB and provide a strong electromagnetic signal for telecoil users. They come with any combination of standard telephone features that a user might want. In addition, most offer options such as a very loud ringer; ringer frequency choices; and a flashing light, strobe, and/or vibrator to announce incoming calls. Some have oversized, easy-to-read, easy-to-push buttons. Many have volume controls, some have tone controls, and a few have controls that mute the handset microphone while the user is listening. Some have a built-in speakerphone, which eliminates feedback from the hearing aid. Some have an emergency call button.

Almost all specialty telephones have one or two headset jacks into which the user can plug a headset, neckloop, silhouette, DAI patch cord, personal communicator, or cochlear implant. Using one of these accessories gives the listener a direct, hard-wired connection to the telephone that eliminates feedback and reduces room noise. Some accessories (for example, headsets and neckloops) allow input to both ears, which can be especially helpful to listeners with hearing loss. Many models also include answering machines. Plugging an accessory device into the telephone's headset jack also allows the listener to hear messages through a direct connection, perhaps with both ears.

Specialty telephones generally accommodate Caller ID, a service offered by telephone service providers for a monthly charge. Although this service may be nothing more than a convenience for people with normal hearing, it can be critically important for people with hearing loss. People who are hard of hearing often have difficulty recognizing voices over the phone. Knowing who's calling can eliminate the initial confusion and provide enough context to make understanding the conversation easier.

Digital Cell Phones

A cell phone offers advantages to people with hearing loss. First, it has a headset jack that allows the user to connect an accessory device (for example, a hearing aid with DAI, a cochlear implant processor, a neckloop, a silhouette, or a personal communicator) to create a direct, hard-wired connection. This allows the phone to be separated from the hearing aid, minimizing feedback and interference. Some cell phones offer Bluetooth capability (see later discussion), which goes a step further and creates a direct, *wireless* connection between a cell phone and hearing aids that are Bluetooth enabled. Most cell phones have volume controls, ringer options, and adjustable ringer volume. In addition, most offer a vibrating signal or flashing screen to announce incoming calls. Some offer email, instant messaging, and text messaging—visual communication options that can be especially helpful to users with hearing loss. Most can accommodate Caller ID (for an extra charge from the service provider). Some have speakerphone capability (again, increasing the distance between the phone and the hearing aid, thereby minimizing feedback and interference).

Cell phones originally were exempt from the Hearing Aid Compatibility Act of 1988. As they became ever more popular, however, people with hearing loss complained of interference when they tried using them with hearing aids. As it turns out, a transmission technology used by *digital* cell phones produces radio frequency (RF) emissions that can be picked up by a hearing aid as buzzing. In 2003, the Federal Communications Commission (FCC) ordered cell phone manufacturers and service providers to begin addressing hearing aid compatibility for cell phones. For cell phones, HAC was defined in terms of RF emissions as well as telecoil compatibility. Today, all major cell phone manufacturers are required to make some models that are HAC.

The FCC requires cell phone manufacturers to rate (1) how well a cell phone works with hearing aids in the microphone (nontelecoil) mode, and (2) how well a cell phone works with telecoils. The rating scale ranges from M1 to M4 for compatibility in the microphone mode and T1 to T4 for compatibility in the telecoil mode. A rating of 1 (M1 or T1) is poor, 2 is fair, 3 is good, and 4 is excellent. Only phones rated 3 or 4 can be labeled HAC.

Newer hearing aids are rated on the same M1 to M4 and T1 to T4 scales. Unfortunately, labeling hearing aids with M and T ratings is not mandated by law. If the hearing aid that you're considering buying doesn't carry a rating, your audiologist may be able to obtain it from the manufacturer.

To select the best cell phone–hearing aid combination, add the M ratings for microphone mode or T ratings for telecoil mode. Look for a combined rating (cell phone + hearing aid) of M5 or M6, or T5 or T6. A rating of 5 should provide good performance; a rating of 6 should provide excellent performance. Despite the best intentions of the FCC and cell phone manufacturers, however, ratings do not *guarantee* performance. It's still necessary to try a cell phone with your hearing aid *before* purchasing it.

Specialty cell phones designed for people with hearing loss are also becoming available. These HAC phones offer up to 50 dB of amplification.

Things to Look for When Shopping for a Digital Cell Phone
- A full-service store owned and operated by a wireless service provider; these stores must allow you to try different cell phones with your hearing aids. Regulations do not require general retailers like Radio Shack, Best Buy, and Wal-Mart to do so.

- A store with a clear return or exchange policy that is provided in writing
- A knowledgeable sales person who can answer your questions about HAC
- Packaging that identifies the cell phone as HAC
- A rating of M3 or M4 if you use hearing aids without telecoils, or T3 or T4 if you use hearing aids with telecoils
- Literature on the cell phone and its HAC
- A cell phone with output jacks and accessories that allow you to listen with both ears
- A cell phone with a volume control
- A cell phone with a vibrating alert or flashing screen in addition to a ringer
- A cell phone with a variety of ringer or tone pattern options
- A cell phone with adjustable ringer volume
- A cell phone with text messaging, instant messaging, and email
- A cell phone with speakerphone capability (increased distance between the hearing aid and telephone reduces feedback and interference)
- A cell phone that can be connected to a teletypewriter (TTY) if the user uses a TTY to make or receive calls (see later discussion)
- A cell phone with video streaming (if needed to communicate with sign language)
- A cell phone with the ability to control backlighting (telecoil users can get interference from things like a phone's backlighting, antenna, keypad display, battery, or circuit board)
- A "flip" or "clam shell" cell phone; this style sometimes works better because the hearing aid is farther from internal sources of interference
- A cell phone with good reception; HAC cannot improve the reception of the phone itself

Bluetooth Solutions

Bluetooth is networking technology that allows electronic devices to find and communicate with one another, without wires, cables, or line-of-sight requirements. Bluetooth technology is inexpensive, power efficient, portable, and highly resistant to most forms of interference. It's a feature that's increasingly found in cell phones and a growing number of other devices, such as fax machines, personal data assistants (PDAs), digital cameras, music players, computers, and computer peripherals (for example, keyboards, mice, and printers). In early 2007, there were more than 1,000 Bluetooth-certified devices on the market.

A Bluetooth-enabled device contains a microchip that makes wireless communication with other Bluetooth-enabled devices possible. The Bluetooth protocol was developed collaboratively by a group of electronics manufacturers in the late 1990s. The working group needed a code name for the technology that was under development. A comparison was made to Viking King Harald Blatand—in English, King Harold Bluetooth. King Bluetooth is remembered for uniting warring factions in what is now Denmark, Norway, and Sweden during the tenth century. The King's ability to connect many different tribes to form his kingdom parallels Bluetooth's ability to connect many different electronic devices. The name Bluetooth stuck.

At this point, Bluetooth is used most often with cell phones. With the user wearing a small (trendy-looking) earpiece, Bluetooth makes it possible to carry on phone conversations using a cell phone that might be tucked away in a purse, briefcase, or pocket. The connection between the earpiece and the cell phone is hands free and wireless.

Hearing aid users can have a wireless connection between their hearing aids and a Bluetooth-enabled phone (which, again, can be in a purse, pocket, or briefcase), free of feedback and interference. There are several ways to accomplish this, and more options will surely follow. One option is to connect a tiny Bluetooth device (shown in Figure 9.11) to the bottom of a compatible BTE hearing aid with a DAI connector. This device allows a wireless connection to be established between the hearing aid and a Bluetooth-enabled cell phone (or another Bluetooth-enabled electronic device). Here's how a cell phone call works. When the phone rings, it's heard through the hearing aid, and the hearing aid microphone automatically shuts off. The call is answered by pressing a button on the little Bluetooth device attached to the end of the hearing aid. The caller's voice is heard through the hearing aid, so it's customized according to the

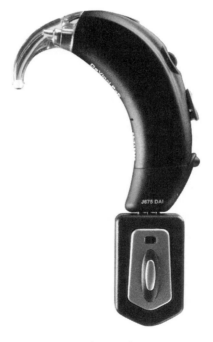

Figure 9.11. Bluetooth Device Attached to a BTE Hearing Aid with a DAI Connector. (Courtesy of Starkey Laboratories, Inc.)

settings programmed by the audiologist. A microphone on the device picks up the user's voice and sends it back to the cell phone. When the call is finished, the Bluetooth connection ends, and the hearing aid microphone is reactivated. The only time that the user needs to touch the phone is to dial. Feedback and interference are eliminated because the phone is separated from the hearing aid. The same device is also designed to receive signals from a wireless microphone/transmitter that can be worn by a companion in a noisy place. This option makes it similar to a personal FM system, but smaller and less expensive. If the user doesn't have a Bluetooth-enabled phone, a Bluetooth adapter can be attached; the same is also true for other audio devices.

If the user's hearing aid doesn't have DAI capability but it has a telecoil, a neckloop with a Bluetooth device allows the cell phone's output to be picked up by the telecoil. The connection between hearing aid and cell phone is still hands free and wireless (Figure 9.12, upper left). This option also allows custom (non-BTE) hearing aids with telecoils to be compatible with Bluetooth-enabled devices.

Alternatively, a hand-held FM transmitter with Bluetooth capability can receive a signal from a Bluetooth-enabled phone and transmit it (using FM radio waves) to BTE hearing aids that are equipped with integrated FM receivers or FM boots (see Figure 9.12, upper right). Again, the problems of feedback and electromagnetic interference are eliminated because the hearing aid is separated from the cell phone. The user speaks directly into the hand-held FM microphone/transmitter, and the caller's voice is heard through the hearing aids. The cell phone is needed only to initiate and terminate calls. The FM microphone/transmitter can also be used as part of a personal FM assistive listening device.

Also available are *streamers* that receive Bluetooth signals from external devices (including cell phones) and wirelessly stream them to the hearing aids that go with them (see Figure 9.12, bottom). The streamer hangs around the user's neck. Some devices offer one channel of sound that goes to both ears; others offer stereo sound.

The future will undoubtedly bring other ways to create wireless connections between hearing aids and Bluetooth-enabled devices. It's even possible that Bluetooth technology may someday be integrated inside hearing aids, eliminating the need for a DAI connector or other accessories. In the shorter term, we're likely to see Bluetooth transmission incorporated into the assistive listening systems found in public facilities.

Devices like the Bluetooth boot adapter, the Bluetooth neckloop, the Bluetooth-enabled FM microphone/transmitter, and the Bluetooth-enabled streamer are innovations designed to allow hearing aids to function as wireless headsets for audio devices (like cell phones). And there are already wireless headsets that function as hearing aids! These headsets have been designed to provide amplification (which can be customized to some extent) when the listener *isn't* talking on the phone or using another electronic device. What's more, high-tech hearing aids

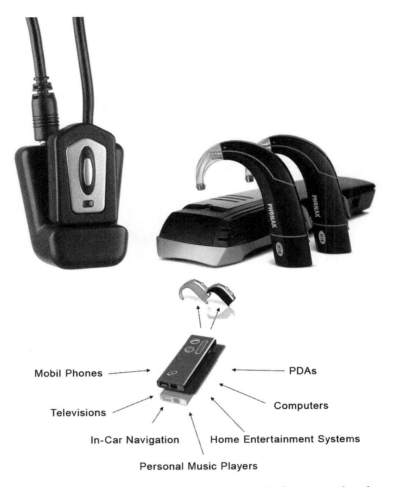

Mobil Phones

Televisions

In-Car Navigation

Personal Music Players

PDAs

Computers

Home Entertainment Systems

Figure 9.12. *Upper left,* Bluetooth device attached to a special neck-loop that makes all hearing aids with telecoils Bluetooth compatible. *Upper right,* Bluetooth-enabled FM microphone/transmitter shown with compatible BTE hearing aids that have FM receivers attached. The Bluetooth signal is picked up from an external source by the microphone/transmitter and sent to the hearing aids via FM. *Bottom,* Bluetooth-enabled "streamer" that transmits the signal from an external source to compatible BTE hearing aids. (Courtesy of Starkey Laboratories, Inc. [*upper left*], Phonak [*upper right*], and Oticon, Inc. [*bottom*].)

and wireless headsets are looking more and more alike—in some cases, even audiologists can't tell them apart.[5] As more people *without* hearing problems wear devices in their ears to communicate with their audio equipment, the distinction between hearing aids and other types of hearing technology is becoming blurred.[6] In fact, we could be seeing the beginning of a convergence between high-tech wireless systems and hearing aids.[7]

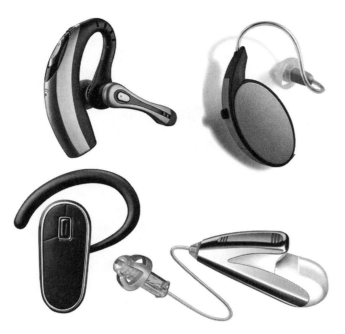

Figure 9.13. Can You Tell Which Are Hearing Aids and Which Are (Wireless) Bluetooth Headsets? (Answer: Upper and lower right are hearing aids; upper and lower left are headsets.) (Courtesy of Plantronics, Inc. [*upper left*], Bernafon, LLC [*upper right*], GN Netcom [*lower left*] and Phonak [*lower right*]).

Listeners with severe and profound hearing loss might need something more, but those with mild or moderate hearing loss might be able to use wireless headsets for the telephone, watching TV, and listening to music, *and* for customized (hearing aid) amplification. Just as some people wear sunglasses that are prescriptive, some people might wear wireless headsets that are prescriptive.[8] Hearing aids will be "hiding in plain sight," and the stigma attached to wearing them should disappear.[9] Perhaps wearing hearing technology is finally becoming fashionable!

Text Telephones

Text telephones are commonly known as *TTYs* (TeleTYpewriters). An older term is *Telecommunication Device for the Deaf* (TTD). This term has been replaced because text telephones are actually used by people with varying degrees of hearing loss. A TTY functions as a typewriter that can send and receive messages over telephone lines. A user types the message to be sent on a TTY keyboard; when a message is received, words print out across a screen or on paper (depending on the model). When both parties are

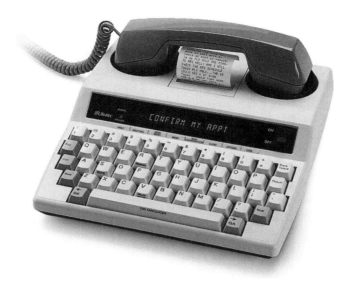

Figure 9.14. Example of a TTY with an Acoustic Connection and Printer (located under the handset). (Courtesy of Ultratec, Inc. and Harris Communications.)

using TTYs, conversations occur in text rather than voice. Many businesses and most government agencies have TTYs for communicating with their patrons who use them; look for a TTY number where the voice telephone number is listed.

There are two types of TTY connections: acoustic and direct. Some TTYs have rubber cups into which the handset of a landline telephone is placed to form an *acoustic* connection. In other cases, a TTY plugs into a phone jack to achieve a direct connection. A *direct* connection eliminates room noise and offers more features, but occasionally there are digital–analog compatibility issues that don't exist with an acoustic connection. Some models accommodate connections of both types.

Dozens of TTY models and feature combinations are available. Some models are designed to work with traditional, corded telephones; some can also be used with cordless phones and TTY-compatible cell phones. Other TTY models are stand-alone units meant to be used in place of a voice telephone.

Some models contain printers, text answering machines with personalized text greetings, and alerting devices to signal incoming calls. Some include a screening system that addresses incoming voice calls. The screener responds to a voice call with a voice message telling the caller that he has reached a TTY and explaining how to contact a Telecommunications Relay Service (see later discussion). Some models offer a 911 emergency dialer that sends a prerecorded voice message informing the operator that the caller has a hearing loss. Some models can accommodate Caller ID. Some are small, lightweight, and designed to be portable.

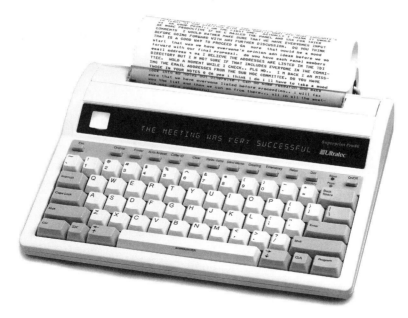

Figure 9.15. Example of TTY with a Direct Connection and Printer. (Courtesy of Ultratec, Inc. and Harris Communications.)

TTY–Computer Communication

Some TTYs (ASCII-equipped) can communicate with any computer; the computer needs no special hardware or software. Alternatively, by adding special software and a special modem, a computer can be modified to function as a TTY (and receive calls from other TTYs).

Telecommunications Relay Services

When both parties have text telephones, messages can be typed and read back and forth. When one party uses a TTY and the other uses a voice telephone, however, a Telecommunications Relay Service (TRS) is needed. Let's say that you're a TTY user and you want to order a pizza (or chat with a friend or call your babysitter). You contact a relay service by dialing 711 (nationwide) and type your message. The message is received by a Communication Assistant (CA) with access to both a voice telephone and a TTY. The CA dials your favorite pizza place and reads your message to the person who answers the phone (converting it from text to voice). The CA then types the pizza person's voice response (converting it from voice to text) and sends it to your TTY. The conversation continues with the CA converting text to voice and voice to text. The CA is required to repeat exactly what has been said or typed and must keep all conversations strictly confidential. Calls can be initiated by either the TTY or voice telephone user.

Title IV of the ADA requires all telephone companies to provide local and long-distance relay services (see Chapter 10). Service providers must make information about their relay services available to the public. The service must allow text telephone users to communicate with people anywhere in the United States at any time (24/7). There can be no restrictions on the number of calls made, the length of calls, or the nature of conversations. Services are free, although typical long-distance charges apply. If you need special equipment or computer modifications (discussed later), they may be free as well; check with your state's agency or commission for deaf and hard of hearing people.

Internet Protocol Relay Service

Internet protocol (IP) relay users connect to a CA using the Internet rather than a telephone. To initiate a call, the user goes to an IP relay center's website and types the number she wishes to reach. A CA dials the number and converts text to voice and voice to text. Because calls are made over the Internet (rather than telephone lines) all calls, even long-distance calls, are free. IP relay is available to anyone with Internet access from a computer or another Internet-enabled device. This eliminates the need to buy or access a TTY. For some, using a computer screen and keyboard is faster, easier, and more familiar than using a TTY.

Video Relay Service

Sign language users can use the Internet to connect to a video relay service. Users typically use a personal computer equipped with a web camera and video conferencing software. The relay center is staffed with sign language interpreters who translate sign language to voice and voice to sign language.

Voice Carry Over Relay Service

Voice carry over (VCO) is a relay option that allows callers to use their own voices to send messages, but to receive messages in writing from a relay service. This makes relay calls quicker and more natural, especially for users who've lost their hearing later in life and have speech that's easy to understand. A VCO call can be made to a person who's using a traditional voice telephone. In this case, the user speaks and the CA converts the other party's voice response to text that's displayed on the screen of the user's VCO phone. A call can also be made to a TTY user, in which case the VCO user speaks and the CA types the conversation for the TTY user. The TTY user types her response directly to the VCO user. A VCO user can also call another VCO user; in this instance, both parties speak and the CA types both sides of the conversation. Special types of VCO arrangements (requiring the user to have two telephone lines) allow the user to hear voice messages as well as read them, although the written message is delayed slightly relative to the voice message.

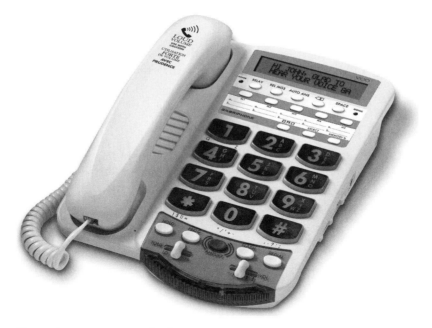

Figure 9.16. A VCO Telephone Allows the User to Communicate by Speaking and Reading. (Courtesy of Clarity, a Division of Plantronics, Inc).

Captioned Telephone Service

This service allows the user to both hear and read the other party's words on a special phone. Speech recognition software is used to create captions in real time. A captioner (at the captioning relay center) repeats what the other party says into a microphone, and speech recognition software converts it into text. Users can listen and read the captions simultaneously or refer to the captions only when clarification is needed.

Internet-based Captioned Telephone Service

More recently, Internet-based captioned telephone services have become available. In this case, a user can read captions on a web browser while listening to the caller's words on a telephone. No special equipment is needed, just a computer with Internet access and a phone (which may be a cell phone).

Telephones in Public Places

Pay telephones and emergency telephones are required to be HAC, which means they must work with telecoils. For people without telecoils, pay phones with amplification and pay TTYs may be available in places where conventional public telephones are provided (the number required varies with the type of facility). Signs indicating where amplified phones and TTYs can be found are required in public places (see Appendix C).

AUXILIARY AIDS AND SERVICES

The communication aids and services in this category include anything and everything that can make the spoken word accessible to persons with hearing loss. This includes some technologies that are used by people with normal hearing, such as Internet search engines, blogs, chat rooms, email, instant messaging, text messaging, and two-way paging, all of which make it possible to communicate and gather information without relying on hearing.

Captioning

Captions look like subtitles printed across the bottom of a television or movie screen. The first captioned television program was Julia Child's *The French Chef* in 1972. The popularity and demand for captions has been on the rise ever since. In the late 1990s, the Federal Communications Commission (FCC) developed a timetable that required the number of captioned television programs to increase over time. Today, virtually everything shown on television is captioned. DVDs for home viewing are captioned as well.

Captions primarily convey the speakers' words; however, they may also provide information about which speaker is talking and other sounds important for understanding the program, event, or news story. Most captions are prepared before a scripted program is broadcast and then synchronized with the audio and visual aspects of the program.

Unscripted events (live coverage of news events, for example) require real-time captioning. Real-time captioning requires special equipment, special software, and a real-time captioner (or trained court reporter) who can transcribe the speaker's message in virtual real time (with occasional errors). The reporter types phonetic codes on a special keyboard, and the software translates the codes into text. The need for special software and a skilled captioner makes real-time captioning considerably more expensive.

Closed captions cannot be seen without a decoder (as opposed to open captions which are visible at all times). The Television Decoder Circuitry Act of 1990 required that all televisions manufactured for sale in the United States after July 1993 contain built-in decoders (those with screens smaller than 13 inches diagonally were exempt). Captions can be viewed on older televisions using a separate decoder box. If you don't know how to access the built-in decoder function on your television, ask your television service provider or television retailer to show you.

In February 2009, television stations will begin broadcasting *only* digital signals. If you have a digital TV manufactured after 2002 (with a screen larger than 13 inches diagonally), you'll be able to see digital programming and digital captions without a converter box. Digital captions allow the viewer to control the caption display, including the font, text size, text color, and background. If you have an older, analog TV that uses rabbit ears or a roof top antenna, you'll need a digital-to-analog converter box to receive digital signals. The digital-to-analog converter box will enable you to see captions as well as digital programming. Some converter boxes can generate and display *digital* captions, so if you're buying a converter box, ask the retailer to show you one that's equipped to deliver digital captions. Newer technologies such as high-definition TV, TiVo, digital video recorders (DVRs), and direct satellite TV can sometimes make it difficult to use captions.[10] Questions about closed captioning problems can be sent by email to the Federal Communications Commission (see the Resources section for contact information).

Movie theaters are not required to provide captioned films. Although several formats for captioning currently exist, captioned films are almost never shown in movie theaters. This is unlikely to change in the near future, because motion picture screens are gradually being converted from analog to digital technology. Once the transition is complete, the challenge will be to develop technologies that allow captions to be viewed by movie-goers who are deaf or hard of hearing but that cannot be seen by other moviegoers.

Computer-assisted Real-time Transcription

Computer-assisted real-time transcription (CART) is like having a personal real-time captioner. A CART reporter instantly converts spoken words into text—verbatim. Similar to real-time captioning, it requires a trained court reporter, a special keyboard, a laptop computer, and special software to produce the text. The reporter listens to the speaker(s) and types what's being said on the keyboard using special codes. Software translates the codes into text. The text is displayed on the laptop computer or projected onto a screen for a larger audience. The text is saved and available for later review, and hard copies can be printed.

CART is particularly helpful in information-intensive situations like court proceedings or important meetings in which the user needs to receive every word, including complicated and unfamiliar terms. College students who are deaf or hard of hearing find CART especially helpful. The transcript appears on a computer screen in front of them so that they can follow a lecture (as well as the comments and questions of fellow students) in real time, and the saved transcript eliminates the need to take notes.

Because of the time, equipment, and skills required, CART services are expensive. Remote CART services, in which the reporter listens from another location and sends the transcript back to the user's computer (or other Internet-enabled device) in real time, are less expensive and becoming increasingly popular.

Computer-assisted Note-taking

Computer-assisted note-taking (CAN) is much less expensive than CART. It's useful when key words, an outline, or notes are enough to enable a person to follow a lecture or discussion. A typist with good note-taking skills types on a regular computer keyboard. The goal is to convey meaning rather than to type everything that's said verbatim. Some CAN typists use special abbreviation software to increase the amount of information they can provide. The typed notes can be read from a laptop computer or projected onto a screen for a larger audience. Like CART, CAN services can be provided from remote locations, which helps to defray the cost. The transcript is sent to the user's computer or Internet-enabled device. Special software allows the user to control the display and to interrupt the note-taker when clarification is needed.

Written Materials

Using written materials to supplement information that's presented orally is a simple, effective, low-cost way to assist people who are deaf or hard of hearing. Providing written materials minimizes the need to take notes, something that makes speechreading difficult, if not impossible. It also reduces the stress listeners experience when they fear that they'll miss something or hear it incorrectly. When you feel that having information in writing would be helpful, ask for it. Be assertive. Other accommodations are far more expensive and difficult to provide. And of course, using a pad and pencil (or word processor) to communicate is a tried-and-true tool.

Sign Language Translation and Sign Language Interpretation

American Sign Language (ASL) is a distinct language with its own syntax and grammar. In other words, ASL is *not* English that's signed. For listeners who have learned ASL, a sign language translator (more often called a *sign language interpreter*) can translate English into ASL and ASL into English. Most people who lose their hearing as adults do not learn ASL, however. Some of them might learn a form of manually coded English in which ASL signs are used in English word order. When this is the case, a sign language interpreter can provide a simultaneous, visual supplement to spoken communication.

Oral Interpretation

An oral interpreter sits close to the listener and speaks or mouths the words of a speaker who's too far away to be seen clearly. The user must have good speechreading skills to benefit.

ALERTING DEVICES

Alerting devices allow people with hearing loss to be independent and feel safe. They're particularly important for people who live alone. In general, they use flashing lights, strobes, vibration, fans, or very loud noises to substitute for conventional sound signals. The resources included at the end of this book can help you to find products that will address most alerting needs.

The simplest units include a sensor that monitors a single sound source (like a doorbell) and transmits a signal to a receiver that alerts the user. The user can choose how he wants to be alerted. Vibrating receivers can be worn close to the body (for example, around the neck, in a pocket, clipped to a belt, or as a wristwatch), placed under a pillow, or tucked between a mattress and box spring. Other types of receivers activate strobe lights or cause lamps to flash on and off. These receivers can be placed on a table, plugged into an outlet, or mounted on a wall or ceiling.

Larger, integrated systems allow several sounds around the house to be monitored by the same unit. The user chooses what she wishes to monitor (front door, back door, telephone, smoke detector, baby's room, etc.) and the type of alert she wishes to receive. Each sensor has its own code so that the user knows whether someone is ringing the front doorbell or knocking at the back door. This information can be conveyed in a number of different ways, from variations in the pattern of light flashes to message screens and coded light panels.

Dozens of alerting devices are available. The following are examples of the types of sounds that can be monitored and conveyed through light, vibration, or very loud noises.

- Smoke alarm
- Carbon monoxide alarm
- Home intruder
- Doorbell
- Intercom/door buzzer
- Telephone ringer
- Knock at the door (and sometimes a touch on the door knob)

- Baby's cry
- Alarm clock
- Timers and signals on appliances
- Automobile turn signals

A recent research study showed that the typical sound signal used by conventional smoke alarms (a 3,100-Hz tone) failed to wake many people with hearing loss, even though they could hear that particular signal when they were awake.[11] Although strobe lights were useful for alerting people who were awake, they also failed to wake many people. The signal found to be most effective was a 520-Hz square wave, a signal that contains a range of frequency components starting at approximately 500 Hz (remember, low-frequency signals tend to be easiest to hear). Bed and pillow shakers were also highly effective but still less effective than the 520-Hz square wave. Unfortunately, few emergency products with low-frequency signals are available at the present time. Nonetheless, when looking for smoke alarms, carbon monoxide alarms, and other emergency equipment, be sure to look for products with low-frequency alerting signals. Until those products are readily available, bed and pillow shakers are a better choice than conventional alarms.

Some alerting units are portable and work well for travel. In addition, hotels and motels are required by the ADA to provide alerting devices on request. Some offer kits to their visitors who are hard of hearing or deaf. The kit may include a TTY, a telephone signaler, a telephone amplifier, a door knock signaler, a visual/audio smoke detector, and/or a wake-up system (like a bed shaker).

HEARING SERVICE DOGS

Hearing service dogs are specially trained to assist their deaf or hard of hearing companions by alerting them to sounds they cannot hear. These sounds might include the sound of a smoke detector, doorbell, crying baby, knock at the door, telephone, alarm clock, timing device, or intruder in the house. Hearing dogs can also let a companion know when her name is being called or an object drops to the floor. Most hearing dogs make physical contact with their companions and then lead them to the source of the sound. The friendship, sense of security, and increased independence that hearing dogs provide is especially helpful to people who live alone. Some agencies provide hearing dogs free of charge.

My Dad

One evening my mother went out to play bridge and forgot her house key. When she came home, she rang the doorbell, but my dad was watching TV and didn't hear it. She went to a neighbor's house and called him, but he didn't hear the telephone ring either. When she rapped on a window in the room where he was sitting, he didn't *hear* her, but he saw her. Looks like it's time for an alerting device.

CHAPTER 10

Take Charge: Don't Let Hearing Problems Get the Best of You

Listening is not merely not talking . . . it means taking a vigorous human interest in what is being told to us.

A. D. Miller

The preceding chapters have addressed technical solutions for hearing loss: hearing aids, cochlear implants, and hearing assistance technology. As we begin this chapter, remember that the goal is to minimize the impact of your hearing loss and maximize the quality of your life. In that effort, hearing technology is a tremendous tool—it can dramatically improve your ability to *hear* sound. But we *understand* sound with our brains, not with our ears, so technology can't be the entire solution. In other words, technology is necessary, but it might not be sufficient. The missing piece is hearing rehabilitation, the subject of this chapter. Although people with milder degrees of hearing loss may not *require* a hearing rehabilitation program, nearly everyone can benefit from one.

HEARING REHABILITATION

If your audiologist has told you that hearing aids can help, trying them is *the* essential first step. If you can't *hear* speech, then you have no hope of understanding it. Simply buying hearing aids doesn't ensure an improved quality of life, however. To achieve that goal, you have to take full advantage of your hearing aids and develop strategies that complement aided hearing. And that's the purpose of hearing rehabilitation. Hearing rehabilitation is a collection of services designed to help you use hearing technology to its greatest advantage, develop skills that can maximize your ability to communicate, and learn how to cope with hearing loss. Hearing aids are just one part of the larger hearing rehabilitation process. To avoid confusion, hearing rehabilitation is the same as *aural rehabilitation* (aural rehab), and *audiologic rehabilitation*.

Virtually all audiologists provide an orientation as part of a hearing aid fitting. All too often, however, this is where hearing rehabilitation ends, when it's really where it should begin. Think about it. If you were getting a prosthetic device like an artificial leg, you wouldn't expect to put it on, receive instructions, and then start using it all day long. You'd expect to receive physical therapy and counseling over a series of sessions. In short, you'd expect a rehabilitation program. After spending what seems like a small fortune on hearing aids, people are often disappointed to learn that a commitment to rehabilitation is necessary for optimal success. But a hearing aid is a very sophisticated prosthetic device. Like a prosthetic limb, it shouldn't be something you simply start wearing and hope for the best. Learning to use it effectively requires guidance, practice, and support.

Ideally, hearing rehabilitation occurs in a structured program that's broad in its approach, combining information about hearing aids with information about a wider range of topics. This information can be presented in individual sessions, group sessions, or a combination of the two. Group sessions offer extra benefits, because they allow participants to share wisdom and support one another. More experienced participants provide encouragement to newer participants as they become accustomed to living with hearing loss and wearing hearing aids. Group interactions also provide ready-made opportunities to practice the communication strategies that are discussed as part of the program.

Whenever possible, spouses and significant others also should participate in the hearing rehabilitation program. Communication is a two-way street; *you* need to learn what you can do to improve communication, and significant others need to learn what *they* can do. Working together makes you allies as you address hearing-related issues. In a group program, family members gain insight into what it's like to have a hearing loss. At the same time, you can gain insight into what it's like to *live with* someone who has a hearing loss. Hearing rehabilitation groups can be sources of much-needed support for better-hearing spouses and family members.

A hearing rehabilitation program—whether it's structured or unstructured; short-term or long-term; carried out in individual sessions, group sessions, or both—should address the communication difficulties that *you* experience at home, work, and play. Finding solutions to these problems should be the program's ultimate goal and the measure of its success. Possible solutions should be developed, practiced, tweaked, practiced again, and then generalized to other situations.

Although the benefits of participating in a hearing rehabilitation program are clear, too few audiologists offer programs that go beyond informal hearing aid orientation and instruction. The reasons for this gap in hearing health care involve time, money, and a lack of awareness on the part of many consumers. If each person who reads this book were to request a hearing rehabilitation program, it's likely that more services would become available.

Before deciding on the audiologist from whom you'll buy hearing aids, ask about the hearing rehabilitation services he offers. If you have a choice, choose the one who offers a structured program or the most extensive services. If you choose an audiologist who doesn't provide hearing rehabilitation services, ask her to help you find them elsewhere. Remember, the job of an audiologist isn't selling hearing aids, it's helping people and families cope with hearing loss—and hearing aids are only part of that picture. If it's impossible to find a hearing rehabilitation program close to you, this book is a good substitute. Another alternative might be to use an interactive, computer-based program at home (see discussion later).

The lack of emphasis on hearing rehabilitation is a primary reason why many people who buy hearing aids end up feeling disappointed and disillusioned. Often, it's the hearing aids that get blamed and retired to a dresser drawer. Users often don't realize that in addition to buying hearing aids (and learning to use them) they must learn new habits and practice using new strategies that supplement aided hearing.

HEARING REHABILITATION SERVICES

Hearing rehabilitation should really begin at the time of your initial hearing evaluation. That first appointment should include a discussion about the problems you experience and what you hope to accomplish. You (and perhaps your spouse) might be asked to complete self-assessment questionnaires (see Chapter 4) that can help to guide the rehabilitation process and document your progress. Your audiologist should explain the results of your hearing test and, when applicable, your amplification and rehabilitation options (see Chapter 4). The cost of rehabilitative services should be part of the discussion. In some settings, this cost is included in the price of new hearing aids; if that's the case, be sure to ask how many sessions and which services are included in the package. In other settings, the cost is separate. In this case, there may be a flat fee for a multisession program, or you might be charged for each session that you attend. Like hearing aids, rehabilitation services tend not to be covered by insurance; however, many facilities offer a sliding fee scale based on the ability to pay.

The remainder of this chapter is divided into the following sections: hearing rehabilitation services directly related to hearing aids, rehabilitation services beyond hearing aids, support/advocacy groups, and your rights under the Americans with Disabilities Act of 1990. The next two major sections—services related to and beyond hearing aids—describe a menu of services from which your personal hearing rehabilitation program should be created.

HEARING REHABILITATION SERVICES DIRECTLY RELATED TO HEARING AIDS

Developing Realistic Expectations

As noted in Chapter 7, hearing aids have become extremely sophisticated in recent years. They process sounds in ways that could only be imagined a decade ago. Even so, the amplification that they provide won't make you hear normally again. Having realistic expectations—or understanding what hearing aids can and cannot do—is critical to your success as a user.

What are some of the things hearing aids *can* do? In favorable listening conditions, they can make sounds loud enough for you to hear them; in other words, they can give you *access* to the sounds you want to hear. In more difficult conditions (for example, when you're some distance from the speaker or there are multiple conversations in the room), they're less effective. Even in those conditions, however, you can expect to hear better with hearing aids than without them. Even when it's very noisy and you're missing a lot, the additional information provided by hearing aids can make filling in the gaps easier. You should expect to hear *better* (but not perfectly) in nearly all situations. What else can you expect? Expect hearing aids to make listening less exhausting and less stressful. Expect to feel less tired at the end of the day. In general, expect hearing aids to make you feel more connected to your surroundings, more independent, more confident, and more at ease. In a nutshell, hearing aids are the single best way to maximize the hearing that you have.

What are some of the things hearing aids *cannot* do? First, they can't make sounds (like speech) perfectly clear if there's distortion in your auditory system. Depending on the nature of your hearing problem (see Chapter 4), you may be unable to understand everything you hear even with the most advanced hearing aids—but that beats the alternative. You definitely can't understand what you do not hear. Second, unlike young, healthy ears, hearing aids can't focus exclusively on what you want to hear and make everything else fade into the background. High-tech hearing aid features help, but hearing in noisy conditions is more difficult (and less pleasant) than hearing in quiet. Finally, hearing aids tend not to be helpful when you are distant from the speaker. Hearing aid microphones can only pick up sounds within a 6- to 12-foot radius. That means you probably won't be able to carry on a conversation with someone across the room or in another room, and therefore there will be situations in which you miss things. But this doesn't mean that all is lost! It simply means that you need to use other strategies to supplement aided hearing. Using those strategies *and* your hearing aids, you should be able to understand *most* of what *most* people say *most* of the time.

Trying Hearing Aids

Your audiologist will talk with you about "test driving" hearing aids on a trial basis. The trial period should be at least 30 days. During that time, the audiologist can check the fit of the hearing aids (or earmolds) in your ears and fine tune the hearing aid settings based on your feedback. At the end of the trial period, you can buy the hearing aids, opt to start a new trial with different hearing aids, or return the hearing aids and get most of your money back. There will be some nonrefundable costs (for hearing testing and taking impressions of your ears, for example). Be sure to ask for the details of all exchange and return policies in writing at the beginning of the trial period. See Chapter 7 for additional information about a trial period with hearing aids.

Trying Hearing Aids

Be sure to ask your audiologist for *written* information about:

- The length of the trial period (it should be a minimum of 30 days)
- Policies related to the hearing aid trial (for example, what happens if an aid is lost, damaged, or stolen during the trial period)
- Policies for the exchange or return of hearing aids at the end of the trial period
- Nonrefundable costs if you opt *not* to buy hearing aids at the end of the trial period (these should not exceed 10 to 15 percent of the total cost)
- The hearing aid warranty
- Buying insurance for hearing aids

Operating Your New Hearing Aids

Buying hearing aids is a substantial investment, and you need to get the "biggest bang for your buck." That requires learning everything you can about the operation of your new hearing aids. For example, if they have user-controlled features, you'll need to practice adjusting them as listening conditions change. There's no sense paying for special features if you don't know how to use them when you need them.

Operating Your Hearing Aids

After the hearing aid orientation, you should be able to

- Identify the components (or parts) of your hearing aids.
- Tell the right hearing aid from the left.
- Put your hearing aids (or earmolds) in your ears and take them out, something that often requires practice. Because it's difficult to see what you're doing, it can be helpful to take someone with you who can watch and help you at home. An earmold or custom hearing aid that's been properly inserted should fit flush with the side of your face; someone standing directly in front of you should see nothing sticking out. If inserting your hearing aids/earmolds continues to be difficult for you, ask your audiologist for help. (Although hearing aids/earmolds will slide into your ears more easily when they're slippery, resist the temptation to put them in your mouth! They're likely to be covered with bacteria and other microorganisms that can be dangerous if ingested.)
- Operate the on/off switches, if your hearing aids have them. Turn the aids off (or the volume all the way down) while putting them in your ears to prevent feedback, and do the same while removing them. Hearing aids will produce feedback when being handled.
- Adjust the volume, if your hearing aids have manual volume controls (typically, rotating the volume control wheel forward or upward means more volume and rotating it backward or downward means less).
- Change programs to accommodate the listening conditions, if your hearing aids have multiple program options that are manually controlled.
- Operate any other special features that are manually controlled (for example, telecoils, direct audio input [DAI], or directional microphones).
- Use your hearing aids on the telephone.
- Determine when it's time to replace the batteries. Your audiologist can give you a rough idea about the battery life that you should expect, but battery life depends on many factors. If you want to be able to predict when you'll need to change batteries, mark your calendar each time you make the switch (some people put the sticky tab from the battery on their calendar), and watch for a pattern to emerge. Some hearing aids will signal their user when a battery is approaching the end of its life. To test a battery informally, cup your hands around the hearing aid; you should hear feedback. Alternatively, ask your audiologist about a buying a small, inexpensive battery tester.
- Remove the old battery and put in a new one. Always carry spare batteries with you. You'll need to use the correct size (your audiologist will tell you which size to buy). Insert batteries carefully. Every battery has a plus (+) side and a minus (−) side. Generally, the plus (+) side goes up when you place the battery in your hearing aid's battery compartment. Don't open the battery compartment door too far or force it closed because they break easily. If the door won't close, the battery is probably the wrong size or it's been inserted upside down.
- See Appendix A for more information on batteries.

Caring for Your Hearing Aids

Your audiologist will show you how to care for your new hearing aids and how to troubleshoot when problems arise. Daily maintenance can prolong their life (well-maintained hearing aids should last 5 to 7 years). Inexpensive tools can make caring for hearing aids easier and more efficient (for example, a wax removal tool, a battery tester, a dehumidifying kit to remove moisture from the hearing aids). Your audiologist may offer some of these tools; if not, she should be able to tell you where you can buy them.

Hearing Aid Care and Maintenance

Regular care and maintenance keeps your hearing aids working at their best. The better you care for your hearing aids, the longer they will last.

- Always store hearing aids in a safe place, preferably a hearing aid drying kit (see later discussion). They'll be protected, and you'll always know where they are.
- Dogs are attracted by the high-pitched whistling of hearing aids and their owner's scent; hearing aids and earmolds left unprotected often get chewed by man's (and woman's) best friend.
- Hearing aids must be handled carefully. Be sure your hands are clean and dry before touching them. Dropping them or applying too much pressure can break their cases and damage their internal circuitry. It's a good idea to put them in, take them out, clean them, and change batteries over a light-colored towel placed on a flat surface (such as a bed or desk).
- Always keep your hearing aids dry. Moisture from perspiration, humidity, rain, snow, or water of any kind can result in expensive repairs. For this reason, don't store hearing aids in the bathroom. If your hearing aids do get wet, put them in a drying (dehumidifying) kit. See Appendix B for more information about such kits. Never attempt to dry your hearing aids using a hair dryer, oven, microwave, or clothes dryer, because heat is also damaging.
- More than 75% of all hearing aid repairs are caused by earwax, dirt, body oil, or moisture accumulating in the hearing aid (or earmold tubing). Nearly all repairs of this type can be prevented with good maintenance, which means cleaning your hearing aids every time they're removed and storing them in a drying kit. Appendix D provides information about cleaning BTE and custom (that is, ITE, ITC, CIC) hearing aids.
- Extreme temperatures can damage hearing aids. Avoid leaving them in direct sunlight, in a closed car, or near a heating or air conditioning unit. Don't wear your hearing aids while drying your hair with a hair dryer.
- Avoid getting hair products on your hearing aids.

- When hearing aids are not in use, remove the batteries. Leave the battery compartment doors open to allow moisture that might have collected in the hearing aids throughout the day to dry. Removing batteries (or at least opening the battery compartment doors) also prevents battery drain while the aids are not in use. With the battery compartment doors closed, batteries continue to drain even with the hearing aids turned off.
- Never leave a dead battery in a hearing aid, because it could leak and cause damage.
- If your hearing aids are not working properly, troubleshooting before consulting your audiologist could save you time and money. See Appendix E for information about troubleshooting hearing aid problems.
- Consider having your hearing aids cleaned professionally at least once a year.

Adjusting to New Hearing Aids

With the proper guidance, hearing aids should become increasingly helpful as you get used to wearing them; achieving maximal improvement can take several months. Initially, you might be surprised by all the sounds you hear—in fact, you might be *shocked* by all the sounds you hear. Welcome back to the world of sound! Unless your hearing loss was sudden, you gradually became less aware of the sounds around you: everyday things like the rustle of newspaper pages being turned, the clatter of silverware on dishes, the sound of running water. Suddenly, you have hearing aids, and you hear *everything*. "Background" sounds that you had all but forgotten might seem loud—your own voice might sound strange. Take heart; adjustments can be made to the hearing aids, and most people *do* adapt. But it takes some time.

Brains are said to be *plastic*; that is, able to be modified. Plasticity means that a brain can reorganize itself to enable new learning, recover from a brain injury (for example, a mild stroke), or adjust to new input (for example, hearing through electronic devices). If you think that young brains are more plastic than older ones, you're right—but even older brains show remarkable ability to adapt and reorganize. You really *can* teach an old dog new tricks. Research in neuroscience has shown that when the brain receives less input from the auditory system (or from a finger, a foot, an eye, on another area of the body), some of the resources normally devoted to processing that input get reassigned to other functions. Your brain needs time to reorganize when input from the ears is restored. If you're a first-time hearing aid user (or even an experienced user trying new hearing aids), your audiologist might suggest a schedule that allows you to adjust without becoming overwhelmed. Usually this means gradually increasing the length of time that you wear the aids each day and the difficulty of the situations in which you wear them.

People who wear their hearing aids daily get the most out of them. Wearing hearing aids only on special occasions makes it unlikely that you'll know how to operate them to your best advantage. More important, it means that your brain won't have had a chance to adapt to the new type of input. You'll be more successful if listening through hearing aids has become routine for you.

People often think that wearing new hearing aids in challenging situations (like a cocktail party or a noisy restaurant) is the best way to test them during their trial period. That's like saying that the best way to test a new artificial leg is to run a marathon. Neither is a good test. Avoid the most difficult situations until you've had some time to practice and adjust.

Suggestions for Adjusting to New Hearing Aids

- Wear your new hearing aids only as long as they are comfortable the first day. Try wearing them a little longer the next day. Take breaks whenever you feel tired. Aim for a total of 6 to 8 hours a day by the end of the first week. The hours don't have to be consecutive; for example, you might try 1 hour with the aids in and 1 hour with the aids out initially, then 2 hours with the aids in and 1 hour with them out, and so on. Wear your hearing aids in quiet situations at home and when interacting with people who are familiar to you.
- Have a friend or family member read to you so you can practice adjusting the manual controls (if you have them). While you're listening, practice combining what you see on the speaker's face with what you hear.
- Read aloud to yourself each day to get your auditory system and brain working together.[1] Reading aloud allows you to practice hearing sounds through your new hearing aids without having to pay attention to the content of what you hear.
- Pay attention to sounds in the background; once you recognize them, it will be easier to ignore them (just as people with normal hearing do).
- During the second week, try wearing the hearing aids for longer periods (aim for at least 3 hours at a time). Wear them at home and in social situations that are neither too noisy nor too stressful. Practice using the telephone. Dial someone you know or a recording (like weather or time). Practice using your telecoil (if you have one); experiment until you find the right place to put the telephone handset.
- During the third week, try wearing your hearing aids for longer periods (aim for at least 6 hours at a time). Try wearing them in more challenging situations (for example, during a worship service, at a friend's home, or in a quiet restaurant).
- During the fourth week, try wearing your hearing aids all day in all situations. If you feel tired or upset, don't hesitate to take them off and rest. Practice understanding conversations (or someone reading to you) in background noise (you can use the television or radio to create noise). In

challenging situations, practice making adjustments if they're available to you (for example, change your listening program or the volume).

- If you experience discomfort or something doesn't sound right, contact your audiologist right away. The problem might be simple and easily fixed.
- Don't get discouraged; remember, the brain needs time to adjust to hearing sounds in a new way. It won't happen overnight but *with practice* it will happen, and it will happen more quickly if you wear your hearing aids at least part of every day.

HEARING REHABILITATION SERVICES BEYOND HEARING AIDS

The previous section discussed hearing rehabilitation services directly related to hearing aids. This section discusses rehabilitation services that go *beyond* hearing aids. Together, the two sections describe a menu of services from which your personal hearing rehabilitation program should be created. Services included in this section fall into two major categories: learning about a variety of hearing-related topics and practicing strategies that complement aided hearing.

Learning about Hearing and Hearing Loss

It stands to reason that you'll be better at finding solutions to your hearing problems if you know something about hearing and hearing loss. A structured hearing rehabilitation program is likely to cover information about normal hearing, hearing disorders, and the effects of hearing loss. This information can also be found in Chapters 2, 3, 5, and 6 of this book.

Learning How Your Hearing Loss Affects Communication

Different types, degrees, and configurations of hearing loss cause very different problems (see Chapter 4). Most people don't understand how their hearing loss affects their ability to understand speech or to hear other sounds in the environment. Because they're unaware of the difficulties they're likely to encounter in various communication situations, they can't prepare for them. Your audiologist can answer questions about the problems you're likely to experience as a result of your particular hearing loss. For example, if you have a bilateral, high-frequency, sensorineural hearing loss, you probably will have difficulty understanding young children.

Learning about Hearing Assistance Technology (HAT)

For situations in which hearing aids fall short, hearing assistance technology may be the answer. For example, you might find an assistive listening device helpful when you're communicating over the telephone, watching television, or traveling in the car. You might find it helpful to use an assistive listening system when attending meetings, movies, concerts, lectures, or religious services. In the workplace, you might use an amplified telephone, a vibrating pager, or a personal FM system with a conference microphone.

Alerting devices typically substitute flashing lights or vibration for a sound signal (for example, a lamp that flashes when the telephone rings). These devices can increase safety and solve many of the problems experienced by people with hearing loss, especially those who live alone. They can be useful in the home, at work, or during travel.

With or without hearing aids, assistive technology can help you to participate more fully in every aspect of your life. Ask your audiologist if there are devices that might solve your particular problems. Information about assistive listening technology is the subject of Chapter 9.

Learning to Make Adjustments to Your Surroundings

Controlling the listening environment, to the extent possible, is an extremely important strategy. For example, at home you should

- Make rooms as quiet as possible (for example, install carpeting and hang draperies). When you're trying to communicate, minimize background noise (for example, turn off running water, the television, or the washing machine). When eliminating noise is impossible, move your conversation away from it.
- Arrange your furniture so that communication can be close and face to face (for example, if you and your spouse have favorite chairs, draw them together and position them so that you can see one another's faces).
- Be sure the lighting is good; you'll understand better if you can see the speaker's face clearly (for example, arrange seating so that the light shines on your spouse's face).
- Arrange seating so your better ear (if you have one) is pointed toward the conversation (for example, be sure that your spouse sits on the side closest to your better ear).
- Position your favorite chair so that you can see people entering the room.
- If you have directional microphones on your hearing aids, position yourself so the background noise is behind you. For example, at the kitchen table sit with the dishwasher behind you rather than in front of you.
- Install assistive listening technology that allows you to hear the television or use the telephone.

Learning to Make Use of Visual, Contextual, and Linguistic Cues

There will be situations in which the conversation you hear through your hearing aids is incomplete because of poor listening conditions, the distortion caused by your hearing loss, the imperfect fidelity of hearing aids, or some combination of those factors. In these situations, you must apply yourself and use *all* the cues that are available to supplement aided hearing.

- Visual cues are available through lip reading, facial expressions, body language, and gestures. Combining these cues to understand speech is called *speechreading* (discussed later).
- Contextual cues are related to the situation and the people involved in it; for example, someone at a potluck dinner is more likely to be talking about *baking a cake* than *raking a fake*. To demonstrate, ask someone to say any five words without using their voice. Without context, you probably won't be able to speechread all five words correctly. Now ask them to say the names of five numbers (or colors, or fruits). The task will be easier because the words have some context.
- Linguistic cues are the duplicate and overlapping cues embedded in our language that give speech messages some predictability. For instance, the sentence, "The girls are taking their lunches to school" includes several cues about plurality (*girls, are, their,* and *lunches*). If you miss one cue, there's a chance you'll get one or more of the others; in other words, you can afford to miss some information and still understand that there's more than one girl. And knowing that makes understanding the rest of the message easier.

For someone with hearing loss, listening must be active rather than passive. The successful listener learns to use all available cues to fill in what's missed through hearing. A hearing rehabilitation group is the perfect place to practice combining various types of cues.

Speechreading

Speechreading combines lip reading (the use of cues that come from watching the speaker's mouth) with those that come from facial expressions, gestures, and body language. We all rely on speechreading, especially when hearing is difficult. The more challenging the listening situation, the harder we work to see the speaker's face. Experts estimate that combining vision with hearing improves speech understanding by 30 percent or more in difficult listening situations. We've all developed some degree of speechreading skill, although some of us have more talent for it than others.

Speechreading *complements* aided hearing. For example, even people with very limited hearing report that wearing hearing aids improves their ability to speechread. Combining what they hear (even if it's only the rhythm of speech) with what they see improves their ability to understand. Some severely hard of hearing and deaf people successfully rely on speechreading and aided hearing for communication. However, as important as speechreading is to listeners with hearing loss, it can't substitute for hearing. In fact, only 30 to 40 percent of the speech signal can be understood through speechreading *alone*. There are several reasons for this:

- First, 60 to 70 percent of English speech sounds can't be seen on the lips; for example, the production of /h/, /k/, and /r/ are not visible.
- Second, among the sounds that *can* be seen, many look alike (for example, /f/ looks like /v/ and /t/ looks like /d/). As a result, approximately half of all English words look like one or more other words (for example, the words "man," "pan," and "ban" can't be distinguished visually).
- Third, the way sounds are formed depends on which sounds precede and follow them.
- Fourth, unless there's a visible pause between words (which rarely happens), sounds run together and become one long, uninterrupted series of lip movements.

Some speakers make speechreading even more challenging. For example, speakers sometimes talk with their mouths obscured: they put their hands in front of their faces, they talk while chewing or smoking, or they talk with their faces turned away. In some situations the lighting is poor, or the speaker is too far away to be seen clearly. There are also people who barely move their mouths when they talk.

In years past, speechreading drill and practice was a primary focus of hearing rehabilitation programs. Today, it's more likely to be part of a broader program designed to enhance overall communication, maximize the benefits of hearing aids, and promote personal and family adjustment to hearing loss. Practicing speechreading during conversations that occur naturally in group hearing rehabilitation sessions is more effective than doing speechreading exercises in isolation. See Appendix F for speechreading tips.

My Dad

People who can't hear well depend especially on their eyesight, and people who can't see well depend especially on their hearing. Unfortunately, my dad has trouble with both. He suffers from macular degeneration, a condition that's taking away his vision. He misses the critically important speechreading cues that most people use to help them understand speech. With poor vision and only one usable ear, it's hard for him to determine where sounds are coming from or who's talking in a group. Because he has difficulty recognizing faces, he has to rely on hearing to recognize voices (but, of course, he has trouble hearing voices too). It's amazing to me that he remains so engaged, so fun, and so cheerful, given his double disability. Anybody in his little town will tell you that if you ask him how he is, he *always* says, "Terrific!" with a big smile. He's my hero.

Auditory Training

Hearing aids enable people to hear (detect) softer sounds, but they don't necessarily make them better listeners. Unlike *hearing*, listening requires effort and concentration. It's focused and deliberate. Auditory training is formal listening training. Along with speechreading, it was once a primary focus of hearing rehabilitation programs. In more recent years, both have been integrated into broader programs designed to improve communication in real-life situations. New insights based on research in neuroscience have renewed interest in auditory training, however. We've learned that when input from the ears to the brain is reduced by hearing loss, areas of the brain devoted to certain hearing functions get reassigned (as mentioned earlier, this is known as brain *plasticity*). We've also learned that with properly structured practice, brain resources can be reclaimed for functions important to listening and communication. Properly structured practice involves short, frequent training sessions rather than longer, less-frequent ones; active listener participation, as opposed to passive learning (tasks must be interactive); immediate feedback about the accuracy of a listener's responses; and a level of difficulty that "adapts" to keep the listener challenged yet motivated.

Participating in a concentrated (daily), adaptive auditory training program with an audiologist tends to be inconvenient and costly. In contrast, a home-based, interactive computer program enables listeners to do intensive training at their own pace and in the comfort of their own homes. An example of such a program is Listening and Communication Enhancement (LACE).[2] More information about LACE can be found in Appendix G. Your audiologist can assist you in selecting the most appropriate program, setting it up, establishing personal goals, and monitoring progress.

Learning New Strategies for Communication

As mentioned, the focus of hearing rehabilitation programs has shifted from an emphasis on speechreading and auditory training lessons to an emphasis on building confidence and improving communication in a variety of situations. This has been called *communication strategies training*.[3]

All such strategies fundamentally begin with taking responsibility for your hearing difficulty. People are likely to be more helpful if they know that you have a hearing loss than if they believe you're not paying attention. Telling people about your hearing problem also gives you an opportunity to provide specific suggestions about what they can do to help you understand (for example, *"Please speak more slowly; Don't cover your mouth; Face me; Use shorter sentences; Tell me when the topic changes."*). Of course, that means knowing enough about your hearing loss to be able to tell others what would be helpful. It also means reminding people (more than once) about what you need—something that might feel uncomfortable. Communication habits are deeply ingrained, and people easily lapse back into old patterns until new ones have been learned.

Participants also learn how to repair communication when it breaks down. Most often, when a person hasn't understood, she says, "*What?*" or "*Huh?*" This is usually understood as a request for repetition, and the response is often exactly that—the speaker repeats the message word for word. Whichever word(s) or phrase(s) the listener didn't understand the first time, she probably won't understand the second or third time either. It's the least effective repair strategy but the one most commonly used. A better strategy is to ask the speaker to say the message differently: to rephrase it, elaborate on it, or simplify it. Another effective strategy is for the listener to use the information he *did* understand to get the information he missed (for example, "*Your sister lives in* which *city?*"). This allows the listener to confirm the part of the message he heard and clarify the part he didn't. Requests for repetition that are less open ended make it more likely that the listener will understand quickly, minimizing disruption to the conversation. For example, asking "Did you say_____?" usually works better than asking, "What did you say?" In other cases, the best strategy may be to ask for a key word, especially when the topic changes (for example, "*Tell me what you're talking about*"). When all else fails, it may be necessary to ask the speaker to write part of a message. A hearing rehabilitation group is the perfect place for participants to develop new strategies and practice using them with one another.

Learning to deal effectively with communication problems discourages participants from resorting to negative coping behaviors like bluffing (pretending to hear when you don't), dominating the conversation (as long as you have the floor, there's no need to understand anyone else), blaming (you'd hear fine if everyone would just quit mumbling), and social withdrawal.

Conversational Styles

A primary goal of communication strategies training is to help listeners become assertive communicators.[4]

- The *passive communicator* avoids conversations, pretends to hear when he doesn't, or is overly dependent on others. The passive communicator would rather miss out than acknowledge the problem and ask for help.
- The *aggressive communicator* is belligerent or blames others for her communication difficulty. She might dominate the conversation or insist on hearing everything.

- The *assertive communicator* shows respect for the rights of conversational partners while honestly and openly expressing his own needs. He takes responsibility for managing communication problems in a considerate way, which might mean reminding people (more than once) about what he needs if he is to understand them.

A hearing rehabilitation group is a good place to practice *assertive* communication behavior.

Assertive Communication
Assertive communication means:

- Standing up for yourself without being insensitive or disrespectful to others.
- Taking responsibility by acknowledging your hearing loss.
- Not blaming others when they unintentionally make communication difficult for you.
- Telling people how they can help you to understand them.
- Being willing to remind people about what you need (again and again).
- Showing conversational partners appreciation for their efforts.
- Making adjustments to your surroundings (for example, rearranging the seating in a meeting room).
- Responding to problems with a sense of humor.

Personal Adjustment Counseling

The average person waits 7 years before seeking help for hearing loss. During those years, feelings of anger, resentment, isolation, vulnerability, loneliness, or depression can develop. Some people begin using inappropriate coping behaviors like bluffing, blaming others, withdrawing, or monopolizing conversations. Important relationships (within the family and beyond it) can be damaged. Even when the hearing loss is finally addressed, problems like these aren't resolved overnight. When negative feelings and damaged relationships affect a person's self-concept and feelings of self-worth, it can be more harmful than the hearing loss itself. It can be helpful to talk with an audiologist or professional counselor who understands the social, emotional, and psychological ramifications of hearing loss.

Most people lose their hearing gradually; however, people who lose their hearing suddenly are particularly vulnerable to adjustment problems. The abrupt transition from "hearing person" to "deaf person" can set off an emotional crisis. If the services of a professional counselor are needed, an audiologist may know of someone with an understanding of hearing loss.

Counseling Family Members about Your Hearing Loss

Hearing loss never affects just one family member; it affects *all* family members. Rehabilitation is therefore most successful when family members (or other significant others) are also involved. Family members can begin by learning what it's like to have a hearing loss. Your audiologist should be able to demonstrate this with a recorded simulation.

Equally important, family members (particularly spouses) often need support themselves. Everyday conversations with you now require special effort. You might be less interested in socializing than you once were. Communication might make you feel tired and irritable. Better-hearing husbands and wives tend to feel more regret about these changes than their partners with hearing loss. A part of hearing rehabilitation is recognizing when you or your significant others are experiencing feelings of sadness, resentment, or frustration, and exploring ways to resolve them.

People who are important in your life need to learn how to improve their communication with you. Research has shown that speech understanding improves when a communication partner is asked to speak more clearly, and it improves even more when she is formally trained to use "clear speech." An example of the difference between typical speech and clear speech is the difference between "Thekids'r swim'n inthepool" and "The kids [pause] are swimming [pause] in the pool."[5] In a recent study, people with sensorineural hearing loss listened to a speaker who had been trained to use clear speech and a second speaker who had been asked to speak more clearly. Speech understanding improved in both cases. When listening to the speaker who had been *trained*, however, listeners recognized sentences in background noise as well as listeners with normal hearing (that is, scores approached 100 percent). And this was after the talker had received less than 1 hour of training! These results suggest that communication can be dramatically improved when family members are provided with clear speech training (as opposed to simply receiving written or verbal instructions).[6]

Clear Speech
Clear speech is characterized by

- Slowed speaking rate
- More pauses
- Longer pauses
- Precise (but not exaggerated) enunciation
- Emphasis on key words

Learning about Sign Language

People who become deaf sometimes hope that learning to use American Sign Language (ASL) will be the solution to their communication problems. Initially, they may not consider that learning another language is helpful only if the people with whom they want to communicate are willing to learn it too. And often they don't realize that learning ASL is like learning any other foreign language—a big undertaking. Learning to fingerspell and learning some useful signs that can be used in English word order is a great idea, however. Couples (and other family members) can use signs and fingerspelling to communicate when they're in public places, during the night when hearing aids aren't being worn, or in emergency situations.

Learning to Monitor Your Voice Level

People with sensorineural hearing loss often have difficulty monitoring the volume of their voices. The tendency is to be too loud, but someone who's been given that feedback might overcompensate and use a voice that's too soft. A hearing rehabilitation program can address this problem by helping listeners sense when their voice level is inappropriate and teaching significant others to provide visual feedback (such as a subtle hand signal) in public.

SUPPORT/ADVOCACY GROUPS

One of the most effective strategies for coping with hearing loss is getting involved in a support/advocacy group. Participation in a local chapter of a national organization can be a source of information, comfort, and fun. Although there can be some overlap, this type of group differs from a local hearing rehabilitation group offered by an audiologist for a period of weeks or months (see earlier in this chapter). Support/advocacy groups are usually led by fellow group members who have lost some or all of their hearing, and the meetings are on-going. Involvement provides opportunities for exploring solutions to common problems, learning about new technologies, and benefiting from the wisdom of others. Perhaps most important, the depth of understanding and emotional support that people with hearing loss can give to one another is something that can't be matched by professionals. If you're struggling, meeting other people who are coping with similar problems can make you feel less alone. If you aren't interested in attending meetings, Internet organizations provide opportunities to share and communicate on-line.

The Hearing Loss Association of America (HLAA; formerly known as Self Help for Hard of Hearing People, or SHHH) is the nation's largest advocacy organization for people with hearing loss. Founded in 1979, the organization's goal is "to open the world of communication for people with hearing loss through information, education, advocacy, and support." Members include people with hearing loss, their families and friends, and interested professionals. The association has local chapters in all 50 states, the District of Columbia, and Puerto Rico. HLAA's website and publications encourage independence and promote self-esteem. Members receive *Hearing Loss*, the nation's only magazine for people who are hard of hearing. *Hearing Loss* features personal stories as well as articles addressing coping strategies, technological innovations, public policy, and advocacy efforts. Each summer, the organization hosts a convention that's completely accessible through hearing technology and other accommodations. The 3-day meeting includes both educational presentations and social events. Manufacturers and vendors come together to create the country's largest display of information, services, and assistive technology for consumers who are hard of hearing. The convention is an excellent opportunity to look at what's new and ask questions of knowledgeable representatives.

Another support/advocacy organization, The Association of Late-Deafened Adults (ALDA), was founded in 1987. For the most part, its members are adults who grew up hearing but are now unable to understand speech without visual aids such as speechreading, sign language, or captioning. The organization's goal is to advocate for relevant legislation, rehabilitation programs, employment opportunities, and communication services. The organization also provides personal support to late-deafened adults as they adjust to becoming deaf. Networking opportunities are offered through local chapters and an annual conference. The association publishes a quarterly newsletter "that blends humor and sensitivity along with first-hand accounts of the frequent absurdities of deafened life."

THE AMERICANS WITH DISABILITIES ACT OF 1990

The Americans with Disabilities Act (ADA) is a landmark civil rights legislation designed to protect persons with disabilities from discrimination. Basically, it says that no person may be denied "full and equal enjoyment" of the goods, services, and facilities that are available to nondisabled people. It follows in the tradition of the Civil Rights Act of 1964, which prohibited discrimination on the basis of race, color, and national origin, and Title IX of the 1972 Education Amendments, which prohibited discrimination on the basis of gender. However, the ADA does more than other antidiscrimination legislation by incorporating a principle known as reasonable accommodation. This principle requires that employers, government entities, and facilities open to the public provide accommodations that give persons with disabilities *access* to the people, places, and things that they wish to pursue. The most familiar accommodation required by the ADA is the wheelchair ramp.

For people who are deaf or hard of hearing, access means *communication* access. For example, Title II (or Section II) of the ADA requires that all services and facilities offered by state and local governments be accessible to people with disabilities. This includes (but is not limited to) police and fire departments, public schools, libraries, public transportation systems, motor vehicle departments, public hospitals, civic arenas, public parks and recreation programs, public swimming pools, municipal golf courses, social service agencies, courtrooms, and jails. Government agencies and facilities may be required to provide accommodations such as visual safety alarms, amplified telephones, text telephones, or assistive listening devices.

Title III of the ADA ensures communication access in places that are *not* owned or operated by the government but that are open to the public (except when providing accommodations would impose an undue burden). Such places include (but are not limited to) restaurants, theatres, stores, hotels, motels, laundries, hair salons, day-care centers, medical offices, museums, banks, pharmacies, professional offices, private hospitals, private schools, concert halls, sports facilities, stadiums, and privately owned transportation systems. For example, on request, hotels must provide reasonable accommodations such as visual/tactile alerting devices, television captioning, and amplified or text telephones. Religious institutions and private clubs are exempt from ADA requirements.

Title IV of the ADA requires all telephone companies to provide local and long-distance relay services. A telecommunications relay service allows a deaf person using a text telephone (TTY) to dial 711 and reach a communications assistant (CA). The CA receives the TTY user's typed message and relays it (by voice) to someone without a text telephone. The CA then converts the other party's voice response into text for the TTY user, and the conversation proceeds. The relay service must allow text telephone users to communicate with people anywhere in the United States at any time. Relay users cannot be charged more than a voice user would be charged for the same call, and no restrictions can be placed on the length of the call or the nature of the conversation. Relay services are described in greater detail in Chapter 9.

ADA in the Workplace

Title I of the ADA prohibits employers from discriminating against otherwise qualified persons in areas such as job application procedures, hiring, firing, compensation, job training, and advancement. The law does not require employers to give special consideration to such applicants during the hiring process, however; successful applicants must be fully qualified in terms of education, experience, skills, and credentials. If a person is qualified, an employer (with 15 or more employees) must provide reasonable accommodations that enable the applicant or employee to perform the essential functions of his job, and this may include job restructuring. For example, the law would not require an employer to hire a deaf person as a telephone receptionist; however, if answering the phone is a small part of that person's job, the duty could be assigned to someone else. Other accommodations could range from simply making an employee's work area quieter to purchasing equipment such as an amplified telephone, text telephone, vibrating pager, personal FM system, or visual alarm that lets a worker know when a machine is malfunctioning. The employer determines whether an accommodation is "reasonable" on a case-by-case basis.

The law requires the employer to bear the cost of accommodations. In general, accommodating people with hearing loss is less expensive than accommodating people with other types of disabilities. Often, minimal accommodations (for example, providing important information in writing) can enable competent workers who lose their hearing to continue doing their jobs. Rather than hiring someone new, accommodating a proven employee who requires no job training can actually be a bargain for an employer.

It's the employee's responsibility to request accommodations in the workplace. This means acknowledging the hearing loss, understanding the difficulties that it creates, and knowing enough to be able to suggest possible solutions. Here is the perfect opportunity to use all the things that you've learned by reading this book or participating in a hearing rehabilitation program! Enlist your audiologist's help and use the Resources section.

When requesting accommodations, a nonadversarial approach is best. It helps if you can demonstrate that the accommodations you're requesting will make you a more productive worker or improve the work environment for everyone (for example, making the work area quieter or improving the lighting). You might consider looking into tax incentives that could benefit your employer (see the Resources section), but this is not required. If you're requesting equipment, it may help to include information about where it can be purchased and how much it costs (again, the law does not require this). An oral request is acceptable, but making the request in writing allows it to be documented.

The law does not obligate an employer to provide accommodations that would cause undue hardship for the company or fundamentally alter its work (for example, those that would require unreasonable expense or disrupt the work environment). In addition, the employer is not obligated to provide exactly what you request; a similar accommodation can be substituted if it enables you to perform the essential functions of your job. Personal devices, such as hearing aids, are not covered by the ADA.

If you feel your request for a reasonable accommodation has been unjustly denied or you have been discriminated against because of your hearing loss, you might have legal recourse. Contact information for filing complaints is provided in the Resources section.

SUMMARY: GOOD COMMUNICATION HABITS

Good Habits for Those with Hearing Loss

- Be sure that your hearing aids are up to date and in good working order; if you're not doing everything you can to help yourself, you cannot expect the people around you to make an effort.
- Wear two hearing aids if this is recommended by your audiologist and you can afford it.
- Maintain your hearing aids in the best possible condition; always carry spare batteries with you.
- Inform people that you have a hearing loss and ask for their help; explain that hearing what they say is important to you.
- Give people specific suggestions about what they can do to help you understand them (for example, *"Please face me when you talk; Please slow down just a bit; Please rephrase that; Please get my attention before you begin talking to me; Please tell me what you're talking about"*). Remember to give speakers positive feedback when things are going well.
- Be prepared to good-naturedly remind people about your hearing loss and what they can do to help. In most cases, people want to be helpful, but they easily slip back into communication habits that are familiar.
- "Stage manage" your conversations:
  - Minimize background noise to the fullest extent possible, or move conversations away from it.
  - Communicate in a well-lit area; the light should fall on the speaker's face.
  - Decrease the distance between you and the speaker to maximize auditory and visual cues (3–6 feet is ideal).
  - Position yourself for a clear view of the speaker's face.
  - Position yourself so that your better ear (if you have one) is directed toward the conversation.
- Give listening and watching the speaker your full attention.
- Be sure you see well; wear eyeglasses if you need them, and be sure your prescription is up to date.
- Whenever possible, get information about the topic or program ahead of time. Stay informed about current events.
- Accept that you will miss some things; try to relax and get the gist of conversations.
- Don't interrupt too quickly; as a conversation progresses, you might understand more. If you feel lost, however, ask for help.
- When you need help, ask for specific information (rather than saying *"Huh?"* or *"What?"*).
- If you haven't heard completely, don't bluff.
- When details are important, get them in writing; carry a notepad and pen with you.
- Listening and watching can be exhausting; be prepared to take breaks from time to time. Let your communication partners know when you need to "tune out" for awhile.
- Learn about hearing assistance technology.

Good Habits for Communication Partners

- Be sure that you have the listener's attention before you begin speaking.
- Face your listener (don't try to communicate when you're out of sight). Don't turn away while speaking.
- Move to the listener when you want to communicate. Decrease the distance between you to maximize auditory and visual cues (3–6 feet is ideal).
- Don't put anything in your mouth or in front of your face while you're talking, because this makes speechreading difficult (for example, avoid eating, smoking, chewing gum, and putting your hands in front of your face).
- Give the listener the topic and let him know when the topic changes.
- Speak precisely, but don't exaggerate your speech (exaggerated mouth movements actually make speechreading more difficult).
- Speak up, but don't shout (shouting distorts speech, making it more difficult to understand). Shouting also seems rude, and it can be physically painful to listeners with sensory hearing loss).
- Decrease your speaking rate ever so slightly.
- Pause between thoughts (phrases).
- Emphasize key words.
- Use gestures.
- Check for comprehension; confirm details (if necessary, in writing).
- Use a microphone whenever one is available.
- When asked to repeat, *rephrase* what you've said; most likely, repeating the same phrase in the same way will cause it to be misunderstood again.
- In group situations, signal the listener about who is speaking (for example, look/nod/gesture in the speaker's direction). It can take a listener with hearing loss a moment to locate where a voice is coming from; by that time, he might have lost part of the message, and it can be hard to catch up.
- Minimize background noise to the fullest extent possible. For example, when entertaining in your home, don't play background music because it can make communication difficult for some of your guests.
- Talk *to* a person who is hard of hearing, not *about* her.
- Recognize how difficult communicating can be for a person with hearing loss, especially in difficult listening environments, and be sensitive to stress and fatigue.

CHAPTER 11

Prevention of Hearing Loss

The ears were made, not for such trivial uses as men are wont to suppose, but to hear celestial sounds.
A Week on the Concord and Merrimack Rivers, Henry David Thoreau

People usually take their hearing for granted, at least until something goes wrong with it. Most people can't imagine what having a hearing loss would be like. They assume that all sounds would become softer, something like what we experience when we plug our ears with our fingers or use earplugs. But plugging our ears only causes a mild conductive loss (see Chapter 4). A mild conductive loss can certainly make listening hard work (if you have normal hearing, consider wearing earplugs for a whole day—the experience is enlightening). A sensorineural hearing loss, however, is more disabling. Along with making sounds softer, sensorineural loss often causes sounds to be distorted. In addition, missing high-frequency information (which is common with sensorineural loss) makes understanding speech difficult, especially in poor listening conditions. Moderately loud sounds can be uncomfortably loud, and the hearing loss can be accompanied by relentless tinnitus. Once people have a sensorineural loss, they wish they'd taken better care of their hearing—but by then it's too late.

In adults, nearly all hearing loss is sensorineural, and nearly all sensorineural hearing loss is permanent. But there *is* good news: many sensorineural hearing losses are preventable.

PREVENTABLE CAUSES OF HEARING LOSS

Although most of the conditions that cause sensorineural hearing loss in adults are not preventable, there are two notable exceptions. Remarkably, noise-induced hearing loss, which accounts for nearly one third of all permanent hearing losses in this country (approximately 10 million), is almost entirely preventable. Hearing loss caused by exposure to ototoxic substances can also be prevented in many cases. Most of this chapter is devoted to those two conditions.

Preventable Causes of *Congenital* Sensorineural Hearing Loss

Several problems that once caused congenital hearing loss (hearing loss that's present at birth) are now preventable. A good example is maternal rubella (German measles). Rubella is dangerous to an unborn child if the mother becomes infected during pregnancy (especially during the first trimester). The baby can be severely affected even if the mother shows no symptoms herself. The last major rubella outbreak occurred in 1964 and 1965. During that outbreak, 20,000 babies were born with disabilities, including hearing loss; an additional 10,000 pregnancies ended in miscarriage or stillbirth. Since 1969, however, nearly all children have been vaccinated against rubella. As a result, hearing loss due to rubella is now rare.

Another example of a condition that once caused congenital hearing loss is Rh incompatibility between a mother and her unborn child. The *Rh factor* is a protein found on the surface of red blood cells. About 85 percent of us have it (and are Rh positive) and about 15 percent of us do not (and are Rh negative). If a mother is Rh negative and her unborn child is Rh positive, the mother can develop antibodies that build up and attack the Rh proteins in her unborn baby's blood (this generally doesn't happen until the mother's second or third Rh-incompatible pregnancy). This condition can be very dangerous to the fetus, causing severe anemia, jaundice, heart failure, hearing loss, or brain damage. Today, these harmful consequences can be prevented by anticipating the condition and treating the mother before it develops.

There are a few other (less notable) causes of hearing loss that are preventable. A small percentage of hearing losses are caused by trauma. For example, closed head injuries can cause permanent sensorineural hearing loss (see Chapter 5). Some result from unavoidable accidents, but others can be prevented by taking minimal safety precautions (for example, using seatbelts in automobiles and wearing helmets while motorcycling, bicycling, skateboarding, ice skating, horseback riding, skiing, or riding on all-terrain vehicles). Accidents and injuries are more likely to happen when participants are under the influence of alcohol or drugs; head injuries are most common among young men between the ages of 15 and 25. Children should be supervised during activities that are potentially dangerous. In addition to head trauma, traumatic injuries to the ear often result when people insert things (such as cotton swab applicators, toothpicks, or hairpins) into their ears or the ears of their children. Remember: never put anything smaller than your elbow in your ear canal (or the ear canal of someone you love)!

Another condition that's preventable is late-onset auditory deprivation (see Chapter 7). If you have a hearing loss in both ears, using only one hearing aid may cause a permanent deterioration in hearing function. In recent years we've learned a good deal about brain plasticity, or how the brain adapts to changes that result from learning, injury, or deprivation (lack of input). Sophisticated imaging techniques indicate that the brain takes some of the resources once devoted to processing sounds coming from the unaided ear and reassigns them to other functions. You've heard it before: use it or lose it. Hearing sensitivity (the ability to *detect* sounds) doesn't necessarily get poorer, but the ability to understand speech can deteriorate. If a second hearing aid is added later, complete recovery may or may not occur—the outcome is impossible to predict at this time. The length of time that only one hearing aid is worn could be a significant factor in recovery, but again, that's impossible to predict at this time. It's important to note that this particular problem occurs only when *both* ears have a hearing loss, but a hearing aid is worn in just *one* ear. Generally speaking, not wearing hearing aids does not make a hearing loss worse.

Finally, the prevalence of hearing loss among smokers is significantly higher than among nonsmokers and ex-smokers, regardless of age group. Studies suggest that smokers might be twice as likely to suffer from hearing loss. The more cigarettes that a person smokes per day and the more years she smokes, the greater the risk to hearing. Moreover, recent research indicates that the combination of smoking, age, and noise exposure creates a risk that's greater than the risks associated with smoking, age, and noise exposure simply added together.

HEARING LOSS CAUSED BY NOISE EXPOSURE

The American Speech-Language-Hearing Association (ASHA) calls loud sound a hazard to human health and hearing. Nevertheless, our world continues to get louder and louder. Hazardous noise occurs in our workplaces, our homes, and our communities. People of all ages are affected. Because the hazard is odorless, tasteless, invisible, and (usually) painless, people don't understand—or choose to ignore—the danger until it's too late. Perhaps it's unfortunate that damaging noise doesn't make our ears bleed; if it did, people might pay more attention.

After aging, exposure to hazardous noise is the most common cause of permanent hearing loss in this country. In fact, many of the hearing losses we attribute to aging are actually caused, at least in part, by noise exposure. This assumption is based on the observation that people who've spent their lives in natural environments hear better than those who've spent their lives in noisy societies. Such a comparison was made in a very famous research study conducted in 1960, in which the Maabans, a tribe living deep in the bush of Sudan, were studied (see Chapter 5). In the absence of exposure to hazardous noise, older tribe members had better hearing than people of the same age who lived in noisier places. What's more, scientists are now exploring a possible link between the effects of *subhazardous* noise exposure that accumulates over a lifetime and the ear's vulnerability to aging. Even if noise levels are not extreme, a person's lifetime exposure might determine how quickly and to what degree presbycusis (hearing loss due to aging; see Chapter 5) develops.

People of all ages (including infants and children) are vulnerable to the damaging effects of noise; the damage is more noticeable in adults because it's accumulated over more years. According to ASHA, the number of Americans age 3 years and older with some form of hearing disorder has more than doubled since 1971, rising from 13 million to more than 31 million today. By most accounts, more people in our society are developing hearing loss, and they're developing it at younger ages than ever before. Record numbers of baby boomers are being diagnosed with hearing loss in their forties and fifties. In fact, the rate of hearing loss among people in their fifties increased by 150 percent between 1964 and 1994.[1] The most obvious explanation for this phenomenon is that we live in a world that continues to get noisier. Not only are we exposed to hazardous noise at work, we expose ourselves at home and at play, and the effects add up. We do our yard work with gas-powered lawn mowers, leaf blowers, and weed trimmers. We ride on motorcycles, snowmobiles, all-terrain vehicles, and jet skis. We attend loud concerts and sporting events. We listen to iPods and other portable music players for hours on end. According to the National Institute on Deafness and Other Communication Disorders (NICDC), approximately 10 percent of all Americans between the ages of 20 and 69 years have already damaged their ears by exposing them to loud noise.

People differ in their susceptibility to damage from noise. Two people can be exposed to the same noise for the same length of time, and one develops a hearing loss whereas the other does not (or the damage is less severe in one case than the other). A person's vulnerability to noise damage seems to depend on her genetic make-up; however, there are factors that appear to increase susceptibility. For example, exposure to certain drugs or certain chemicals seems to increase the damage that results from hazardous noise.

When is sound considered hazardous? Prolonged or repeated exposure to sound levels greater than 85 dB (roughly the level of a gas-powered lawn mower) is hazardous. Exposure is defined by both the level of the noise and the duration of the exposure. As the sound level increases, the length of safe exposure time decreases. Guidelines published by the National Institute for Occupational Safety and Health (NIOSH), one of the National Institutes of Health (NIH), state that a person's daily exposure should not exceed the equivalent of 85 dB for 8 hours a day.[2] The guidelines also incorporate an *exchange rate* of 3 dB; each time the noise level increases by 3 dB, safe exposure time is cut in half. For example, exposure to 85 dB is permissible for 8 hours, exposure to 88 dB is permissible for 4 hours, exposure to 91 dB is permissible for 2 hours, and so on. Exposure to levels of 115 dB or greater is extremely dangerous and should be avoided altogether. The 3 dB exchange rate used by NIOSH is more conservative than the 5 dB exchange rate used by the Occupational Safety and Health Administration (OSHA). OSHA regulations govern permissible noise exposure in the workplace; see later in this chapter. Both NIOSH and OSHA guidelines are designed to prevent noise-induced hearing loss in the "average" person and will *not* protect persons who are more susceptible than average.

"Safe" Noise Exposures

According to NIOSH, your daily exposure to noise should not exceed the equivalent of

- 85 dB for 8 hours
- 88 dB for 4 hours
- 91 dB for 2 hours
- 94 dB for 1 hour
- 97 dB for 30 minutes
- 100 dB for 15 minutes
- 103 dB for 7½ minutes
- 106 dB for 3¾ minutes
- 109 dB for < 2 minutes
- Avoid exposure to levels of 115 dB and greater for *any* length of time

The louder the noise, the shorter the permissible exposure time. See Appendix I for examples of everyday sound levels.

There are two distinct types of hearing loss related to noise exposure (see Chapter 5). One type results when an extremely loud impulse noise (for example, a gunshot or explosion) occurs close to the ear. This is known as *acoustic trauma*. A single, intense sound can cause structures within the ear to be ripped apart. The resulting hearing loss is immediate, typically permanent, and often accompanied by tinnitus (ringing in the ears).

The more common type of noise-induced hearing loss begins gradually and gets worse over time. The offending noise levels are less extreme, but the exposure is prolonged or repeated (for example, repeated exposure to job-related noise, chain saw noise, or loud music). With this type of exposure, hair cells within the cochlea die as a result of metabolic exhaustion (see Chapter 5). Some people (but not *all* people) experience warning signs before this type of damage results in permanent hearing loss. If you've been exposed to noise that's loud enough to damage *your* hearing (remember, susceptibility to damage varies from person to person), you may have experienced *temporary threshold shift* (TTS). Following exposure, sounds may have seemed muffled or you may have had trouble understanding speech. You may have experienced ringing in your ears; in fact, you may have been more aware of the ringing than the temporary hearing loss. If you've experienced TTS, you've already damaged hair cells in the cochlea. TTS is your body's way of telling you that you've exposed yourself to more noise than your ears can handle. Listen to your body's message and don't repeat that kind of exposure!

With repeated exposure, the temporary hearing loss (and maybe the tinnitus) can become permanent. You probably won't be aware of it at first. The loss begins gradually and starts at the high frequencies—a high-frequency hearing loss prevents you from hearing soft consonant sounds like /s/, /f/, /sh/, and /th/. In other words, you're able to *hear* speech, but it's less clear, especially in noisy conditions. With continued exposure, the loss can affect more frequencies, and speech will become increasingly difficult to understand. But by the time you're aware of it, nothing can be done to undo the damage. No medicine, no surgery, no hearing aid can bring back hearing that's been damaged by noise. Hearing aids can help, but they can't bring back normal hearing.

For most people, noise exposure varies throughout the day—but the exposures add up. Even if your exposure at work is within permissible limits, stopping at a noisy health club on the way home or taking a motorcycle ride in the evening can make your total daily noise "dose" unsafe. Until recently, determining daily noise exposure was difficult and complex. A personal noise dosimeter is now available at a reasonable price (approximately $100). This portable device measures sound levels for 16 hours and calculates the cumulative noise exposure dose, alerting the user to the need for hearing protection.

When Is Noise Too Loud?

In the workplace, your employer has a legal obligation to measure noise levels that might be dangerous; however, there are no regulations to protect you against hazardous noise outside the workplace. As a rule of thumb, noise is potentially dangerous if

- You have to shout to be heard by someone an arm's length (or less) away.
- Your ears hurt during or after exposure.

- Your ears ring during or after exposure.
- Sounds seem muffled or speech is hard to understand during or after exposure (that is, you experience temporary threshold shift).

Because noise-induced hearing loss develops gradually, people sometimes believe that they've built up a tolerance or immunity to loud noise. However, there's no such thing; you can't "toughen up" your ears. If noise no longer bothers you, it's probably because it's already damaged your hearing. But make no mistake; your hearing will continue to get worse as long as exposure continues.

Occupational Noise Exposure

The most common cause of noise-induced hearing loss is exposure to occupational noise. According to NIOSH, 30 million American workers are exposed to potentially hazardous noise on a regular basis; however, not all of them have daily noise doses that exceed safe limits (for example, they might be exposed to noise levels greater than 85 dB, but for only part of the day). For as many as 9 million workers, the daily noise dose *does* exceed safe limits. As a result, noise-induced hearing loss is considered the most common occupational "disease." Workers whose jobs put them at increased risk include (but are not limited to) farmers; miners; construction workers; highway workers; factory workers; utility workers; pilots; dentists; firefighters; police officers; disc jockeys; subway workers; musicians; music teachers; rock stars; industrial arts teachers; lawn maintenance workers; cab, truck, railway, and bus operators; and military personnel. Many of these workers work in industries that aren't adequately covered by the federal regulations designed to protect hearing.

Farming Can Be Hazardous to Your Hearing

On the farm, exposure to engine noise, loud animals, or power tool motors can damage hearing. A recent screening of New York farmers found that 77 percent had hearing loss. The magazine *Iowa Farmer Today* reported that the noise levels produced by tractors range from 74 to 112 dB, those produced by combine harvesters range from 80 to 115 dB, and the squeals of pigs—particularly pregnant sows—range from 85 to 115 dB.[3]

An additional 9 million workers are exposed to industrial chemicals, like solvents and heavy metals, which can also damage hearing. In some cases, chemicals act synergistically with noise exposure to increase hearing damage (that is, the combined effect is greater than the effects of noise exposure and chemical exposure simply added together). The occupational health community pays little attention to the risks these chemicals pose to hearing, and the potential for hearing damage is rarely considered when chemical exposure limits are set.

The most effective way to prevent occupational hearing loss is to limit employee exposure through engineering and administrative controls. Engineering controls reduce noise at its source and include things like machine modification (for example, installing mufflers on equipment), machine isolation (for example, building sound barriers around machines), and worker enclosures (for example, isolating workers from noise in sound-treated environments). Administrative controls include things like moving workers away from noise, dividing noisy tasks among several employees so that no employee's exposure exceeds safe limits, and replacing noisy equipment with quieter alternatives. When these controls are not feasible or they fail to make workers' exposures safe (that is, when workers are exposed to the equivalent of 85 dB or more for 8 hours a day), OSHA regulations require that the employer provide a hearing loss prevention (hearing conservation) program.[4] The program must include noise exposure monitoring; engineering and administrative noise controls; baseline hearing testing with annual retests; a program for selecting, fitting, training, and supervising the use of personal hearing protectors; educational programming for both management and workers about the effects of noise; recordkeeping; and analysis of program effectiveness. In addition, documented cases of occupational hearing loss must be reported to OSHA.

The OSHA regulations are designed to prevent noise-induced hearing loss in the "average" person. They will *not* protect people who are more susceptible to noise damage than average (those with so-called tender ears). According to the Centers for Disease Control, one in four workers exposed to noise levels that comply with OSHA criteria will develop a hearing loss.[5] This means that even with adequate hearing conservation programs in place, noise-induced hearing losses will continue to occur. Many (if not most) programs offered by employers are *not* adequate, however. And, unfortunately, the enforcement of OSHA regulations isn't either. For example, according to a well-known audiologist, hearing conservationist, and author, when a worker develops a hearing loss, the company can use its poor recordkeeping and/or lack of precise measurements (of both noise levels and the employee's hearing) to avoid responsibility. If a baseline hearing test wasn't performed before the worker was exposed at work, the company can claim that the hearing loss was preexisting or caused by recreational noise exposure (a good program includes a worker education component that warns against recreational noise exposure). It's ironic that companies often spend more money litigating and paying workers' compensation claims than it would cost to put a good hearing conservation program in place.[6]

The bottom line: if you're exposed to noise at work, take responsibility for your own hearing. Be sure your initial baseline audiogram is preceded by at least 14 hours of quiet (TTS can make your preemployment hearing appear poorer than it really is, thereby making it more difficult to demonstrate a change as a result of work-related exposure). Because OSHA allows industries to substitute wearable hearing protectors for more effective engineering and administrative controls, you must be conscientious about using them. Don't depend on your employer to *make* you use hearing protection; ask for it and use it whenever it's appropriate. Be sure you receive information about the types of protectors that are available and which ones might be best for you. Your employer should offer you a choice, but all too often hearing protectors are ordered by purchasing agents on the basis of cost. They're sometimes uncomfortable, which means they're not worn—and protectors that aren't worn can't protect hearing. Be sure that your hearing conservation program also includes instruction about how to *insert* hearing protectors, and then take care to put them in properly. Protectors that aren't inserted properly can't protect hearing either.

Serving Your Country Can Be Hazardous to Your Hearing

Soldiers sent to battle zones are at least fifty times more likely to suffer noise-induced hearing loss than soldiers who don't see combat. As of mid-2008, 58,000 troops had returned from Iraq and Afghanistan with hearing loss.[7] According to a 2003–2004 study at the U.S. Army Center for Health Promotion and Preventative Medicine,[8] thousands of these hearing losses could have been prevented. Initially, the supply of earplugs was inadequate, there was a failure to provide unit commanders with information about the importance of hearing protection, and, in many cases, baseline hearing testing was not performed before deployment. Later improvements included a greater effort to test the hearing of all new soldiers, broadened distribution of ear protectors and increased training regarding their use, and the deployment of audiologists to a hospital in Baghdad.[9]

Overall, at least 10 percent of military personnel suffer noise-induced hearing loss,[10] making it the most common occupational hazard associated with military service. In 2006, 2.5 million veterans received disability payments for hearing loss or tinnitus.

Working at the Mall Can Be Hazardous to Your Hearing

Employees whom you might not have considered at risk for hearing loss are the salespeople at a chain of stores notorious for playing loud, pulsing dance music. Every store in the chain plays the same music and receives instructions about how loud it should be played. This retailer regularly gets complaints from their customers as well as from mall operators and other mall tenants. OSHA has also received a number of complaints. Although the exposure of customers is usually relatively brief, the noise levels could be hazardous to employees.

Nonoccupational Noise Exposure: Living Loud

Noise-induced hearing loss is caused by exposure to hazardous noise in the workplace, exposure to hazardous noise outside the workplace, or a combination of the two. It doesn't matter if the offending noise comes from a stamping press in a manufacturing plant, a symphony orchestra, a jet ski, or an iPod. Examples of hobbies that can be dangerous to hearing include target shooting and hunting; driving or riding in "boom cars"; riding on motorcycles, snowmobiles, all-terrain vehicles, and motorboats; attending auto races, sporting events, concerts, video arcades, health clubs, and movies; flying airplanes; and using (power) woodworking tools. Examples of household tools and appliances that can be dangerous to hearing include vacuum cleaners; gas-powered lawn mowers, leaf blowers, and weed-trimmers; snow blowers; chain saws; and (power) shop tools. Passing boom cars, sirens, car alarms, and traffic add to the noisy background of our lives. Prolonged exposure to any one of these noise sources has the potential to cause hearing loss, but exposure to different noises adds up. And, unlike occupational noise exposure, nonoccupational exposure isn't controlled by federal regulations.

Rock and Roll Can Be Hazardous to Your Hearing

For the past 20 years, an organization called Hearing Education and Awareness for Rockers (H.E.A.R.) has worked to raise awareness of music-related hearing problems. Its executive director and co-founder, Kathy Peck, formed H.E.A.R. after noticing hearing problems following a 1984 concert in which her band, the Contractions, opened for Duran Duran at Oakland Stadium. Surprised by the lack of hearing care for musicians, Peck teamed up with Flash Gordon, MD at the Haight-Ashbury Free Clinic to set up a hearing center. Pete Townshend of The Who donated $10,000 to get H.E.A.R. off the ground. Over the years, the organization has evolved into an advocacy group, producing public-service announcements and helping to pass a San Francisco ordinance that requires entertainment venues to distribute free earplugs. Their website contains interesting and helpful information (see the Resources section).

Portable Music Players

In a discussion about recreational noise exposure, portable music players like Apple iPods and other MP3 players deserve special mention. These devices are revolutionizing the way we listen to music, yet there's concern about their potential to harm hearing. But portable music players have been around for a long time—why all the fuss now?

Before digital technology, playing music at very loud levels caused distortion, and that tended to put a natural cap on volume. Digital technology, however, has made it possible to play music at potentially dangerous levels without distortion. In addition, iPods and other MP3 players make it possible to listen for dangerously long periods of time. An audio tape or compact disk (CD) is relatively short, naturally limiting exposure time, but iPods can hold thousands of songs and play for hundreds of hours. Remember: risk is determined by both the level of the sound and the duration of the exposure.

For these reasons, portable music fans are being cautioned about their listening habits. For example, iPod manuals have always carried a warning that states, "Permanent hearing loss may occur if earbuds (earphones) or headphones are used at high volume." In France, the maximum output of portable music players (like iPods) has been legally capped at 100 dB, and elsewhere in Europe the cap is 104 dB. However, these levels should be considered "safe" only for very short periods: 15 minutes or less at 100 dB and roughly 6 minutes or less at 104 dB. Some users may be unaware that listening responsibly involves a trade-off between exposure time and sound level. No such caps exist in this country. Since April 2006, Apple has provided a free download that allows users to limit the maximum volume on newer iPod models. More recently, Apple has applied for a patent for software-based technology that tracks a user's sound exposure over time and imposes recovery periods during which volume is reduced, giving the ears a chance to recover.

How do you use a portable music player safely? The length of time that you can listen varies with the volume setting. The type of portable music player and the type of earphone you use are also important factors. For example, using stock (over-the-ear) headphones, an *average* user can safely listen to a *CD player* for 60 minutes or less at 60 percent of maximum volume (the so-called 60/60 rule).

Today, more than 100 million people use MP3 players (including iPods) to listen to music. The table below shows maximum "safe" listening times (per day) for a range of volume levels and earphone styles used with these devices.[11] For example, an *average* person using stock iPod earphones (earbuds) can listen safely for 4.6 hours per day at 70 percent of full volume. (To find 70 percent, look for the visual volume display on your device.) Using the same earphones, a typical user can safely listen for 1.2 hours a day at 80 percent of maximum volume. However, listening at full volume for more than just 5 minutes per day (with the same earphones) would put the average user at risk. Remember that not all listeners are "average." Some are less susceptible to noise damage, but some are more susceptible. Listeners with so-called tender ears might incur hearing loss even when these guidelines are followed. And, unfortunately, there's no way to predict who might be more prone to damage.

The table also shows that at the same volume setting (say, 70 percent), safe listening times differ for various earphone styles. For example, as a general rule, earbuds produce higher sound levels than "supra-aural" earphones (over-the-ear headphones). However, a research study showed that

Table 11.1. Maximum "Safe" Listening Time for MP3 Players

Percent of Volume Control	Maximum Listening Time per Day[a]			
	Supra-Aural[b]	Earbud[c]	iPod Stock Earphones[d]	Isolator[e]
10–50	No limit	No limit	No limit	No limit
60	No limit	No limit	18 h	14 h
70	20 h	6 h	4.6 h	3.4 h
80	4.9 h	1.5 h	1.2 h	50 min
90	1.2 h	22 min	18 min	12 min
100	18 min	5 min	5 min	3 min

[a] Using NIOSH damage-risk criteria
[b] Supra-aural earphones (over-the-ear headphones) sit on top of the ears.
[c] An earbud is similar to an earplug that goes into the ear canal.
[d] The stock earphones that come with iPods are earbuds.
[e] "Isolator" earphones block out background noise; they can be earbuds or headphones; those used in the study were earbuds.

in quiet, most people tended to adjust volume to roughly the same level, regardless of the type of earphone they used.[12] It was in *noisy* environments that listeners were more likely to increase volume to dangerous levels.[13] This happened less often when listeners used sound-isolating ("isolator") earphones that blocked out background noise. This suggests that investing in sound-isolating earphones (either earbuds or over-the-ear headphones) is a great way to enjoy your MP3 player more safely.

Listening to Portable Music Players Can Be Hazardous to Your Hearing

Enjoying your favorite tunes on a portable music player is likely to be safe if you

- Pay attention to the volume.
  - As you increase the volume, decrease the length of time you listen.
  - *Do not* listen at full volume (and if you absolutely *must*, listen for less than 5 minutes).
  - Set the volume in a quiet environment, and don't increase it to overcome noise in a poor listening environment.
  - Set the volume once, and don't increase it as you adapt to the sound level.
  - Check to be sure you can hear a person talking (not shouting) from 3 feet away while listening through earphones.
- Pay attention to the length of time you listen.
  - If you want to listen all day, don't increase the volume beyond 60 percent, and give your ears a 5-minute break at least once every hour.
- Invest in better earphones (earbuds or headphones).
  - Earphones that block out background noise allow music to be enjoyed at less dangerous levels.

- High-fidelity earphones allow you to appreciate music without making the volume dangerously loud.
- *Change* your listening habits if you experience ringing or sense that speech is muffled after listening.
  - Give your ears a longer rest between exposures.
  - Next time you listen, decrease both volume and listening time.
- Remember that hearing loss begins very gradually; by the time you notice a problem, the damage has already been done.

Tell a friend or family member about the safe use of portable music players. Refer young children to the "Listen to Your Buds" consumer awareness campaign sponsored by ASHA (see the Resources section).

Movies Can be Hazardous to Your Hearing

Movie-goers often complain that movies have become too loud—and they *are* loud, especially the peak levels that are reached during action scenes. Digital technology now allows the volume to be cranked up without distortion. Previews seem even louder than feature films, although the Trailer Audio Standards Association has lowered permissible levels to 85 dB. Luckily, exposure duration is relatively brief, and that's half of the equation. Most movies last less than 3 hours, including previews. For that duration, exposure (*if it indeed meets industry standards*) probably isn't dangerous to the average person.

Making Music Can Be Hazardous to Your Hearing

Making music—whether as part of a rock band, philharmonic orchestra, jazz ensemble, or school marching band—can be dangerous to your hearing. Surprisingly, studies indicate that the prevalence of noise-induced hearing loss is greater among classical musicians than rock or pop musicians. There are several reasons for this, including the duration of exposure. The classical musician may play 5 to 10 hours a day, including performances, rehearsals, and teaching. Rock musicians are more likely to play two or three nights a week. Other factors contributing to increased exposure include the size of modern orchestras (much larger than the chamber-sized orchestras of Mozart's day), the way in which orchestra members are arranged relative to one another, and the positions in which instruments are held (often close to the ear).[14]

Just a few of the famous baby boomer musicians who've spoken publicly about their music-induced hearing losses or tinnitus include Jeff Beck, Bono, Cher, Eric Clapton, President Bill Clinton, Phil Collins, Mick Fleetwood, Ted Nugent, Sting, Pete Townshend, and Neil Young.

Hearing Protectors

Hearing protectors prevent some portion of a dangerously loud sound from entering the ear and damaging fragile hair cells within the cochlea; they don't shut out *all* sound. In other words, the offending noise, warning signals, or people talking can still be heard, but at a softer level. Generally, the level of sound entering the ear is reduced (attenuated) enough to make it safe, but occasionally noise levels are so great even the best hearing protectors are inadequate. Dozens of hearing protectors are available.

Hearing protectors (except those that are custom made) are given a noise reduction rating (NRR) by the Environmental Protection Agency (EPA). The NRR is a measure of how much attenuation (noise reduction) the hearing protector provides under *ideal* conditions. Generally, the NRR ranges from 10 dB to 35 dB. Let's say, for example, that you're operating a chain saw, which produces a buzz of approximately 110 dB. A hearing protector with an NRR of 30 dB *should* reduce the noise to a safe level of 80 dB. However, the amount of attenuation a protector *actually* provides depends on proper use. Most workers get only a fraction of the NRR because of poor fit or poor insertion. In fact, OSHA assumes that the average user gets less than half of the attenuation indicated by the protector's NRR. Using the example of the chain saw, OSHA would assume attenuation of less than 15 dB, which would only reduce the noise to a level of 95 dB, which is still potentially dangerous. Poor fit and poor insertion of hearing protectors are leading causes of occupational hearing loss.

When choosing a hearing protector, you can't rely on the NRR to accurately represent the amount of attenuation that *you'll* receive (however, the EPA *is* considering proposals that would make its method of testing hearing protectors more similar to real-world usage). Nevertheless, it's a good idea to look for an NRR so that you know the product has been tested and was designed to be used as a hearing protector. Although more isn't always better, when in doubt, choose the protector with the highest NRR.

There are two major types of hearing protectors: earplugs and earmuffs. Choosing the one that's best for you is a matter of personal preference. Products in both categories can provide roughly the same protection when used properly, and they're generally comparable in price. Wearing *both* earplugs and earmuffs at the same time provides about 5 dB more attenuation than whichever protector has the higher rating, and this should be done whenever noise levels exceed 100 dB (about 97 percent of industrial exposures are less than 100 dB). To buy hearing protectors for use outside the workplace, check hardware stores, home improvement stores, drug stores, sporting goods stores, gun stores, music stores, and the Internet.

Earplugs

An earplug fits into the outer portion of the ear canal. The fit needs to be snug enough to seal the canal completely. When that doesn't happen,

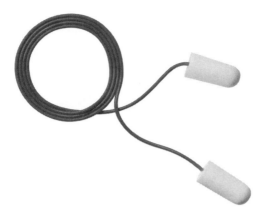

Figure 11.1. Example of Foam Earplugs. (Courtesy of E-A-R.)

sound can find its way into the ear (similar to water, sound can leak through any opening). An earplug that doesn't fit well or isn't inserted properly probably will not provide adequate protection and can also irritate the ear canal. There are a two ways to check informally for proper fit and insertion. First, listen to your own voice. With a good fit, it should sound louder and deeper than usual because of the occlusion effect—like when you plug your ears with your fingers (see Chapter 7). Second, listen to the noise around you. After inserting your earplugs, cup your hands tightly over your ears while listening to a continuous noise. If your earplugs fit properly and are inserted correctly, you shouldn't hear much difference with your ears covered versus uncovered.

There are several different types of earplugs. Foam earplugs (which are compressible or squishy) should be rolled into a thin, crease-free cylinder between your thumb and fingers or across your palm. No-roll foam products are also available. At least one half of the plug's length should be inserted into the ear canal. Reach over your head with one hand and pull up on the opposite ear. Use your other hand to insert the plug with a gentle rocking motion until it's in as far as it can go. The plug will then expand to fit the size and shape of your ear canal. Foam earplugs are effective, inexpensive, and disposable (designed for one-time use). Some have tapered ends, some are attached to cords, and some come with stems so there's no need to touch the part that goes into the ear with dirty hands.

Premolded earplugs come in a variety of sizes, shapes, and materials. Many have flanges or sealing rings to hold them in place. Finding the right size usually takes some trial and error, and it's not unusual to need a different size for each ear (some plugs are a different size on each end, so that reversing the plug changes its size). Premolded plugs are inserted like moldable (squishy) plugs, except that rolling is unnecessary (an advantage in less-than-clean environments). Some premolded plugs are meant for

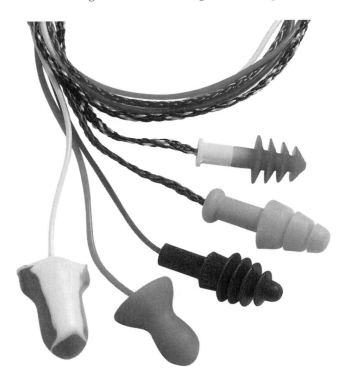

Figure 11.2. Examples of Premolded Earplugs. (Courtesy of Sperian Hearing Protection, LLC.)

one-time use (disposable), whereas others are designed to be washed and reused. They're convenient to carry and relatively inexpensive. Again, some are attached to cords, and some have stems so that there's no need to touch the part that goes into the ear.

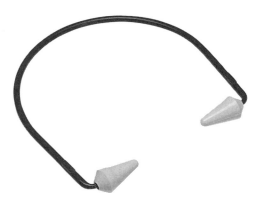

Figure 11.3. Example of Banded Earpods/Earplugs. (Courtesy of E-A-R.)

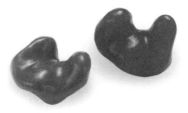

Figure 11.4. Examples of Custom Earplugs (these are color-coded for right [red] and left blue]). (Courtesy of Westone Laboratories, Inc.)

Banded earplugs or earpods are occasionally called *canal caps*. A lightweight, spring-loaded band holds them in place, making insertion quick and easy. They're especially convenient for people who work or play around intermittent noise and need to use hearing protection on and off (for example, airport workers who guide airplanes on the tarmac). When it's quiet, the band can be left hanging around the neck; when hazardous noise resumes, the plugs can quickly be put into place. When in use, the band can be worn over the head, behind the neck, or under the chin. Banded earplugs tend to provide less attenuation than do conventional earplugs or earmuffs.

Custom earplugs are made to fit your ears from impressions taken by an audiologist. The process is very much like having custom earmolds or custom hearing aids made. Custom plugs should be more comfortable and provide better protection; however, a perfect fit sometimes requires adjustments. Custom earplugs are more expensive than noncustom products.

Some premolded and custom earplugs are activated by dangerous noise levels but provide little or no attenuation when noise levels are *not* dangerous. Noise-activated earplugs are ideal for law enforcement and military personnel who can unexpectedly be exposed to gunfire and explosions but must be able to hear the sounds around them, such as the footsteps of an approaching enemy. Some earplugs use a system of valves, whereas others use a filter system to provide instant protection against dangerous sound levels. One plug is reversible; inserting one end provides protection against high-level, impulse noise without attenuating other sounds. When the plug is reversed, all sounds are attenuated, including ongoing high-level noise. This type of "tactical earplug" is used by the Army and the Marines.

Conventional earplugs attenuate the high frequencies more than other frequencies. This makes sounds softer, but it also gives them a muffled quality. There are times when it's important to hear sounds exactly as they are, only quieter, as when listening to music or working on an engine. Using earplugs that reduce all frequencies by the same amount makes listening more natural and more enjoyable. Earplugs that provide uniform attenuation across the frequencies are referred to as *musician's earplugs*

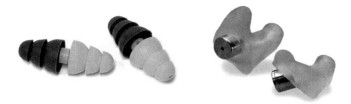

Figure 11.5. Examples of Noise-activated Earplugs. *Left*, Premolded, reversible Earplugs. Inserting one end provides protection against high-level, impulse noise (like gunfire or explosions), yet allows the user to hear other sounds (footsteps, rifle bolts being drawn) without attenuation. Inserting the other end provides more conventional protection against continuous noise that's potentially dangerous; *all* sounds are attenuated. *Right*, Custom Earplug with a Sonic Valve. The sonic valve also protects against impulse noise without attenuating other sounds. (Courtesy of E-A-R [left] and Westone Laboratories, Inc. [right].)

or *high-fidelity earplugs*. For example, Etymotic Research offers plug-in, interchangeable filters for custom earplugs that provide 9, 15, or 25 dB of *flat* attenuation (the ER9, ER15, and ER25, respectively). This means that the user can choose different attenuators for different situations (each attenuator is bought separately). The user may even choose different attenuators for each ear (depending, for example, on her position relative to other musicians). Custom high-fidelity earplugs work very well, but they're expensive, ranging in price from $150 to $200 per set. For musicians and others on a budget, noncustom, high-fidelity ETY-Plugs provide 20 db of flat attenuation and sell for about $12 a set (including neck cord and carrying case). They come in two sizes.

Finally, electronic earplugs (digital or analog) provide electronic circuitry for both amplification and hearing protection. In other words, these are hearing protectors with circuitry that enables them to provide generic amplification. The circuitry prevents hazardous sounds from entering the ear; it also prevents sounds from being amplified to dangerous levels. These devices are available in BTE, ITE, and ITC styles.

Earmuffs

Earmuffs can be purchased with different types of ear cushions and ear cups of different sizes. Over-the-head, behind-the-head, or under-the-chin headbands accommodate face shields, hard hats, and other protective equipment. Alternatively, many ear cups can be snapped onto hard hats. Ear cushions must form a seal around the entire ear to prevent sound from entering the ear canal. Eyeglasses, caps that go over the ears, behind-the-ear hearing aids, pencils behind the ear, and long hair can prevent a

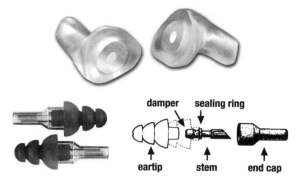

Figure 11.6. *Top,* Example of Custom, High-fidelity Musician's Earplugs. *Lower left and right,* Noncustom, High-fidelity ETY Earplugs. (Courtesy of Etymotic Research, Inc.)

good seal. Headband tension must be adequate to hold earmuffs firmly around the ear; adjusting the band to make it more comfortable is likely to reduce the protection that earmuffs provide. Some people prefer earmuffs to earplugs because they don't require insertion, whereas others just don't like wearing anything in their ears. On the other hand, some people find earmuffs hot and heavy.

Noise-activated earmuffs allow nonharmful sounds to pass through but suppress hazardous noises (they're sometimes used by hunters). *Noise cancellation* earmuffs rely on active noise reduction. Circuitry within the earmuff detects a noise and reproduces it 180 degrees out of phase; sounds

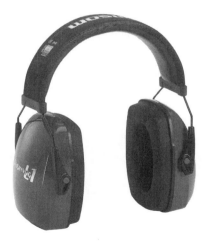

Figure 11.7. Example of Earmuffs on Headband. (Courtesy of Sperian Hearing Protection, LLC.)

that are identical but opposite in phase cancel each other. This technology is effective for reducing continuous, low-frequency noise like the roar of a lawn mower or engine noise during air travel, but it's not particularly useful in industrial situations. *Electronic earmuffs* provide both amplification and hearing protection. Dangerous impulse noises are blocked but electronic circuitry amplifies sounds picked up by microphones that are mounted on the ear cups. Amplified sound is prevented from exceeding a safe level (82 dB). Some electronic earmuffs come with a built-in AM/FM radio. Again, all sounds (including those from the radio and those coming through the microphones) are prevented from reaching dangerous levels.

My Friend, Jim

Jim, a lifelong dairy farmer and avid hunter, has a hearing loss that's worse in his left ear than in his right (in other words, his loss is asymmetric). There are two likely reasons for the asymmetry. First, when driving a tractor (or similar equipment), Jim turns to his right to look behind him, which means that his left ear is more exposed to the engine noise in front. Second, when right-handed people shoot a rifle, the right shoulder protects the right ear when the gun is fired. The noise comes from the muzzle, and the unprotected left ear is more likely to be damaged.

Nowadays, Jim wears hearing protection while he works (and in one ear when he hunts). According to Jim, the first thing he noticed when he started wearing earplugs was that he got much less tired while working. He says that it wasn't until he wore hearing protection that he realized how exhausting the noise was, and the difference was remarkable.

If you already have a hearing loss, it's even more important that you protect the precious hearing that you have left. In fact, having a hearing loss may make you particularly vulnerable to further damage. Neither hearing aids nor earmolds are designed to be used as hearing protectors. Many have tiny holes, called *vents*, which are intended to allow air into the ear canal (see Chapter 7); however, Vents also allow harmful noise to enter the ear canal. Even without vents, hearing aids and earmolds don't provide adequate hearing protection.

If you wear hearing aids and spend time in noisy environments, you should talk with your audiologist about possible solutions. For example, if it's not necessary to hear well while you're in a noisy setting, removing your hearing aids might be the simplest solution. Hearing aids worn in noise levels that exceed 85 dB can further damage hearing and aren't of much benefit anyway. If you want to wear earmuffs over your (custom) hearing aids, consider earmuffs with flat attenuation. Another possibility is to use electronic earmuffs that can substitute for hearing aids while you're in a noisy setting. Microphones outside the cups and speakers inside the cups allow the earmuffs to act as generic hearing aids that amplify soft and moderately loud sounds. If you have a hearing loss, hearing protection is an issue that should be discussed with your audiologist.

Remember, the effects of noise add up. Your total noise "dose" for the day includes exposure at home (for example, leaf blowing), at play (for example, listening to loud music), *and* at work. It's important to wear hearing protectors when exposed to dangerous noise *in any setting*. Carry them with you at all times as you would sunglasses. Be sure to try several devices to see what works best for you. Different protectors work better for different people and in different situations. Whatever you choose, a good fit is important for protection and comfort. Never rely on cotton or tissue, because the protection that they provide is minimal.

Other Dangers of Noise

William Stewart, MD, former Surgeon General of the United States (1965–1969), once said, "Calling noise a nuisance is like calling smog an inconvenience. Noise must be considered a hazard to the health of people everywhere."[15] In addition to damaging our hearing, noise affects our physical health and sense of well-being. It can increase blood pressure, pulse, and breathing rates. It can affect the cardio-vascular system, changing the way the heart beats and perhaps increasing the risk of heart attack. It can increase stomach acid, sometimes leading to stomach upset, digestive problems, and ulcers. Sleep can be disrupted, reducing efficiency, contributing to the development of chronic health conditions, and affecting mood. Noise can create physical and mental strain, resulting in fatigue, anxiety, irritability, and depression. It can interfere with communication, contribute to accidents and injuries, and reduce productivity. It can degrade job performance by reducing attention to tasks, and this includes the performance of children in school. Several research studies have demonstrated the negative effects of noise on student achievement. Children in classrooms located close to railroad tracks, airports, and noisy streets don't perform as well as their counterparts in quieter classrooms.

Noise and Society

The epidemic of noise-induced hearing loss has been called "a disease of civilization." It's a result of the mismatch between the natural world for which our bodies were designed and the civilization that we have built. There are no sounds in nature are loud as the ones we've created.

Not only are noise levels greater than ever before, the noise is more constant. Noise is almost everywhere, almost all the time. There's simply less quiet these days. An ever-present, noisy background means that there's less time for our ears to rest and heal between high-level exposures. This may cause delicate hair cells within the cochlea to wear out at an earlier age. As mentioned earlier, there appears to be a link between a person's lifetime noise exposure—even to "nonhazardous" sound levels—and the amount of hearing loss that he will experience with age.

Noise has been described as the most pervasive pollutant in America. It's been compared to second-hand smoke because it damages our health and invades our personal space without our consent. Noise pollution affects our quality of life and our sense of community by causing people to be less patient, less helpful, and more irritable.[16] In 2005, New York City Mayor Michael Bloomberg sought to overhaul his city's noise statute (the federal Noise Control Act of 1972 gives responsibility for regulating community noise to cities and states). Mayor Bloomberg declared "excessive and un-reasonable noise to be a menace to public health, comfort, convenience, safety, welfare, and the prosperity of the people." The mayor reported that 410,000 noise complaints had been made to a citizen hotline during the previous 14 months, making noise the most common complaint. In fact, noise pollution was described as the city's number one quality-of-life issue. Proposed revisions to the statute included, among other things, new limits on noise at construction sites, bars, clubs, and cabarets, and common sense standards for car stereos, loud music, barking dogs, and loud mufflers.[17] The new regulations took effect July 1, 2007.

Dozens of grass-roots organizations have sprung up to advocate for quieter communities. Only a handful are mentioned here, but if you visit their Web sites, you will find links to many more. The Noise Pollution Clearinghouse (NPC) says, "Good neighbors keep their noise to themselves." The NPC's mission is "to create more civil cities and more natural rural and wilderness areas by reducing noise pollution at the source." The NPC's goals include raising awareness, strengthening laws and governmental efforts to control noise pollution, and assisting antinoise pollution activists. The NPC actively supports persons and groups opposed to noise pollution by providing access to sound-level monitoring equipment and helping them prepare for presentations before planning commissions, zoning boards, city councils, and judges. The organization helps people to network with others involved in similar projects and connects them with experts in the field. A variety of resources are available on the NPC website, including information about quiet products and services. You can also subscribe to the NPC newsletter, *The Quiet Zone*, or link to other antinoise groups, resources, and newsletters at the website (see the Resources section).

The federal government is doing some advocacy of its own. Healthy Hearing 2010 is a national campaign to improve the hearing of all Americans through prevention, early detection, treatment, and rehabilitation. It's part of a larger campaign called *Healthy People 2010*, a national prevention program coordinated by the U.S. Public Health Service. Healthy Hearing

2010 challenges people and communities to take specific steps to ensure healthy hearing. Schools and other local organizations are encouraged to launch Healthy Hearing projects. To find more information about how your state or community can join the campaign, see the Resources section.

There are several other national campaigns aimed at hearing loss prevention through education. The purpose of these campaigns and others like them is to reduce noise-induced hearing loss and tinnitus by increasing awareness, shaping attitudes, and changing behaviors, particularly among school-aged children. One example is Wise Ears!, which represents a national effort to educate the public about hearing protection. It was launched by a coalition of federal and state agencies, public interest groups, businesses, industries, and unions. Another example is Dangerous Decibels, a public health partnership for the prevention of noise-induced hearing loss. The Resources section lists both websites.

Want to Contribute to a Quieter World?

Noise Free America is another national group dedicated to fighting all noise pollution, but particularly that associated with boom cars, car alarms, leaf blowers, and motorcycles with illegally loud exhaust systems ("loud pipes"). The group reports that noise levels have risen sixfold in major U.S. cities over the past 15 years. Its website offers a variety of resources, including an "Ask an Expert" section and links to other antinoise groups and resources. Some of the more interesting features on the website include a monthly "Noisy Dozen" award that recognizes major noise polluters, a large collection of boom car ads "in which electronics companies encourage boom car boys to engage in violence and misogyny," and an "I Like Noise" section that gives boom car and motorcycle fans a chance to respond to the group's antinoise message in their own words.

Noise Free America offers a "personal checklist" of suggestions for making the world quieter. Here's an adapted version:

- Don't use power leaf blowers, hedge trimmers, or weed trimmers, and don't hire a gardener who uses them.
- Don't mow your lawn before 9:00 am or after 9:00 pm.
- Don't use a keyless car entry system.
- Don't use a noisy car alarm; there are other kinds of security systems.
- Keep your car muffler in good working order.
- Avoid revving your car or motorcycle engine unnecessarily; while waiting, turn off your engine instead of idling.
- Use your car horn only in emergencies; don't announce your arrival by honking.
- Don't blast your car stereo or radio; keep your car windows closed when playing either one.

- Ride your bike or walk as much as possible.
- Use headphones when listening to music (and keep the volume low to protect your hearing).
- When you buy appliances (for example, washing machines, air conditioners, or vacuum cleaners), choose the quietest model available (some carry noise ratings).
- If you live in an apartment or condominium, keep the volume of your home entertainment (television or music) as low as possible, especially at night. Keep the bass at an extremely low level.
- Train your dog not to bark unnecessarily; never leave your dog alone for long periods.
- Warn your neighbors if you're going to be making noise. If you're having a party, invite them.
- Be considerate when using your cell phone.
- Make it known that music and televisions are not always welcome in public places and commercial establishments.
- If you own a store, restaurant, or other business, closely monitor noise levels.
- Ask local government officials for more stringent noise ordinances and to enforce existing ones.
- Ask managers of movie theaters, restaurants, stores, dance clubs, and exercise centers to turn down the volume. If you're curious about noise levels, electronics retailers offer relatively inexpensive sound-level meters.
- Treat complaints about *your* noise seriously and respectfully.
- Insist on your right to quiet and give others the same courtesy.

Tips for Preventing Noise-induced Hearing Loss

- Avoid loud noise. If you need to shout to be heard by someone an arm's length (or less) away, the noise is *too loud*.
- Turn it down. Turn down the volume on your car radio and CD player. Turn down television volume. Turn down the volume on your portable music player. If other people can hear music coming from your earphones, it's too loud. Buy a device with an automatic volume limiter.
- Limit your exposure time. When you can't avoid loud noise, make your exposure time as brief as possible.
- Give your ears a break. When you can't avoid loud noise, take breaks as often as you can (at least 5 minutes every hour). Your ears have some ability to recover from noise exposure if you give them a chance.
- Get some distance. When you can't avoid loud noise, get as far away from the source as possible (for example, stay away from the speakers at a concert).
- Protect yourself. When you can't avoid loud noise, wear adequate hearing protection and use it properly. Remember, hearing protection isn't only for

the workplace. Wear it when you mow the lawn, run the vacuum cleaner, shoot a gun, or ride a motorcycle.

- Buy better earphones. Instead of turning up the volume to overcome background noise, buy noise-blocking earphones.
- Listen to what your body is telling you. If you experience temporary hearing loss, ringing, or pain after exposure to loud noise, don't expose yourself to that much noise again. You've already done some damage to your ears.
- Don't smoke. It increases the risk of hearing loss by restricting blood flow and increasing the production of free radicals (see later discussion).
- Eat a healthy diet. A healthy diet increases antioxidants, which protect hearing against noise damage.
- Be a responsible consumer. Buy quieter products. Look for noise ratings when you buy recreational equipment, appliances, power tools, or lawn equipment. If the manufacturer doesn't provide a noise rating, ask for one. Promote labeling standards that allow consumers to "buy quiet."
- Be a responsible parent or grandparent. Look for noise ratings on toys; inspect them for noise danger just as you would inspect them for small pieces that could be swallowed. Cap guns, power horns, fireworks, model airplanes, toy vehicles with horns and sirens, walkie-talkies, musical instruments, and toys with cranks can be dangerously loud, especially at close range (remember, a child's arms are short, so she will hold toys closer to the ear). Don't allow children to participate in dangerously loud activities without hearing protection. Don't allow them to listen through earphones for prolonged periods or to blast the television volume. Teach your children to value and protect their hearing.
- Make your home a haven of quiet. Use carpeting, rugs, and window treatments to reduce noise. Place pads under noisy appliances. Don't use more than one noisy appliance at the same time. Seal doors and windows to shut out traffic noise.
- Know your hearing. Have your hearing tested annually if you're exposed to loud noise or every 3 years if you're not.
- Remember, when you make decisions about exposure to dangerous noise, consider: How loud? How long? How close?[18]

"dB Drag Racing" Can Be Hazardous to Your Hearing[19]

"dB Drag racing" is a "sport" in which the aim is to create the loudest sound possible and capture it inside a car (the ultimate in boom cars). Unimaginably loud sound is measured on a drag racing–style meter in real time, with the owner of the loudest system declared the winner. To the sport's credit, the "dB Drag Racing Creed" includes commitments to "never operate my system in a manner that will disturb those around me" and "never operate my system in a manner that could result in injury."

Stats from the 2008 "dB Drag Racing" season (9/20/07–9/18/08):
   Total Events: 552
   Average dB level: 141.9 dB (comparable to the roar of a Boeing 747 taking off at close range)
   Maximum dB level: 180.6 dB (comparable to firing a shell from an artillery piece at close range)

HEARING LOSS RESULTING FROM OTOTOXICITY

Drugs known to damage delicate hair cells within the inner ear are often used to fight life-threatening infections and cancer (see Chapter 5). Aminoglycoside antibiotics and cisplatin are two examples. Physicians use aminoglycoside antibiotics to treat serious infections because they're highly effective, and few people have developed resistance to them. Cisplatin, the most ototoxic drug in common use, is a chemotherapy agent widely used to treat cancer.[20] These and other medications have the potential to cause hearing loss, tinnitus, or vestibular (balance) dysfunction that can be temporary or permanent.

Ototoxic drugs first damage hearing at the *ultrahigh frequencies*. These frequencies (pitches) are higher than those tested during a hearing evaluation and higher than those shown on an audiogram (that is, higher than 8,000 Hz). What's important is that they're higher than the frequencies important for speech understanding (the frequencies that make up speech are *lower* than 8,000 Hz). In other words, ototoxic drugs first damage hearing at frequencies that we can afford to lose. With continued exposure, however, damage spreads to frequencies we *cannot* afford to lose. Whether (or how much) damage occurs in a given person depends on several factors, including dosage, duration of use, and method of administration. The amount of damage also depends on a person's susceptibility—what causes hearing loss in one person might not in another—and there's no way to predict who's more susceptible at the present time.

Nonetheless, there *is* an opportunity for prevention. When patients are taking potentially ototoxic drugs, their hearing should be monitored (ideally, at the ultrahigh frequencies). If a change in hearing is detected, it may be possible for the physician to switch to another drug, reduce the dose, or somehow alter treatment to prevent further loss of hearing. If treatment cannot be changed, hearing at frequencies important to speech understanding can be damaged, and the damage can be permanent. Unfortunately, this simply can't be avoided in some cases.

Whenever possible, hearing should be tested 24 hours before the first dose of a potentially ototoxic drug is given. The results of this test serve as a baseline against which future results will be compared. When preexposure testing is not practical, testing should be done as after treatment is initiated as possible (within 24 hours). Hearing should then be monitored on a regular basis (at least once or twice each week for patients receiving ototoxic antibiotics, or before each chemotherapy treatment).[21] Because ototoxic hearing loss can begin months after a drug has been discontinued, hearing should be monitored periodically for 6 to 12 months after treatment ends.

If the patient is responsive (able to raise a hand or finger, press a button, or give a verbal response), behavioral hearing thresholds can be obtained. If not, *otoacoustic emissions* (OAEs), a physiologic response produced by the cochlear hair cells (see Chapter 4), are also highly sensitive to ototoxicity and require no response from the patient. It might be possible to detect a change in OAEs before a change in behavioral thresholds is observed; however, OAEs require healthy middle ear function and relatively normal hearing (thresholds better than about 40 dB) to be useful, and this can limit their utility with someone who has a preexisting hearing loss.

If you or someone you love is treated with chemotherapy to fight cancer or with powerful antibiotics to fight infection, ask your physician if the drugs can damage hearing. If the drugs are potentially ototoxic, ask that your hearing (or that of your loved one) be closely monitored by an audiologist. It might be possible to prevent damage (or further damage) to hearing.

If you have a sensorineural hearing loss or suffer from tinnitus, always remind your doctor when new medications are prescribed. Ask if these medications have the potential to be ototoxic. Read labels and ask your pharmacist about the possible effects of over-the-counter medications on hearing (and tinnitus). Be aware of the early warning signs of ototoxicity (for example, onset or worsening of tinnitus, loss or further loss of hearing, balance problems, or a feeling of fullness in the ears), and let your doctor know immediately if you experience any of them. Never stop taking a prescribed medication without consulting your physician first, however.

FUTURE TRENDS IN HEARING RESTORATION AND HEARING LOSS PREVENTION

Hair Cell Regeneration

Aging, exposure to hazardous noise, disease, ototoxic drugs, and trauma are some of the things that can damage delicate hair cells within the cochlea. In fact, hair cell damage is responsible for nearly all permanent hearing loss. In humans, hair cells that have been destroyed are lost forever. We can't bring them back, and we can't grow new ones. The damage is irreversible. This is not true of all species, however. Just two decades ago, scientists discovered that birds are able to replace hair cells that have been damaged or destroyed. We now know that all vertebrates, except mammals, are able to regenerate hair cells.[22] In some cases, the supporting ("nonsensory") cells that surround hair cells divide, and some of the new cells become hair cells. In other cases, supporting cells transform themselves ("transdifferentiate") into new hair cells. When regrowth is adequate, the regeneration process shuts itself off, and hearing is restored. In contrast, the damaged hair cells of humans and other mammals do not replace themselves, and permanent hearing loss results.

Today, researchers are hard at work trying to learn how the regeneration process works in animals and how to make a similar process occur in humans. One promising approach involves the manipulation of specific genes. For example, scientists recently coaxed new hair cell growth in adult guinea pigs (who, like humans, are mammals) by inserting a particular gene into the cochlea. In the *developing* cochlea, this gene is found in cells that ultimately become hair cells, but it is not found in those that become other types of cells within the inner ear. Therefore, it appears that when this gene is present, it instructs developing cells to become hair cells. When it's absent, cells develop into nonsensory cells. When scientists transferred the gene into the cochleae of *mature* guinea pigs in whom hair cells had been destroyed by large doses of ototoxic drugs, nonsensory cells developed into new, immature hair cells. Subsequent studies have shown that the technique not only causes the regrowth of hair cells, it actually restores hearing in deafened adult guinea pigs. In other laboratories, scientists are taking a different approach. These scientists are working to encourage the growth of new hair cells by "turning off" genes that *prevent* regeneration. In other words, they're working to "suppress the suppressor."

Another promising line of research involves the use of stem cells in the cochlea. Unlike other cells in the body, stem cells are unspecialized and retain their ability to develop into different types of cells. Under certain conditions, they can be coaxed into becoming cells with special functions. Embryonic stem cells have the ability to develop into any type of cell, but their use is controversial and fraught with obstacles. In contrast, adult stem cells exist in many body tissues, but usually can develop into only the cell types found in their tissue of origin (for example, stem cells in the liver can only develop into new liver cells). Adult stem cells have been identified in the cochlea, and it's possible that they can be converted into hair cells. If that's actually the case, stem cells might someday play a role in the regeneration of damaged hair cells in the human cochlea.[23]

The successful regeneration of cochlear hair cells in mammals was an enormous accomplishment. Although many obstacles remain to be overcome, it's quite possible that scientists will someday use regenerative techniques to at least partially restore hearing in humans.

Otoprotective Agents

Believe it or not, scientists have come up with a pill that helps to protect hearing from damage caused by noise exposure (more about that later).

Scientists are actually studying several *otoprotective agents,* some of which are likely to receive approval from the U.S. Food and Drug Administration (FDA) long before cochlear hair cell regeneration becomes a viable treatment option. Although both areas of research hold great promise, hair cell regeneration and otoprotection are quite different. Hair cell regeneration could one day reverse some types of existing hearing loss, whereas otoprotective agents could one day *prevent* some types of hearing loss. These agents could protect hearing against the effects of harmful noise and ototoxic drugs, or prevent damage from becoming permanent if taken soon after exposure. As such, it's *possible* that otoprotective agents might one day help to prevent hearing loss in large numbers of people.

Many of the most promising otoprotective agents are actually micronutrients that are consumed as part of a healthy diet, although generally not in amounts sufficient to protect hearing against harmful noise and ototoxins. Nonetheless, because these agents are already present in the foods that we eat, they're not foreign to the human body. Some are available as nutritional supplements, but none has received FDA approval for use as a prevention or treatment for hearing loss.

In the case of noise exposure, otoprotective agents supplement rather than replace wearable hearing protection. There are situations in which noise-induced hearing loss occurs even when hearing protectors are used properly. For example, because the noise levels on the decks of aircraft carriers are so great (approximately 120–140 dB), even the best hearing protectors cannot make them safe. In other military situations, hazardous noise can occur without warning. In the future, it's likely that people exposed to extreme noise levels in any setting will be able to take an otoprotective pill in addition to wearing hearing protection. The potential applications seem almost endless: for example, otoprotective agents might be given to patients who must take ototoxic drugs to fight cancer, to members of a high school marching band, or to people who've already sustained some noise-induced hearing loss and might be exceptionally vulnerable to further damage. However, these agents will be used to *supplement* rather than replace wearable hearing protection.

Taken before exposure, these agents may prevent the hair cell damage that leads to hearing loss. However, there's also reason to believe that taking them hours (or perhaps even days) after exposure might prevent damage from becoming permanent (or at least reduce the amount of damage). This means they could be used to treat damage associated with unanticipated noise exposures such as air bag deployment, gunfire, and explosions. It's also possible that these agents could prevent or reverse damage when monitoring indicates that an ototoxic drug has begun to affect hearing.

Scientists have learned that many disorders (for example, stroke, fibromyalgia, cardiovascular disease, Parkinson's disease, Alzheimer's disease, and some forms of cancer) involve what are known as oxidative processes. Oxidation occurs when a molecule loses an electron. This "oxidated" molecule (also known as a *free radical*) is unstable until it steals an electron from another molecule. This changes the *other* molecule into a free radical, setting off a chain reaction as the process repeats itself. Aggressive free radicals steal electrons from almost any nearby molecule, often causing damage to the other molecule in the process.

Oxidation is a natural process; free radicals are produced as cells go about doing the work that cells do (routine metabolism). Our bodies are exposed to tens of thousands of free radicals every day; however, they're usually balanced by antioxidants and specialized enzymes. Antioxidants donate electrons to free radicals, stabilizing them and preventing damage to other cells. Cell damage occurs when the number of free radicals produced exceeds the number that can be neutralized.

Free radicals build up in virtually all body tissues over the course of a lifetime, causing wear and tear at the cellular level. The accumulation of damage done by free radicals over the years contributes to aging. Damage caused by free radicals also underlies some types of hearing loss, most notably hearing loss that results from aging, noise, and ototoxins. Exposure to noise or ototoxins causes the production of too many free radicals. Antioxidants come to the rescue by neutralizing free radicals. They protect or rescue hair cells, thereby reducing the harmful effects of age, noise, and ototoxic substances. The body's natural antioxidant defenses can be overwhelmed, however. Wherever there are too many free radicals—or too few antioxidants to counteract them—cells can suffer damage or die. The result could be a new wrinkle on your face, or a loss of hair cells in the cochlea.

People vary in their susceptibility to damage from noise and ototoxins. Susceptibility is due in part to a person's genetic make-up, something that can't be altered. However, a person's oxidative state at the time of exposure might also have an impact on susceptibility, and that can be influenced by lifestyle choices. For example, smoking increases the formation of free radicals, and a poor diet can result in low antioxidant levels. Both have been shown to increase the risk of noise-induced hearing loss in animal studies.

Our body's defenses against free radicals can be strengthened by eating healthy foods. As mentioned, many of the otoprotective agents being studied are antioxidants normally consumed as part of a healthy diet, although usually not in quantities sufficient to protect hearing. For example, research has shown that guinea pigs given a combination of Vitamins A, C, and E, with magnesium, were less vulnerable to noise-induced hearing loss. (Researchers at the University of Michigan have launched a start-up company, OtoMedicine, that's developing the "ACE-magnesium" combination.) Eating a healthy, well-balanced diet that includes fruits, vegetables, whole grains, nuts, low-fat dairy products, lean meat, fish, and poultry (along with some red wine or grape juice) is always a good idea and can help to protect hearing.

It's possible that our defenses against free radical damage can be further strengthened by taking certain nutritional supplements, many of them antioxidants. Animal studies have already demonstrated the ability of antioxidants to protect against noise-induced hair cell damage. For example, researchers blasted guinea pigs with noise at 115 dB for 5 hours, resulting in a hearing loss of up to 50 dB in the unprotected guinea pigs. Guinea pigs given an otoprotective agent before exposure showed only minimal hearing loss. Similarly, another otoprotective agent under study appears to protect against cisplatin- and aminoglycoside-induced ototoxicty.[24]

Nevertheless, eating huge quantities of specific foods or using dietary supplements to protect hearing is *not* recommended. Until an agent has been approved by the FDA specifically for the prevention or reversal of hearing damage, supplements should not be used for that purpose. Even if approved, the use of supplements should be discussed with a physician who is familiar with your medical history and the medications that you take. Nutritional supplements have the potential to interact with medications and create negative side effects.

Why Is Cochlear Hearing Loss Typically Greatest at the High Frequencies?

There are probably several reasons. However, scientists have observed that most oxidative damage occurs in the basal turn of the cochlea, the area responsible for high-frequency hearing. Scientists have not yet determined whether there's more oxidative stress in that area, or if the hair cells there are less able to defend themselves against it. In any case, sensory hearing loss is almost always greatest at the high frequencies.

"The Hearing Pill"

A controlled clinical trial that examined the ability of a commonly available nutritional supplement called N-acetylcysteine (NAC) to prevent noise-induced hearing loss was conducted near the end of 2004 at the Marine Corps training facility at Camp Pendleton, California.[25] NAC reduces oxidative stress by helping the body to produce antioxidants. Nearly 1,000 recruits volunteered to participate in the study for approximately 1 month during their routine training. The Marines were exposed to 300 rounds of M-16 gunfire over the course of 1 week. In addition to the standard earplugs that *all* recruits wore, approximately 600 participants also took NAC three times a day. The remaining participants were given a placebo (something that looked the same but contained no NAC). The study's design was ideal because noise exposure could be tightly controlled. There was no opportunity for participants in either group to increase their exposure with noisy recreational activities in the evening. In addition, researchers could be certain that participants were actually taking their NAC doses. Recruits received their final hearing tests 10 days after their exposure to noise was finished. Compared with the placebo, NAC reduced permanent hearing loss in the ear closest to the gunfire by about 25 percent. Additional studies are under way to determine the ideal dose.

The U.S. Navy holds the patent on the NAC formulation used in this study, but the government requires that such work be made available to the public. Accordingly, the Navy has a cooperative research and development agreement with a commercial firm that sells the compound as a hearing supplement over the Internet. No prescription is required. The supplement has not been approved by the Food and Drug Administration (FDA), nor is it undergoing review for such approval.

Other companies are also developing compounds to protect against hearing damage. In all cases, however, these compounds are meant to *supplement*, and not *replace*, hearing protectors.

Appendices

APPENDIX A

Hearing Aid Batteries

- Today, nearly all hearing aid batteries are the zinc air type. Each zinc air battery comes from the factory with a sticker on it. Removing the sticker turns the battery on. Once the battery has been activated, it continues to discharge even if the sticker is replaced.
- As long as they're stored properly and the stickers have not been removed, zinc air batteries have a shelf life of one or more years, depending on the manufacturer. Nonetheless, you should buy high-quality batteries where you know they'll be fresh.
- It's necessary to use the battery size that's correct for your hearing aid. Batteries come in standard sizes, although a given size may be labeled differently by different manufacturers. Fortunately, manufacturers use a standardized color code on their sticky tabs and packaging that makes it easy to find the correct size.
- Generally speaking, a battery costs about $1.00 (or less if purchased in quantity) and will last anywhere from a few days (CIC) to a few weeks (BTE). This may sound like a short life compared to something like a watch battery; however, a hearing aid performs far more work than a watch and therefore requires more power. Battery life depends on the power of the hearing aid, the size of the battery, the type of circuitry in the hearing aid, the volume setting at which the aid is worn, the number of hours the aid is worn each day, and environmental conditions such as temperature and humidity.
- Batteries should be stored at room temperature. Heat and cold shorten battery life.
- Batteries should be stored in a dry place—not in the refrigerator. Cold, moist air from the refrigerator can cause condensation to form under the sticker, and that can cause the battery to discharge before you're ready to use it.
- Don't carry batteries in a purse or pocket where they might contact metal objects like keys, coins, or other batteries. This could cause a battery to discharge,

leak, or even rupture. Keep new batteries in their original packaging until needed.

- Because hearing aid batteries are small, they can be difficult to see and handle. Look for packages that dispense one battery at a time, or batteries with longer sticky tabs that make them easier to use.
- Batteries are harmful if swallowed, so they must be kept away from infants, children, pets, and people with poor eyesight who might mistake them for pills. If a battery is swallowed, consult the National Button Battery Hotline at 202-625-3333 (collect calls accepted). Your physician or emergency room staff may also wish to call this number.
- Batteries that have been fully discharged can be disposed of in your regular trash, but be sure to discard them where they can't be found by infants, children, or pets.

APPENDIX B

Hearing Aid Drying Kits (Dehumidifiers)

Moisture of any type is harmful to hearing aids and can result in expensive repairs (or worse). Sources of moisture include perspiration and humidity, as well as accidental dips in the pool and unexpected downpours. Storing your hearing aids in a dehumidifier when they're not in use improves their performance and prolongs their life. Simple, inexpensive dehumidifiers typically consist of silica crystals (or another desiccant) in an airtight container. Hearing aids are placed in the container, and the crystals absorb the moisture that has accumulated in them. After many uses, the crystals become saturated with moisture, and this is signaled by a change in their color. The crystals can usually be reactivated by heating them in an oven.

You may want to consider investing in an electronic dehumidifier. These offer features like a desiccant that absorbs moisture and dries earwax, germicidal lights that disinfect and sanitize, and fans that circulate warm air to dry the hearing aid's components. Batteries should also go into the dehumidifier, because removing moisture from a battery can extend its life a bit. Of course, electronic dehumidifiers cost more than the simple, nonelectronic versions.

APPENDIX C

The International Symbol of Access for Hearing Loss

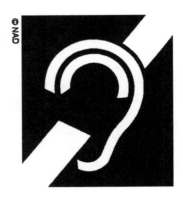

Figure AC.1. The International Symbol of Access for Hearing Loss.

This symbol identifies locations where communication access for people with hearing loss is provided. For example, it's used to identify public TTYs or telephones that have amplification, and meeting rooms, theatres, and churches that have assistive listening systems.

APPENDIX D

Care and Maintenance of Hearing Aids

CARE AND MAINTENANCE OF BEHIND-THE-EAR (BTE) HEARING AIDS

A BTE hearing aid attaches to a custom earmold that holds the aid on the ear and directs amplified sound into the ear canal (see Chapter 7). The earmold should fit snugly but comfortably.

- Your BTE hearing aid should be wiped off each day with a soft, dry cloth (never use anything damp).
- Check for earwax in the earmold's sound bore (the hole where the sound comes out) each morning. Waiting until morning allows the wax to harden a bit, making it easier to remove. If the wax is close to the surface, gently lift or brush it out using the wax removal tool from your audiologist. Be careful not to push the wax farther into the earmold (to prevent wax from going in rather than coming out, try holding the earmold upside down over a soft surface while cleaning it).
- The earmold itself should be cleaned each day using a disinfectant recommended by your audiologist (for example, a disinfectant towelette made especially for hearing aids). Do *not* use alcohol, because it can ruin the earmold's surface. If you do not use a disinfectant, you should regularly remove the earmold from the hearing aid and wash it (but discuss this with your audiologist first). To remove the earmold, grasp the earhook of the hearing aid (rather than the hearing aid itself) with one hand and *gently* twist the earmold tubing off the earhook with the other. Do *not* separate the tubing from the earmold or the earhook from the hearing aid. Once the earmold has been disconnected from the hearing aid, wash the earmold (but not the hearing aid!) with soap and warm (not hot) water. Be sure the tubing and earmold are completely dry before reattaching them to the earhook of the hearing aid. To be sure, blow through the tubing or, better yet, use a rubber bulb to squeeze air through it (a tool like this can be obtained by

your audiologist). When you reattach the earmold, be sure to orient it in the correct direction relative to the hearing aid. (Holding it in your hand, assume that you're looking at your head and the earmold from the rear. Envision the long [canal] portion of the earmold pointing toward your ear canal, and the hearing aid going behind your ear.) If you wear two hearing aids, it's a good idea to wash, dry, and reattach the earmolds one at a time so you don't confuse them.

- When your earmold tubing becomes hard, cracked, or stretched, it must be replaced by your audiologist; check daily to be sure it's in good condition and doesn't contain droplets of moisture.
- Some of the new BTEs used with open canal fittings have a slim tube attached to a tiny eartip that delivers sound into the ear canal. Both the tube and eartip need to be cleaned daily. The tube (and the eartip attached to it) should be removed from the hearing aid and wiped with a damp cloth. A cleaning rod or reamer should be used to push wax and debris all the way through the tube. Be cautious about using water, because it may become trapped inside the tube.

CARE AND MAINTENANCE OF CUSTOM HEARING AIDS

There are no separate earmolds with "custom" hearing aids: in-the-ear (ITE), in-the-canal (ITC), and completely-in-the-canal (CIC) hearing aids (see Chapter 7). With these styles, the hearing aid itself fits into the ear. Like earmolds, custom hearing aids should fit snugly but should not be uncomfortable.

- Each day, you should clean your hearing aids with a disinfectant recommended by your audiologist. Do not use alcohol, and *never* get them wet.
- Check for earwax in the microphone and sound bore (the hole where the sound comes out) each morning. Earwax is a constant problem with custom hearing aids and *the* major reason for repairs. Waiting until morning allows the wax to harden a bit, making it easier to remove. If the wax is close to the surface, gently lift or brush it out using the wax removal tool from your audiologist. Be careful not to push the wax farther into the hearing aid (to prevent wax from going in rather than coming out, try holding the aid upside down over a soft surface while cleaning it).
- Ask your audiologist about the advisability of using a guard to protect your hearing aid from wax.

APPENDIX E

Troubleshooting Hearing Aid Problems

If your hearing aid isn't working properly, try these things before calling your audiologist (it could save you time and money):

- Read the information that came with your hearing aid; there might be a simple solution to the problem.
- If your hearing aid or battery is very cold or very hot, allow it to return to room temperature.
- Try a fresh battery. Be sure the battery is the right size for your hearing aid and that you have inserted it correctly (usually, the + side goes up). If you're uncertain about the status of your batteries, invest in an inexpensive battery tester (see your audiologist). Properly dispose of old batteries so they don't get mixed up with new ones.
- Be sure the battery compartment door is completely closed (but don't force it).
- If your hearing aid has an on/off switch, be sure it's turned on. Some hearing aids have an M/T/O switch. In this case, M means microphone, T means telephone, and O means off. Unless you're using the telephone, the switch should be in the M position.
- If your hearing aid has a volume control, be sure it's set properly. Generally, the volume should not be set at full-on.
- If your hearing aid has a button that allows you to switch programs, be sure you have selected the correct program.
- Using a magnifying glass and a bright light, look for wax in the sound bore (the hole where the sound comes out) of the hearing aid or earmold. If you see wax, carefully remove it with your wax removal tool.
- Similarly, check for wax in the microphone opening.
- Remove excess wax from your ear canals. Too much wax can cause hearing aids to whistle, amplification to seem weak, or your voice to sound hollow. You can

remove wax with an over-the-counter product designed to soften it, but consult your physician first.

- Check the earmold tubing (if you have a BTE) for moisture. When warm air from inside your ear reaches the outside where it's cooler, water vapor condenses and can collect in the tubing. Remove the earmold from the hearing aid and blow the moisture out.
- If the tubing has become hard or cracked, have it replaced (see Appendix C).
- Check to be sure the tubing isn't being twisted when you position the hearing aid behind your hear.
- Check to be sure the hearing aid or earmold is sitting in your ear properly. An improperly inserted hearing aid/earmold will reduce the amplification that reaches your ear.
- Check to be sure that you aren't trying to put the right hearing aid (or earmold) into the left ear or vice versa.
- Use a dehumidifying kit to remove any moisture from the hearing aid (see Appendix B).
- Check the battery contacts for corrosion; if the contacts look dirty or corroded, gently clean them with a cotton swab and a tiny bit of alcohol (but *not* enough to get the hearing aid wet).
- If feedback is the problem, try to determine its cause. Hearing aids whistle temporarily when something (like your hand) covers them, trapping amplified sound and causing it to be reamplified. Persistent feedback, however, can suggest that the hearing aid (or earmold) no longer fits or isn't inserted properly. Remove the hearing aid (or earmold) from your ear and place your finger tightly over the sound bore. If the feedback stops, fit or insertion is the likely problem. If the feedback continues, the hearing aid itself might need repair. Feedback can also mean the hearing aid's volume is set too high, the ear canal is plugged with wax, or there's a problem with the earmold tubing (it's cracked, blocked by earwax, or contains moisture).

If you try these things and the hearing aid still isn't working, call your audiologist. Do not attempt to make repairs yourself; that could violate the hearing aid's warranty.

APPENDIX F

Speechreading

TIPS FOR IMPROVING SPEECHREADING WHEN YOU ARE THE LISTENER

- Face the speaker and get as close as possible (3–6 feet is usually ideal).
- Look directly at the speaker; watch her lips, facial expressions, gestures, and body language.
- Be sure the light is on the speaker's face rather than behind him.
- Tell the speaker what she can do to help you speechread, and be specific.
- Ask for the topic, and ask the speaker to let you know when the topic changes.
- When conversing with several people, ask each of them to signal (by nodding or raising a finger, for example) when they begin to speak. This will help you to locate the person who is speaking more quickly.
- Don't try to get every word; instead, try to relax and get the gist of the message (words or phrases that come later may help to clarify things you missed earlier).
- When you miss something, ask the speaker to rephrase rather than repeat.
- Stay abreast of current events; this improves your ability to benefit from context.
- Wear your hearing aids; it will improve your ability to speechread. There's a synergistic relationship between hearing ability and speechreading ability; the ability to hear improves the ability to speechread and vice versa. Interestingly, many of the sounds that are hardest to hear (for example, weak, high-frequency consonants like /s/, /f/, and /th/) are easiest to see, whereas many of the sounds that are hardest to see (for example, more powerful, low-frequency vowels) are easiest to hear. This is one of the ways in which hearing and speechreading complement one another.
- Take breaks as needed (this is hard work!).

ADDITIONAL TIPS FOR IMPROVING SPEECHREADING WHEN YOU ARE THE SPEAKER

- Look directly at the listener.
- Don't begin speaking until the listener is looking at you.
- Don't obscure your face with your hands, the newspaper, or other objects.
- Don't eat, chew, or smoke while talking.
- Don't turn away while talking.
- Don't exaggerate lip movements, talk too fast, or shout.

APPENDIX G

The Listening and Communication Enhancement (LACE) Program

To communicate effectively, you must have good listening skills, be able to process speech rapidly, and have the ability to remember what you hear (auditory memory). These abilities can be degraded by hearing loss and the natural aging process. LACE is a computer training program designed to strengthen those abilities through auditory training. Just as physical therapy can strengthen muscles to compensate for physical weakness or injury, LACE can strengthen skills and strategies to compensate for hearing loss. The program requires 30 minutes of training each day, 5 days a week, for 4 weeks. It's home based, self-paced, and interactive. It's intended to supplement rather than replace the counseling you receive from your audiologist.

The auditory training exercises are designed to improve your auditory memory, the speed at which you process information, your understanding of speech when several people are talking, and your ability to use contextual cues. In addition, LACE provides information about hearing loss and offers communication tips for you and the people with whom you interact. It helps train the brain to fill in the gaps that occur even *with* hearing aids and demonstrates that it's possible to comprehend a message without understanding every word. The program is designed to help you feel more confident about what you *think* you heard.

LACE training is adaptive, meaning that it's never too difficult on too easy (when a response is correct, the next item will be slightly more difficult; when a response is incorrect, the next item will be slightly less difficult). In other words, training intensifies as skills improve. The user receives feedback after each response and at the end of each session; the information is transmitted confidentially to the audiologist.

In a 2007 study that tracked 625 people who bought new hearing aids during a 6-month period, users who used LACE were four times more likely to be satisfied with their hearing aids than those who did not. Statistical analysis indicated that there were no significant differences between the two groups other than LACE participation.[1]

LACE runs on almost any version of Microsoft Windows and can also be used on an Apple Macintosh (Mac) computer. It's designed for computer novices.

APPENDIX H

Communicating When You Are Not at Home

IMPROVING YOUR ABILITY TO FUNCTION IN THE WORKPLACE

- Wear hearing aids that are up to date and in good working order; wear two hearing aids if that's what your audiologist recommends and you can afford it.
- Be assertive about your needs; ask your employer for appropriate accommodations. For example
  - Move your work to a quieter area, or make your work area more quiet (avoid photocopiers, heating/cooling systems, busy areas where people congregate to talk, and other sources of noise).
  - Use a telephone with an amplifier or a text telephone.
  - Use flashing lights or vibration to signal fire, the telephone ringing, or the end of machine cycles.
  - Use an assistive listening device at meetings; ask for important information to be conveyed in writing.
- Explain your hearing loss to supervisors and coworkers. Give them specific suggestions about how they can help you (for example, by getting your attention before they speak, speaking clearly, moving closer and facing you, speaking one at a time, minimizing background noise, and using email instead of the phone to convey information).
- Help your coworkers to understand that hearing aids help, but they don't make hearing normal; explain that speechreading also has limitations, and that hearing is more difficult in some situations than others.
- Because functioning with a hearing loss can be hard work
  - Schedule less demanding tasks between more demanding ones
  - Keep difficult situations and difficult people in perspective; give people the benefit of the doubt
  - Keep your self-confidence and your sense of humor!

IMPROVING HEARING IN THE CAR

- Turn off the radio or CD player.
- Close the windows to minimize traffic and wind noise.
- If you have a better ear, sit with it facing the center of the car.
- If you wear two hearing aids, reduce the volume on the one closest to the window.
- Invest in an assistive listening device.

IMPROVING HEARING IN RESTAURANTS

Restaurants pose special problems for people with hearing loss (and sometimes for people with normal hearing). Noise is a common complaint, ranking close to poor service. A noise rating system would be helpful, but until that happens, here are a few tips for making dining out more pleasurable:

- Whenever possible, choose restaurants with less noise and good acoustics.
- Restaurants with low ceilings, carpeting, tablecloths, fabric-covered furniture, and window treatments made of soft materials are likely to be less noisy.
- Smaller restaurants with fewer tables, or restaurants with tables arranged in several small rooms rather than one large one, are likely to be quieter. In general, more upscale restaurants tend to be less noisy.
- Look for places that do not play recorded background music, and definitely avoid those with live entertainment if you want to have conversation. If recorded music is playing, explain your problem to the manager and ask her to turn it off while you're dining (be assertive!). Be aware that you are not alone; the disturbance caused by recorded music is a common complaint among diners.
- Choose to dine before or after the crowd; restaurants are quieter when they are not busy.
- Call ahead and request a "quiet" table in a well-lit area (away from the restaurant's entrance, bar, kitchen, fountain, heating/cooling system, and sound system speakers).
- Ask for a booth or a table in a corner, rather than in the middle of the room.
- If you have directional microphones on your hearing aids, sit with the background noise behind you. If you do not have directional microphones, it's usually best to sit with your back to the wall (to minimize noise coming from behind).
- At the table, position yourself where you can hear and see best (for example, sit with your better ear directed toward the conversation, do not look into light coming from a window, and so forth).
- Dining with a group is challenging; if possible, choose a round table rather than a rectangular one so you can see the faces of your companions. Ask your companions to speak one at a time.
- Look for a restaurant with adequate lighting to facilitate speechreading.
- Move tall objects (flowers, candles, menus) that obscure your view of others.
- Read the specials as you come in, rather than relying on your ability to hear the waiter when he describes them (or ask for them in writing at your table).

- Read the menu carefully so that you can anticipate the choices you will be asked to make (for example, if you must choose a salad dressing, read the list of alternatives ahead of time).
- Consider investing in an assistive listening device (for example, a personal FM system).
- Let your dining companions know what they need to do to help you understand them (be assertive!).

IMPROVING HEARING IN AUDITORIUMS, THEATERS, OR MEETING ROOMS

- Contact the facility ahead of time to ask if it has an assistive listening system for its patrons who are hard of hearing. Most public facilities are required by law to provide such a system at no charge.
- If the facility does not have a system, ask why. If you believe the law requires a system, let them know. To find out, read the Public Accommodations section of the "ADA Questions and Answers" brochure available at www.ADA.gov/publicat.htm, or call the ADA Information Line at 1-800-514-0301. Make suggestions about what you find most helpful at other facilities. Volunteer to help as a "consumer consultant."
- If an assistive listening system is available, become familiar with it. Make arrangements to meet with someone knowledgeable, preferably the person responsible for the system. Other employees may have little or no experience with it (in some cases, even the person who has been assigned responsibility for it has limited experience).
- When it's not possible to visit the facility ahead of time, arrive early. Inquire at the ticket window or look for the "International Symbol of Access for Hearing Loss," which will direct you to the facility's assistive listening system (see Appendix C).
- If you are *not* using the assistive listening system, arriving early gives you time to find a seat where you can see *and* hear best, for example, away from background noise, as close to the speaker(s) as possible, with your better ear directed toward the speaker(s), with your back to the light source, etc.
- Learn as much as possible about the program that you are attending ahead of time.

IMPROVING HEARING IN PLACES OF WORSHIP

- If your place of worship does not have an assistive listening system, ask for one (consider volunteering to do the research); the system should work in all rooms where people communicate.
- If there's already a system in place, volunteer to help maintain it, make others aware of it, and teach others how to use it.
- Ask all speakers to use the system at all times.
- If it's not possible to get an assistive listening system that everyone can use, consider buying an assistive listening device for your own use.
- Sit as close to the front as possible.

- Sit with a friend who can tell you about announcements or changes that are not printed in the bulletin or program.
- Ask for a copy of the sermon/homily/message ahead of time.

IMPROVING HEARING DURING TRAVEL

- When making hotel reservations, request accommodations for your hearing loss. In the United States, hotels with more than five rooms are legally obligated to provide minimal accommodations in at least some of their rooms. Accommodations may include an amplified telephone, a TTY, alerting devices, and so forth.
- Use closed captions on your television to avoid disturbing other guests.
- Invest in an assistive listening device (for example, a personal FM system or a personal communicator) for car travel.
- When traveling by airplane, ask someone working at the gate to let you know about changes announced over the PA system. Ask someone sitting near you to do the same. On the plane, tell the flight attendant and your seatmate that you may be unable to hear announcements.
- Invest in an assistive listening device for guided tours and activities; sit or stand as close to the guide as possible; ask for information in writing ahead of time.
- In case of emergency, carry a card (available from the Hearing Loss Association of America) explaining your hearing problem.

IMPROVING HEARING DURING HOSPITAL STAYS

A hospital stay can be especially difficult for a patient with hearing loss. Some of the reasons include

- At best, you're not feeling well (and at worst, you could be gravely ill).
- You may not be wearing your hearing aids (you may not feel well enough to put them on or they may whistle when you lie down).
- To make matters worse, you may not be wearing your eyeglasses either.
- Hospital rooms are filled with hard surfaces, making the acoustics poor.
- People tend to speak in low voices so that they don't disturb other patients.
- Hospitals have become very noisy places. According to researchers at Johns Hopkins University, between 1960 and 2006, average noise levels rose from 57 dB to 72 dB during the day and from 42 dB to 60 dB in the evening.[1]
- You may be awakened at all hours by well-meaning nurses and aides who sometimes talk in the dark, with their faces turned away, or while wearing masks.
- Nurses may use the intercom to respond to the call button, making it difficult for you to understand.
- You may be unable to hear the telephone or television (at least without disturbing others).
- If you are unable to hear a knock on a closed door, your privacy may be invaded.
- You may feel anxious about missing instructions or announcements.
- You may have difficulty understanding your doctor, whose visit may be very brief and who might use terms that are unfamiliar to you.

Here are a few things that can help:

- Whenever possible, inform hospital staff about your hearing problem ahead of time; of course, you will need to remind them when you arrive.
- Let hospital staff know that you may have trouble understanding when you're not wearing your hearing aids, if personnel are wearing masks, or when messages come over the intercom. Tell them how they should communicate with you. For example, ask to have important information provided in writing.
- By law, hospitals must provide accommodations (at no charge) that enable people with hearing loss to communicate with doctors, nurses, and other personnel (private practitioners are obligated to do the same). Explain the type of accommodations that will be helpful (for example, a personal communication device, an amplified telephone with visual alert, or a personal FM device).
- Ask that the International Symbol of Access for Hearing Loss be posted on your door and in your medical records to indicate that you have a hearing loss (see Appendix C).
- Store your hearing aids safely to guard against loss or damage.

Appendix I

Sound Levels of Recreational, Occupational, and Military Noise Sources

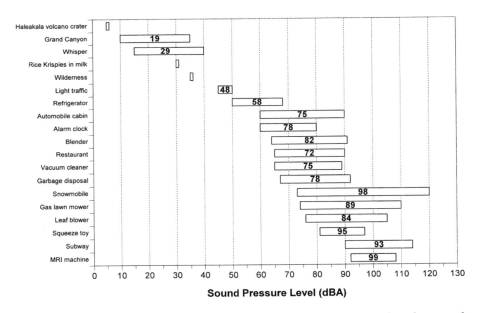

Figure AI.1. Means and Ranges for Sound Levels of Recreational and Natural Noise Sources. (From the Noise Navigator Database; with permission from Elliott Berger, Senior Scientist, Auditory Research, E-A-R/Aearo Technologies.)

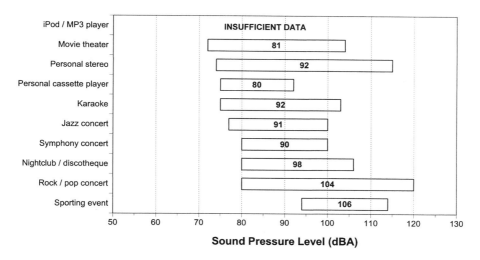

Figure AI.2. Means and Ranges for Sound Levels of Entertainment Noise Sources. (From the Noise Navigator Database; with permission from Elliott Berger, Senior Scientist, Auditory Research, E-A-R/Aearo Technologies.)

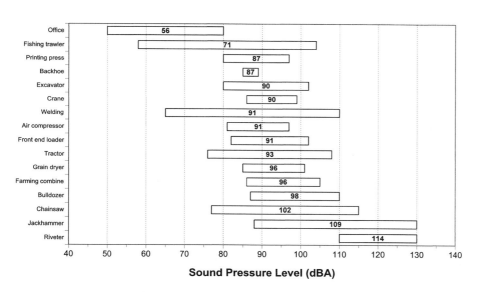

Figure AI.3. Means and Ranges for Sound Levels of Occupational Noise Sources. (From the Noise Navigator Database; with permission from Elliott Berger, Senior Scientist, Auditory Research, E-A-R/Aearo Technologies.)

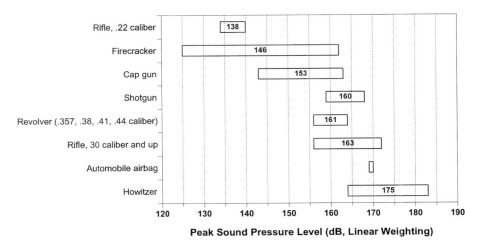

Figure AI.4. Means and Ranges for Sound Levels of Common Weapons and Explosive Devices. (From the Noise Navigator Database; with permission from Elliott Berger, Senior Scientist, Auditory Research, E-A-R/Aearo Technologies.)

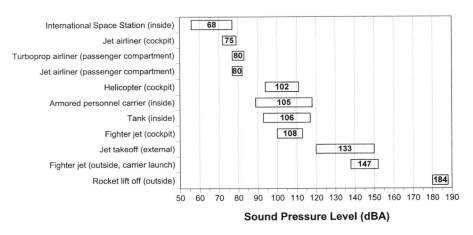

Figure AI.5. Means and Ranges for Sound Levels of Military Equipment and Aircraft. (From the Noise Navigator Database; with permission from Elliott Berger, Senior Scientist, Auditory Research, E-A-R/Aearo Technologies.)

Notes

CHAPTER 2

1. Nance, W. E. and Dodson, K. "Relevance of Genetics to Audiology," *Audiology Today* 19, no. 5 (2007): 18–27.

2. Love, J. K. *Helen Keller in Scotland: A Personal Record Written by Herself* (London: Methuen & Company, 1933), 68.

3. See Love, p. 68.

4. Ramsdell, D. A. "The Psychology of the Hard-of-Hearing and Deafened Adult," in *Hearing and Deafness* 4th ed., Davis, H. and Silverman, S. R. (eds.) (New York: Holt, Rinehart and Winston, 1978), 499–510.

5. Kochkin, S. and Rogin, C. M. "Quantifying the Obvious: The Impact of Hearing Aids on Quality of Life," *The Hearing Review* 7, no. 1 (2000): 8–34.

6. Hnath Chisolm, T., Johnson, C. E., Danhauer, J. L, Portz, L. J. P., Abrams, H. B., Lesner, S., McCarthy, P. A., and Newman, C. W. "A Systematic Review of Health-related Quality of Life and Hearing Aids: Final Report of the American Academy of Audiology Task Force on the Health-related Benefits of Amplification in Adults," *Journal of the American Academy of Audiology* 18, no. 2 (2007): 151–183.

7. See Hnath Chisolm et al.

8. See Kochkin and Rogin.

9. Kochkin, S. *The Impact of Untreated Hearing Loss on Household Income* (Alexandria, VA: Better Hearing Institute, 2007). Available at http://www.betterhearing.org/research/.

10. Kübler-Ross, E. *On Death and Dying* (Riverside, NJ: Simon and Schuster, 1977).

11. Kochkin, S. "Publications—Quotes," BHI, http://www.betterhearing.org/research/quotes.cfm.

12. American Speech-Language-Hearing Association. "Hearing Aids for Adults," ASHA, http://www.asha.org/public/hearing/treatment/adult_aid. html.

CHAPTER 4

1. U. S. Food and Drug Administration. "Hearing Aid Devices: Professional and Patient Labeling and Conditions for Sale," *Federal Register* 42, no. 31 (1977): 9286–9297.
2. Kochkin, S. "MarkeTrak VII: Hearing Loss Population Tops 31 Million," *Hearing Review* 12, no. 7 (2005): 16–29.
3. Bess, F. H. and Tharpe, A. M. "Unilateral Hearing Impairment in Children," *Pediatrics* 74, no. 2 (1984): 206–216.

CHAPTER 5

1. American Academy of Otolaryngology—Head and Neck Surgery. "Why Do Ears Itch?" AAO-HNS, http://www. entnet.org/HealthInformation/ swimmersEar.cfm.
2. Nance, W. E. and Dodson, K. "Relevance of Genetics to Audiology," *Audiology Today* 19, no. 5 (2007): 18–27.
3. Rosen, S., Bergman, M., Plester, D., El-Mofty, A., and Satti, M. "Presbycusis Study of a Relatively Noise-Free Population in the Sudan," *Annals of Otology, Rhinology and Otolaryngology* 71 (1962): 727–743.
4. Hain, T. C. "Ototoxic Medications," http://www.dizziness-and-balance. com/ disorders/bilat/ototoxins.html.

CHAPTER 6

1. Audiology Awareness Campaign. "Tinnitus," AAC, http://www.audiology awareness.com/hearinfo_tinnitus.asp.
2. Sinopoli, T., Davis P. B., and Hanley, P. "Tinnitus: Addressing Neurological, Audiological, and Psychological Aspects with Customized Therapy," *The Hearing Review* 14, no. 9 (2007): 32–35.
3. McKenna, L. and Andersson, G. "Changing Reactions to Tinnitus," *The Hearing Review* 14, no. 9 (2007); 12–21.
4. Foehl, A. "New Ratings Proposed for Veterans' TBI," *The ASHA Leader* 13, no. 3 (2008): 1, 4, 6.
5. See Foehl.
6. Dupriest, J. "Tinnitus Research Escalates," *Advance for Audiologists* 10, no. 1 (2008): 73–74.

CHAPTER 7

1. American Academy of Audiology. "Hearing Aid FAQs," AAA, http://www. audiology.org/aboutaudiology/consumered/guides/hearingaids.htm.
2. VIP Notes. "Oticon Sets New Hearing Aid Distribution Guidelines," *Advance for Audiologists* 10, no. 1 (2008): 16.

3. Ross, M. "Premium Digital Hearing Aids," *Hearing Loss Magazine* 29, no. 2 (2008): 22–25.

4. Johnson, E. E. "Survey Finds Higher Sales and Prices, Plus More Open Fittings and Directional Mics," *The Hearing Journal* 60, no. 4 (2007): 52–58.

5. Audiology Awareness Campaign. "Hearing Aid Warranties," AAC, http://www.audiologyawareness.com/ha_warranty.asp.

6. Nabelek, A. K., Tucker, F. M., and Letowski, T. R. "Toleration of Background Noises: Relationship with Patterns of Hearing Aid Use by Elderly Persons," *Journal of Speech and Hearing Research* 34 (1991): 679–685.

CHAPTER 8

1. Miller, M. H. "Auditory Nerve Implant May Deliver a Wide Range of Sounds," *The Hearing Review* (July 2007): 60–62.

2. SHHH (now the Hearing Loss Association of America). "Questions for Adults to Ask the Surgeon When Being Evaluated for a Cochlear Implant" (consumer booklet).

3. SHHH (now the Hearing Loss Association of America). "Cochlear Implants: When Hearing Aids Aren't Enough" (consumer booklet).

CHAPTER 9

1. Ross, M. "Supplement Your Hearing Aids with Hearing Assistive Technologies (HAT)," *Hearing Loss Magazine* (Nov/Dec 2006).

2. Myers, D. G. "In a Looped America, Hearing Aids Would Be Twice as Valuable," *The Hearing Journal* 59, no. 5 (2006): 17.

3. See Myers, pp. 17–22.

4. Myers, D. G. "Let's Loop America," http://www. hearingloop.org.

5. Dybala, P. D. "ELVAS Sightings—Hearing Aid or Headset?" Audiology Online, Article 1542 from http://www. audiologyonline.com (2006).

6. Dybala, P. D. "ELVAS Sightings: Cochlear Implants and Hearing Aids Get Wired," *The Hearing Journal* 59, no. 3 (2006): 10–15.

7. See Dybala, *The Hearing Journal*.

8. See Dybala, Audiology Online.

9. See Dybala, Audiology Online.

10. Linke-Ellis, N. "Going to Captioned Movies," *Hearing Loss Magazine* (Jan/Feb 2008): 15–17.

11. Bruck, D. and Thomas, I. "Waking Effectiveness of Alarms (Auditory, Visual and Tactile) for Adults Who Are Hard of Hearing," Report for the Fire Protection Research Foundation for the 2006–2007 U.S. Fire Administration Grant (2007).

CHAPTER 10

1. McSpaden, J. B. "Open Letter to Patients: Hard Truths and 'Straight Talk' on Hearing Better," *The Hearing Review* 15 no. 2 (2008): 32.

2. Sweetow, R. W. and Henderson Sabes, J. "The Need for Development of an Adaptive Listening and Communication Enhancement (LACE)

Program," *Journal of the American Academy of Audiology* 17 (2006): 538–558.

3. Tye-Murray, N. *Foundations of Aural Rehabilitation: Children, Adults, and Their Family Members* 2nd ed. (Clifton Park, NY: Thomson Delmar Learning, 2004), 41–80.

4. See Tye-Murray.

5. Cassie, R., McNutt Campbell, M., Frenette, W. L., Scott, L., Howell, I., and Roy, A. "Clear Speech for Adults with a Hearing Loss: Does Intervention with Communication Partners Make a Difference?" *Journal of the American Academy of Audiology* 16 (2005): 157–171.

6. Greer Clark, J. and English, K. *Counseling in Audiologic Practice* (Boston: Allyn and Bacon, 2004), 202.

CHAPTER 11

1. Sherman, B. D. "Losing Your Ears to Music: The Hearing Loss Epidemic and Musicians," *Early Music America* (2000). Available at http://www.bsherman.org/hearingloss.htm.

2. National Institute for Occupational Safety and Health (NIOSH). "Criteria for a Recommended Standard: Occupational Noise Exposure—Revised Criteria," Publication No. 98-126 (Cincinnati: NIOSH, 1998). Available at http://www.cdc/gov/niosh/docs/98-126/chap1.html.

3. American Speech-Language-Hearing Association. "Squealing Pigs a Noise Hazard," *The ASHA Leader* (July 12, 2005): 5.

4. Occupational Safety and Health Administration (OSHA). "Occupational Noise Exposure: Hearing Conservation Amendment; Final Rule," *Federal Register* 48 (1983): 9738–9785.

5. Kirkwood, D. H. "Largest Gathering of Audiologists Ever Brings a New Rap Home from Denver," *The Hearing Journal* 60, no. 6 (2007): 42–52.

6. Lipscomb, D. M. "An Exercise in Futility: Frustrations of a Hearing Conservationist (A Historical Review and Summary of Hearing Conservation Issues)," Audiology Online, www.audiologyonline.com/articles/article_detail.asp?article_id=1371.

7. Battat, B. "From the Executive Director's Desk," *Hearing Loss Magazine* (May/June 2008): 6.

8. Helfer, T. M., Jordan, N. N., and Lee, R. B. "Postdeployment Hearing Loss in U. S. Army Soldiers Seen at Audiology Clinics From April 1, 2003, through March 31, 2004," *American Journal of Audiology* 14 (2005): 161–168.

9. American Speech-Language-Hearing Association. "Hearing Loss Rises among U. S. Soldiers in Iraq," *The ASHA Leader* 11, no. 4 (2006): 5, 19.

10. Bloom, S. "New Hearing Conservation Initiatives: Small Steps with Great Potential," *The Hearing Journal* 59 (2006): 23–30.

11. Portnuff, C. D. F. and Fligor, B. J. "Sound Output Levels of the iPod and Other MP3 Players: Is There Potential Risk to Hearing?" (Paper presented at Hearing Loss in Children at Work and Play conference, Cincinnati, Ohio, October 19, 2006).

12. Fligor, B. J. "Hearing Loss and iPods: What Happens When You Turn Them to 11?" *The Hearing Journal* 60, no. 10 (2007): 10–16.

13. See Fligor.

14. Naquin Shafer, D. "Hearing Protection Proposed for UNGC Music Students," *The ASHA Leader* 11, no. 4 (2006): 11.

15. The Right to Quiet Society. Home page, http://www. quiet.org.

16. The American Speech-Language-Hearing Association. "Noise and Hearing Loss," ASHA, http://www.asha.org/public/hearing/disorders/noise.htm.

17. City of New York, Office of the Mayor. "Mayor Bloomberg Calls on City Council to Pass Noise Code," www.nyc.gov/portal/site/nycgov/menuitem. c0935b9a57bb4ef3daf2f1c701c789a0/index.jsp?pageID=mayor_press_release &catID=1194&doc_name=http%3A%2F%2Fwww.nyc.gov%2Fhtml%2Fom% 2Fhtml%2F2005b%2Fpr320-05.html&cc=unused1978&rc=1194&ndi=1.

18. National Institute on Deafness and Other Communication Disorders. "Crank it *Down*," NIDCD, http://www.nidcd.nih.gov/health/inside/sum06/ pg1.asp.

19. dB Drag Racing: Car Stereo Competition. Home page, http//:www.termpro. com/dbdrag/.

20. Campbell, K. C. M., Larsen, D. L., Meech, R. P., Rybak, L. P., and Hughes, L. F. "Glutathione Ester But Not Glutathione Protects against Cisplatin-induced Ototoxicity in a Rat Model," *Journal of the American Academy of Audiology* 14, no. 3 (2003): 124–133.

21. Konrad-Martin, D., Helt, W. J., Reavis, K. M., Gordon, J. S., Coleman, L. L., Bratt, G. W., and Fausti, S. A. "Otoxoxicity: Early Detection and Monitoring," *The ASHA Leader* (May 24, 2005): 1, 11–14.

22. Rubel, E. W. "Promising Research on Hair Cell Regeneration," *The Hearing Review* (October 2004). Available at http://www.hearingreview.com/ issues/articles/2004-10_01.asp.

23. Lonsbury-Martin, B. "Advances in Audiology Research: An Overivew," *The ASHA Leader* 11, no. 4 (2006): 1, 15, 22.

24. Campbell, K. C. M., Kelly, E., Targovnik, N., Hughes, L., Van Saders, C., Bendix Gottlieb, A., Dorr, M. B., and Leighton, A. "Audiologic Monitoring for Potential Ototoxicity in a Phase I Clinical Trial of a New Glycopeptide Antibiotic," *Journal of the American Academy of Audiology* 14 (2003): 157–168.

25. Naquin Shafer, D. "A Magic Pill? Compound Could Mediate Noise-induced Hearing Loss," *The ASHA Leader* (June 14, 2005): 5, 30.

APPENDIX G

1. Martin, M. "Software-based Auditory Training Program Found to Reduce Hearing Aid Return Rate," *The Hearing Journal* 60, no. 8 (2007): 32–35.

APPENDIX H

1. American Speech-Language-Hearing Association. "Hospital Noise Stresses Patients and Staff," *ASHA Leader* 11, no. 3 (2006): 6.

Resources

Some of the entries in this section are companies that sell products. Inclusion does not imply endorsement, nor does it imply preference over those that have not been included. The contact information listed here was current as of October 2008.

Professional Associations (and sources of consumer information)

American Academy of Audiology (AAA)
11730 Plaza America Drive, Suite 300
Reston, VA, 20190
Voice Telephone: (703) 790-8466; Toll-free: (800) 222-2336
TTY: (703) 790-8466
Fax: (703) 790-8631
E-mail: info@audiology.org
Website: www.audiology.org

American Speech-Language-Hearing Association (ASHA)
10801 Rockville Pike
Rockville, MD, 20852
Voice Telephone: (301) 897-5700; Toll-free: (800) 638-8255
TTY: (301) 897-0157
Fax: (301) 571-0457
E-mail: actioncenter@asha.org
Website: www.asha.org *and* www.asha.org/public/hearing/

American Academy of Otolaryngology-Head and Neck Surgery
  (AAO-HNS)
One Prince Street
Alexandria, VA, 22314-3357
Voice Telephone: (703) 836-4444
TTY: (703) 519-1585
Fax: (703) 683-5100
E-mail: entinfo@entnet.org
Website: http://www.entnet.org/healthinformation/

Support/Advocacy/Self-help Organizations for People with Hearing Loss

Hearing Loss Association of America (HLAA) (formerly Self Help for Hard
  of Hearing People [SHHH], this organization is the source of *Hearing
  Loss* magazine)
7910 Woodmont Avenue, Suite 1200
Bethesda, MD, 20814
Voice Telephone: (301) 657-2248
TTY: (301) 657-2248
Fax: (301) 913-9413
E-mail: info@hearingloss.org
Website: www.hearingloss.org

Association of Late-Deafened Adults (ALDA)
8038 MacIntosh Lane
Rockford, IL 61107
Toll-free Voice Telephone or TTY: (866) 402-2532
E-mail: info@alda.org
Website: www.alda.org

Other Sources of Consumer Information

Better Hearing Institute (BHI)
515 King Street, Suite 420
Alexandria, VA 22314
Voice Telephone: (703) 684-3391
Fax: (703) 684-6048
Email: mail@betterhearing.org
Website: www.betterhearing.org *and*
www.betterhearing.org/hearing_solutions/qualityOfLife.cfm

Deafness Research Foundation (DRF) (DRF is the source of *Hearing Health*
  magazine)
641 Lexington Avenue FI 15
New York, NY 10022

Voice Telephone: (212) 328-9480
E-mail: info@drf.org
Website: www.drf.org

House Ear Institute
2100 W. Third Street
Los Angeles, CA 90057
Voice Telephone: (213) 483-4431; Toll-free: (800) 388-8612
TTY: (213) 484-2642
Fax: (213) 483-8789
E-mail: info@hei.org
Website: www.hei.org/education/health/health.htm *and*
www.hei.org/news/facts/facts.htm

National Institute on Deafness and Other Communication Disorders
   (NIDCD)
National Institutes of Health
31 Center Drive, MSC 2320, Bldg. 31, Room 3C-35
Bethesda, MD 20892-2320
Voice Telephone: (301) 496-7243; Toll-free: (800) 241-1044
Fax: (301) 402-0018
E-mail: nidcdinfo@nidcd.nih.gov
Website: www.nidcd.nih.gov/health/hearing

CHAPTER 2

General Information about the Deaf Community and Deaf Culture

National Association of the Deaf (NAD)
8630 Fenton Street, Suite 820
Silver Spring, MD 20910-3819
Voice Telephone: (301) 587-1788
TTY: (301) 587-1789
Fax: (301) 587-1791
E-mail: nadinfo@nad.org
Website: www.nad.org

CHAPTER 3

General Information about How the Ear Works

American Academy of Otolaryngology-Head and Neck Surgery (refer to
the listing under Professional Associations for complete contact information [above])
Visit: www.entnet.org/HealthInformation/earWorks.cfm

House Ear Institute (refer to the listing under Other Sources of Consumer
Information for complete contact information [above])
Visit: www.hei.org/education/health/health.htm

General Information about the Vestibular System

National Institute on Deafness and Other Communication Disorders
(NIDCD) (refer to the listing under Other Sources of Consumer Information for complete contact information [above])
Visit: www.nidcd.nih.gov/health/balance/balance_disorders.asp *and*
www.nidcd.nih.gov/health/balance/baldizz.htm *and*
www.nihseniorhealth.gov/balanceproblems/toc.html

Organization for People Affected by Vestibular Disorders

Vestibular Disorders Association
P.O. Box 13305
Portland, OR 97213-0305
Voice Telephone: (503) 229-7705; Toll-free: (800) 837-8428
Fax: (503) 229-8064
Website: www.vestibular.org

CHAPTER 5

General Information about Conditions Affecting
the Ear or Hearing

American Academy of Otolaryngology-Head and Neck Surgery (refer to
the listing under Professional Associations for complete contact information [above])

National Institute on Deafness and Other Communication Disorders
(NIDCD) (refer to the listing under Other Sources of Consumer Information for complete contact information [above])

Visit:
www.entnet.org/HealthInformation/earwax.cfm (Earwax)
www.entnet.org/HealthInformation/swimmersEar.cfm (Swimmer's Ear)
www.entnet.org/HealthInformation/perforatedEardrum.cfm (Eardrum
    Perforations)
www.entnet.org/HealthInformation/otosclerosis.cfm (Otosclerosis)
www.nidcd.nih.gov/health/hearing/otosclerosis.asp (Otosclerosis)
www.entnet.org/HealthInformation/Earaches.cfm (Otitis Media)
www.entnet.org/HealthInformation/earsAltitude.cfm (Eustachian Tube
    Function, Barotrauma)

www.entnet.org/HealthInformation/Ear-Tubes.cfm (Tympanostomy
   Tubes)
www.entnet.org/HealthInformation/cholesteatoma.cfm (Cholesteatoma)
www.entnet.org/HealthInformation/Genes-and-Hearing-Loss.cfm
   (Genetic Hearing Loss)
www.nidcd.nih.gov/health/hearing/older.asp (Age-Related Hearing
   Loss)
www.nidcd.nih.gov/health/hearing/presbycusis.asp (Age-Related
   Hearing Loss)
www.entnet.org/HealthInformation/hearingProtection.cfm
   (Noise-induced Hearing Loss)
www.nidcd.nih.gov/health/hearing/noise.asp (Noise-induced Hearing
   Loss)
www.nidcd.nih.gov/health/balance/meniere.asp (Ménière's Disease)
www.nidcd.nih.gov/health/hearing/sudden.asp (Sudden Idiopathic
   Sensorineural Hearing Loss)
www.entnet.org/HealthInformation/autoimmuneInnerEar.cfm
   (Autoimmune Inner Ear Disease)
www.nidcd.nih.gov/health/hearing/neuropathy.asp (Auditory
   Neuropathy/Auditory Dys-synchrony)
www.nidcd.nih.gov/health/hearing/acoustic_neuroma.asp (Acoustic
   Tumors of CN VIII)

Organization for People Affected by Ménière's Disease

Ménière's Network
The EAR Foundation
2000 Church Street, P.O. Box 11
Nashville, TN 37236
Voice Telephone and TTY: (615) 627-2724; Toll-free: (800) 545-4327
Fax: (615) 627-2728
E-mail: info@earfoundation.org
Website: www.earfoundation.org/programs.asp?content=menieres_
network

Organization for People Affected by Acoustic Tumors of CN VIII

Acoustic Neuroma Association
600 Peachtree Pkwy., Suite 108
Cumming, GA 30041
Voice Telephone: (770) 205-8211; Toll-free: (877)-200-8211
Fax: (770) 205-0239; Toll-free: (877) 202-0239
Email: info@anausa.org
Website: www.anausa.org

Warm Air Ear Dryers

Sahara DryEar
3315 E. Russell Road, A4-920
Las Vegas, NV 89120
Toll-free Voice Telephone: (800) 570-6096
E-mail: CustomerService@dryear.net
Website: www.dryear.net/How_the_DryEar_Ear_Dryer_Works_s/26.htm

Mack's EarDryer
Mack's Ear Care
McKeon Products, Inc.
25460 Guenther
Warren, MI 48091
Voice Telephone: (586) 427-7560
Fax: (586) 427-7204
Website: www.macksearplugs.com

CHAPTER 6

Organization for People Affected by Tinnitus

American Tinnitus Association (ATA)
P.O. Box 5
Portland, OR 97207-0005
Voice Telephone: (503) 248-9985; Toll-free: (800) 634-8978
Fax: (503) 248-0024
E-mail: tinnitus@ata.org
Website: www.ata.org

General Information about Tinnitus

American Academy of Otolaryngology—Head and Neck Surgery (refer to
the listing under Professional Associations for complete contact information [above])
Visit: www.entnet.org/HealthInformation/tinnitus.cfm

National Institute on Deafness and Other Communication Disorders
(NIDCD) (refer to the listing under Other Sources of Consumer Infor-
mation for complete contact information [above])
Visit: www.nidcd.nih.gov/health/hearing/noiseinear.asp

Oregon Health and Science University Tinnitus Clinic
NRC04
Oregon Health Sciences University
3181 S.W. Sam Jackson Park Road
Portland, OR 97239-3098

Voice Telephone: (503) 494-7954
TTY: (503) 494-0910
Fax: (503) 494-5656
E-mail: ohrc@ohsu.edu
Website: www.ohsu.edu/ohrc/tinnitusclinic

Cognitive Behavioral Therapy (CBT)

Association for Behavioral and Cognitive Therapies
305 7th Avenue, 16th Floor
New York, NY 10001
Voice Telephone: (212) 647-1890
Fax: (212) 647-1865
Website: www.aabt.org

Neuromonics Tinnitus Treatment

Neuromonics Tinnitus Treatment
2810 Emrick Boulevard
Bethlehem, PA 18020
Toll-free Voice Telephone: (866) 606-3876
Fax: (484) 214-0166
Email: customerservice@neuromonics-usa.com
Website: www.neuromonics-usa.com/index.htm

Tinnitus Retraining Therapy (TRT)

Emory Tinnitus & Hyperacusis Center
Department of Otolaryngology
1365-A Clifton Road, NE
Atlanta, GA 30322
Voice Telephone (clinic): (404) 778-3109
E-mail: Pawel_Jastreboff@Emory.Org
Website: www.tinnitus-pjj.com

Tinnitus Masking Devices

Refer to the listings under Companies That Sell Assistive Listening Devices, Telephones and Telephone Accessories, Signaling Devices, or Tinnitus Maskers in the Resources section for Chapter 9 (below).

General Information about Hyperacusis

American Academy of Otolaryngology—Head and Neck Surgery (refer to
the listing under Professional Associations for complete contact information [above])

Visit: www.entnet.org/HealthInformation/hyperacusis-
increasedsensitivity.cfm

CHAPTER 7

Major Hearing Aid Manufacturers (and sources of consumer information)

Resound
8001 Bloomington Freeway
Bloomington, MN 55420
Voice Phone: (952) 769-8000; Toll-free: (800) 248-4327
Fax: (952) 769-8001
E-mail: customerexperience@gnresound.com
Website: www.gnresound.com

Phonak Hearing Systems
4520 Weaver Parkway
Warrenville, IL 60555-3927
Voice Telephone: (630) 821-5000; Toll-free: (800) 679-4871
Fax: (630) 393-7400
E-Mail: info@phonak.com
Website: www.phonak-us.com

Oticon, USA
29 Schoolhouse Road
Somerset, NJ 08875-6724
Voice Telephone: (732) 560-1220; Toll-free: (800) 526-3921
Fax: (732) 560-0029
E-mail: webmaster@oticonus.com
Website: www.oticonusa.com

Siemens, USA
10 Constitution Ave, PO Box 1397
Piscataway, NJ 08855-1397
Voice Phone: (732) 562-6600; Toll-free: (800) 766-4500
Fax: (732) 562-6640
Website: www.usa.siemens.com/hearing

Sonic Innovations, Inc.
2795 E. Cottonwood Parkway, Ste. 660
Salt Lake City, UT 84121
Voice Telephone: (801) 365-2800; Toll-free: (888) 678-4327
Fax: (801) 365-3000
E-mail: info@sonici.com
Website: www.sonici.com

Starkey Laboratories, Inc.
6700 Washington Avenue S
Eden Prairie, MN 55344-3476
Voice Telephone: (952) 941-6401; Toll-free: (800) 328-8602
Fax: (952) 828-9262
Website: www.starkey.com

Widex Hearing Aid Company
35-53 24th St.
Long Island City, NY 11106
Voice Phone: (718) 392-6020; Toll-free: (800) 221-0188
Fax: (516) 739-5261
E-mail: info@widexusa.com
Website: www.widex.com

Middle Ear Implants

Vibrant Soundbridge
MED-EL Corporation (refer to the listing under Cochlear Implant Manufacturers in the Resources section for Chapter 8 for complete contact information [below])
Visit: www.vibrantmedel.us/archive/layout/splash.asp

Bone Conduction Devices

Bone Anchored Hearing Aid (Baha®)
Cochlear Americas (refer to the listing under Cochlear Implant Manufacturers in the Resources section for Chapter 8 for complete contact information [below])
Visit: www.cochlearamericas.com/Products/2013.asp

TransEar
Ear Technology Corporation
P.O. Box 1516
Johnson City, TN 37605
Toll-free Voice Telephone: (888) 382-9327
Fax: (423) 928-0515
E-mail: info@eartech.com
Website: www.transear.com

Financial Assistance for the Purchase of Hearing Aids

Audient Alliance for Accessible Hearing Care
Northwest Hearing Care
901 Boren Ave., Suite 810

Seattle, WA 98104-3534
Voice Telephone: (206) 838-7194; Toll-free: (877) 283-4368
Fax: (206) 838-7195
E-mail: info@audientalliance.org
Website: www.audientalliance.org

Lions Affordable Hearing Aid Project (AHAP)
Lions Clubs International Foundation
300 West 22nd Street
Oak Brook, Illinois 60523-8842
Voice Telephone: (630) 571-5466, ext. 615
E-mail: LionsAHAP@lionsclubs.org
Website: www.lionsclubs.org/EN/content/lcif_gr_ahap.html

The Starkey Hearing Foundation (Hear Now)
6700 Washington Ave South
Eden Prairie, MN 55344
Toll-free Voice Telephone: (800) 769-2799
Fax: (952) 828-6946
Website: www.sotheworldmayhear.org

Travelers Protective Association Scholarship Trust for the Deaf and
    Near-Deaf
3755 Lindell Boulevard
St. Louis, MO 63108
Voice Telephone: (314) 371-0533
Fax: (314) 371-0537
E-mail: support@tpahq.org
Website: www.travelersprotectiveasn.com/deaf_scholarships.htm

Buying Hearing Aids on Credit:

CareCredit
901 East Cerritos Ave.
Anaheim, CA 92805
Voice Telephone: (714) 490-4833; Toll-free: (800) 300-3046
Fax: (714) 758-3691
Website: www.carecredit.com

Citi Health Card
541 Sid Martin Road
Gray, TN 37615
Toll-free Voice Telephone: (866) 832-8762
Fax: (866) 352-5204
Website: www.healthcard.citicards.com

The Helpcard
P.O. Box 829
Springdale, AR 72765
Toll-free Voice Telephone: (888) 750-6795
Fax: (800) 245-7491
Website: helpcard.com

Hearing Aid Warranties (that supplement those offered by hearing aid manufacturers)

Discovery Hearing Aid Warranties
4318 Downtowner Loop N, Suite K
Mobile, AL 36609
Toll-free Voice Telephone: (800) 525-7936
Fax: (251) 342-2158
Website: www.discoverywarranties.com

Hearing Aid Insurance

ESCO (Ear Service Corporation)
3215 Fernbrook Lane North
Plymouth, MN 55447-5325
Toll-free Voice Telephone: (800) 992-3726
E-mail: info@earserv.com
Website: www.earserv.com

Midwest Hearing Industries, Inc.
4510 West 77th Street, Suite 201
Minneapolis, MN 55435
Toll-free Voice Telephone: (800) 821-5471
Fax: 952-835-9481
Website: www.mwhi.com

CHAPTER 8

General Information about Cochlear Implants

American Academy of Otolaryngology—Head and Neck Surgery (refer to the listing under Professional Associations for complete contact information [above])
Visit: www.entnet.org/HealthInformation/cochlearImplants.cfm

Cochlear Implant Manufacturers

Advanced Bionics Corporation
25129 Rye Canyon Loop

Valencia, California 91355
Toll-free Voice Telephone: (877) 829-0026
Toll-free: TTY: (800) 678-3575
Fax: (661) 362-1500
Email: customerservice@advancedbionics.com
Website: www.bionicear.com

Cochlear Americas
400 Inverness Parkway, Suite 400
Englewood, CO 80112
Voice Telephone: (303) 790-9010; Toll-free: (800) 523-5798
Fax: (303) 792-9025
E-mail: info@cochlear.com
Website: www.cochlear.com

MED-EL Corporation (North America)
2222 E. Highway 54, Suite B-180
Durham, NC 27713
Voice Telephone: (919) 572-2222; Toll-free: (888) 633-3524
Fax: (919) 484-9229
E-mail: implants@medelus.com
Website: www.medel.com/ENG/US/

CHAPTER 9

General Information about Assistive Listening Systems

U.S. Architectural and Transportation Barriers Compliance Board
The Access Board
1331 F Street, NW #1000
Washington, DC 20004
Voice Telephone: (202) 272-5434; Toll-free: (800) 872-2253
TTY: (202) 272-5449; Toll-free: (800) 993-2822
Fax: (202) 272-5447
Website: www.hearingresearch.org/BulletinConsumers.htm

General Information about Induction Loops

Let's Loop America!
E-mail: myers@hope.edu
Website: www.hearingloop.org

Hearing Aids with Integrated Ear-level FM

Phonak Hearing Systems
4520 Weaver Parkway

Warrenville, IL 60555-3927
Voice Telephone: (630) 821-5000; Toll-free: (800) 679-4871
Fax: (630) 393-7400
E-Mail: info@phonak.com
Website: www.phonak-us.com/ccus/consumer/products_us/fm/whatisfm.
  htm

Companies That Sell Assistive Listening Devices, Telephones and Telephone Accessories, Signaling Devices, or Tinnitus Maskers

ADCO Hearing Products, Inc.
4242 South Broadway
Englewood, CO 80113
Voice Telephone or TTY: (303) 794-3928; Toll-free: (800) 726-0851
Fax: (303) 794-3704
Website: www.adcohearing.com

ALDS-Distributing Inc.
P.O. Box 12118
Murrayville RPO
Langley, Canada
Voice Telephone: (604) 514-0053; Toll-free (866) 845-2537
Fax: (604) 514-0037
Website: www.alds.com

Ameriphone
213 West 35th St. #2W
New York, NY 10001
Toll-free Voice Telephone: (888) 449-0444
E-mail: info@onlinephonestore.com
Website: ameriphone.com

Assistech, Inc.
2738 N. Campbell Ave.
Tucson, AZ 85719-3141
Toll-free Voice Telephone or TTY: (866) 674-3549
Fax: (520) 883-3172
Website: www.assistech.com

Assisted Access, Inc.—NFSS Communications
822 Preston Court
Lake Villa, IL 60046
Toll-free Voice Telephone or TTY: (800) 950-9655
Fax: (847) 265-8044

E-mail: assistedaccess-nfss@comcast.net
Website: www.nfss.com

Audex
710 Standard Street
Longview, Texas 75604
Toll-free Voice Telephone: (800) 237-0716
Fax: (800) 283-3974
Website: www.audex.com

AudioLink Services
Toll-free Voice Telephone: (800) 516-6955
Website: www.audiolinks.com

Beyond Hearing Aids, Inc.
463 Erlanger Rd., Suite 1
Erlanger, KY 41018
Toll-free Voice Telephone or TTY: (800) 838-1649
Fax: (859) 342-4979
Website: www.beyondhearingaids.com

Centrum Sound Systems
572 La Conner Drive
Sunnyvale, CA 94087
Voice Telephone: (408) 736-6500
Fax: (408) 736-6552
E-mail: sales@centrumsound.com
Website: www.centrumsound.com

Clarity
4289 Bonny Oaks Drive, Suite 106
Chattanooga, TN 37406
Toll-free Voice Telephone: (800) 426-3738 or (800) 552-3368
Fax: (800) 325-8871
E-mail: clarity@plantronics.com
Website: www.clarityproducts.com

ClearSounds Communications
8160 S. Madison Street
Burr Ridge, IL 60527
Voice Telephone: (630) 654-9200; Toll-free: (800) 965-9043
Fax: (888) 654-9219
E-mail: customersolutions@clearsounds.com
Website: www.clearsounds.com

COMTEK Communications Technology, Inc.
357 West 2700 South
Salt Lake City, UT 84115
Voice Telephone: (801) 466-3463; Toll-free: (800) 496-3463
Fax: (801) 484-6906
Website: www.comtek.com

Conversor Limited
The Lansbury Estate
102 Lower Guildford Road
Knaphill, Woking,
Surrey GU21 2EP
United Kingdom
E-mail: info@conversorproducts.com
Website: www.conversorproducts.com

Cordless Workz
1135 Kildaire Farm Rd., Suite 200
Cary, NC 27511
Voice Telephone: (919) 342-5055; Toll-free: (800) 516-4279
Fax: (919) 287-2996
Website: www.cordlessworkz.com

General Technologies
7417 Winding Way
Fair Oaks, CA 95628
Toll-free Voice Telephone: (800) 328-6684
Fax: (916) 961-9823
E-mail: devices4less@hotmail.com
Website: www.devices4less.com

Global Assistive Devices, Inc.
4950 North Dixie Highway
Fort Lauderdale, FL 33334
Voice Telephone: (954) 776-1373; Toll-free: (888) 778-4237
Fax: (954) 776-8136
E-mail: info@GlobalAssistive.com
Website: www.globalassistive.com

HARC Mercantile
1111 West Centre Ave.
Portage, MI 49024
Voice Telephone or TTY: (269) 324-1615; Toll-free: (800) 445-9968
Fax: (269) 324-2387

E-mail: info@harc.com
Website: www.harc.com

Harris Communications
15155 Technology Drive
Eden Prairie, MN 55344
Voice Telephone: (952) 906-1180; Toll-free: (800) 825-6758
TTY: (952) 906-1198; Toll-free: (800) 825-9187
Fax: (952) 906-1099
E-mail: info@harriscomm.com
Website: www.harriscomm.com

HATIS (Hearing Aid Telephone Interconnect Systems)
231 Market Place, Suite 377
San Ramon, CA 94583
Voice Telephone: (925) 736-7984
Fax: (925) 736-1524
E-mail: uhearme@hatis.com
Website: www.hatis.com

Hear-More
42 Executive Blvd.
Farmingdale, NY 11735
Toll-free Voice Telephone: (800) 881-4327
Toll-free TTY: (800) 281-3555
Text Messaging Service: (631) 752-3277
Fax: (631) 752-0689
Website: www.hearmore.com

Hear-Tronics International
7431-34 West Atlantic Ave., P.O. Box 167
Delray Beach, FL 33446
Voice Telephone: (561) 495-9898; Toll-free: (800) 453-3561
Fax: (561) 495-4020
E-mail: info@hear-tronics.com
Website: www.hear-tronics.com

Hearing Resources
4311 NE Tillamook Street
Portland, OR 97213
Voice Telephone: (503) 774-3668; Toll-free: (800) 531-2139
Fax: (503) 774-7247
E-mail: info@earlink.com
Website: www.earlink.com

HITEC Group
8160 S. Madison Street
Burr Ridge, IL 60527
Toll-free Voice Telephone: (800) 288-8303
Toll-free TTY: (800) 536-8890
Fax: (888) 654-9219
E-mail: customersolutions@hitec.com
Website: www.hitec.com

LS&S (Learning, Sight & Sound Made Easier)
1808-G Janke Dr.
Northbrook, IL 60062
Toll-free Voice Telephone: (800) 468-4789
Toll-free TTY: (866) 317-8533
Fax: (877) 498-1482
Website: www.lssproducts.com

Life with Ease
P.O. Box 302
Newbury, NH 03255
Toll-free Voice Telephone: (800) 966-5119
E-mail: questions@lifewithease.com
Website: www.lifewithease.com

Marilyn Electronics
6 Feener Circle
Randolph, MA 02368
Voice Telephone or TTY: (781) 961-1034; Toll-free: (800) 622-9558
FAX: 781-961-6962
Website: www.marilynelectronics.net

Oval Window Audio (home induction loops)
33 Wildflower Court
Nederland, CO 80466
Voice Telephone or TTY: (303) 447-3607
Fax: (303) 447-3607
E-mail: info@ovalwindowaudio.com
Website: www.ovalwindowaudio.com

Potomac Technology
One Church Street, Suite 101
Rockville, MD 20850-4158
Toll-free Voice Telephone or TTY: (800) 433-2838
Fax: (301) 762-1892

E-mail: info@potomactech.com
Website: www.potomactech.com

Pure Direct Sound (home induction loops)
7788 N.E. Yeomalt Pt. Dr.
Bainbridge Island, WA 98110
Voice Telephone: (206) 842-5124
E-mail: amco@mindspring.com
Website: www.puredirectsound.com

Pure White Noise (tinnitus masking)
6219 Whittondale Drive
Tallahassee, FL 32312
E-mail: sales@purewhitenoise.com
Website: www.purewhitenoise.com

Silent Call Communications
5095 Williams Lake Road
Waterford, MI 48329
Voice Telephone or TTY: (248) 673-7353; Toll-free (800) 572-5227
Fax: (248) 673-7360
E-mail: CustomerService@SilentCall.com
Website: www.silentcall.com

Sleepsonic Speaker Pillow for Tinnitus
303 First Street SE, Ste #2 PMB 75
Yelm, WA 98597
Toll-free Voice Telephone: (866) 468-0820
Website: www.sleepsonic.com/tinnitus_pillow.html

Sound Clarity, Inc.
359 North 1st Ave.
Iowa City, IA 52245
Toll-free Voice Telephone or TTY: (888) 477-2995
Fax: (319) 354-5851
Website: www.soundclarity.com/shopcustcontact.asp

Soundbytes
P.O. Box 9022
Hicksville, NY 11802
Toll-free Voice Telephone: (888) 816-8191
TTY: (516) 937-3546
Fax: (516) 938-1513
E-mail: info@soundbytes.com
Website: www.soundbytes.com

TecEar
30215 Woodgate Drive
Southfield, MI 48076
Voice Telephone: (248) 867-2759
E-mail: info@tecear.com
Website: www.tecear.com

Teltex, Inc.
1081 West Innovation Drive
Kearney, MO 64060
Voice Telephone: (816) 628-1949; Toll-free: (888) 515-8120
Toll-free TTY: (888) 515-8120
Fax: (816) 635-4043
E-mail: info@teltex.com
Website: www.teltex.com/

TV Ears, Inc.
2810 Via Orange Way, Suite A
Spring Valley, CA 91978
Toll-free Voice Telephone: (888) 883-3277
Fax: (888) 958-7899
E-mail: info@tvears.com
Website: www.tvears.com

Ultratec, Inc.
450 Science Drive
Madison, WI 53711
Toll-free Voice Telephone or TTY: (800) 482-2424
Fax: (608) 238-300
E-mail: service@ultratec.com
Website: www.ultratec.com

United TTY Sales and Service
21004 Brooke Knolls Rd.
Laytonsville, MD 20882
Toll-free Voice Telephone or TTY: (866) 889-4872
Fax: (301) 963-0785
Website: www.unitedtty.com/index.htm

Weitbrecht Communications
926 Colorado Avenue
Santa Monica, CA 90401-2717
Toll-free Voice Telephone or TTY: (800) 233-9130
Fax: (310) 450-9918
E-mail: sales@weitbrecht.com
Website: www.weitbrecht.com

Williams Sound
10321 W. 70th Street
Eden Prairie, MN 55344-3446
Voice Telephone: (952) 943-2252; Toll-free: (800) 328-6190
Fax: (952) 943-2174
E-mail: info@williamssound.com
Website: www.williamssound.com

Companion Mics

Etymotic Research, Inc.
61 Martin Lane
Elk Grove Village, IL 60007
Voice Telephone: (847) 228-0006; Toll-free: (888) 389-6684
Fax: (847) 228-6836
E-mail: customer-service@etymotic.com
Website: www.etymotic.com/ephp/compmic.aspx

Bluetooth Wireless Technology and Hearing Aids

ELI DirX Ear-Level Instrument
Starkey Laboratories Wireless Products (refer to the listing under Major
Hearing Aid Manufacturers in the Resources section for Chapter 7 for
complete contact information [above])
Visit: www.elihearing.com/UnitedStatesENG/Docs/Features1.htm

SmartLink SX
Phonak Hearing Systems (refer to the listing under Major Hearing Aid
Manufacturers in the Resources section for Chapter 7 for complete contact
information [above])
Visit: www.phonak-us.com/ccus/consumer/products_us/fm/smartlink.htm

Epoq Streamer
Oticon, USA (refer to the listing under Major Hearing Aid Manufacturers
in the Resources section for Chapter 7 for complete contact information
[above])
Visit: www.myoticon.com/Streamer/Default.aspx

General Information about Telecommunication Relay Services

Federal Communications Commission
445 12th Street SW
Washington, DC 20554
Toll-free Voice Telephone: (888) 225-5322
Toll-free TTY: (888) 835-5322

Fax: (866) 418-0232
E-mail: fccinfo@fcc.gov
Website: www.fcc.gov/cgb/consumerfacts/trs.html

National Institute on Deafness and other Communication Disorders
(NIDCD) (refer to listing under Other Sources of Consumer Information
for complete contact information [above])
Visit: www.nidcd.nih.gov/health/hearing/telecomm.asp

General Information about Captioning

National Captioning Institute
National Help Desk
1900 Gallows Road, Suite 300
Vienna, VA 22182
Voice Telephone or TTY: (703) 917-7600; Toll-free: (800) 374-3986
Fax: (703) 917-9878
E-mail: mail@ncihelpdesk.org
Website: www.ncicap.org *and* www.ncihelpdesk.org

Federal Communication Commission (refer to the listing under Telecommunication Relay Services in the Resources section for this chapter for
complete contact information [above])
E-mail: closedcaptioning@fcc.gov (for questions about closed captioning
    problems)
Visit: www.fcc.gov/cgb/consumerfacts/dtvcaptions.html *and*
    www.fcc.gov/cgb/consumerfacts/CC_converters.html

State Telephone Equipment Distribution Programs

Telecommunications Equipment Distribution Program Association
    (TEDPA) (state programs vary widely, but some provide free or low-
    cost telephone equipment to eligible residents)
301 West Preston Street
Suite 1008
Baltimore, MD 21201
Website: www.tedpa.org/interiorPage.php?pageID=111&viewType=sm

General Information about Hearing Aid Compatibility
with Telephones

CTIA—The Wireless Association
1400 16th Street NW, Suite 600
Washington, DC 20036
Voice Telephone: (202) 785-0081

TTY: (202) 736-3880
Fax: (202) 785-3684
Website: www.accesswireless.org *and*
www.accesswireless.org/product/hearing.cfm

Federal Communications Commission (refer to the listing under Telecommunication Relay Services in the Resources section for this chapter for complete contact information [above])
Visit: www.fcc.gov/cgb/consumerfacts/hac_wireless.pdf *and*
    www.fcc.gov/cgb/consumerfacts/hac_wireline.pdf

Directory of Service Dog Schools (by state)

Wolf Packs, Inc.
PO Box 3195
Ashland, OR 97520
Voice Telephone: (541) 482-7669
Website: www.wolfpacks.com/serviced.htm

CHAPTER 10

The Americans with Disabilities Act (ADA)

U.S. Department of Justice (ADA Home Page)
950 Pennsylvania Avenue, NW
Washington, DC 20530-0001
Voice Telephone: 202-514-2000
E-mail: AskDOJ@usdoj.gov
Website: www.ada.gov

Job Accommodation Network (JAN), U.S. Department of Labor Office of Disability Employment Policy (information about reasonable accommodations in the workplace)
P.O. Box 6080
Morgantown, WV 26506-6080
Voice Telephone: 304-293-7186; Toll-free: (800) 526-7234
Toll-free TTY: (877) 781-9403
Fax: 304-293-5407
Website: www.jan.wvu.edu *and* www.jan.wvu.edu/soar/disabilities.html
    and www.jan.wvu.edu/soar/hear.html *and*
    www.jan.wvu.edu/soar/hearing/deaf.html

U.S. Department of Justice, Civil Rights Division, Disability Rights Section (Tax Incentives Packet for employers complying with the ADA)
950 Pennsylvania Avenue, NW
Washington, DC 20530-0001

Toll-free Voice Telephone: (800) 514-0301
Toll-free TTY: (800) 514-0383
Website: www.ADA.gov/taxpack.htm

Filing ADA Violation Complaints

The U.S. Equal Employment Opportunity Commission (ADA violation
   complaints relevant to Title I)
1801 L Street, N.W.
Washington, D.C. 20507
Voice Telephone: (800) 669-4000
TTY: (800) 669-6820
E-mail: info@ask.eeoc.gov
Website: www.eeoc.gov *and* www.eeoc.gov/policy/ada.html *and* www.
   eeoc.gov/facts/deafness.html   *and*   www.eeoc.gov/charge/overview_
   charge_filing.html *and* www.eeoc.gov/facts/fs-fed.html

Federal Transit Administration (ADA violation complaints relevant to
   Title II)
East Building
1200 New Jersey Ave SE
Washington, DC 20590
Toll-free Voice Telephone: (866) 377-8642
Toll-free TTY: (800) 877-8339
Toll-free VCO: (877) 877-6280
E-mail: FTA.ADAAssistance@dot.gov
Website: www.fta.dot.gov/civilrights/civil_rights_2360.html

United States Access Board (ADA violation complaints relevant to Title II)
1331 F Street, NW, Suite 1000
Washington, DC 20004-1111
Toll-free Voice Telephone: (800) 872-2253
Toll-free TTY: (800) 993-2822
E-mail: info@access-board.gov
Website: www.access-board.gov/enforce.htm

Federal Communications Commission (ADA violation complaints relevant
to Title IV) (refer to the listing under Telecommunication Relay Services
in the Resources section for this chapter for complete contact information
[above])
Visit: http://www.fcc.gov/cgb/dro/title4.html

Hearing Rehabilitation Materials

Hear Again, Inc.
37 Grandview Drive

Latham, NY 12110
Voice Telephone: (518) 786-3573
Fax: (518) 785-6905
E-mail: info@hearagainpublishing.com
Website: www.hearagainpublishing.com

Listening and Communication Enhancement (LACE)
Neurotone Auditory Solutions
2317 Broadway, Suite 250
Redwood City, CA 94063
Voice Telephone: (650) 839-0260; Toll-free: (800) 409-5223
Fax: (650) 839-0200
E-mail: info@neurotone.com
Website: www.neurotone.com

CHAPTER 11

Companies That Sell Noise-blocking or Noise-canceling Headphones or Earbuds

Bose Corporation
The Mountain
Framingham, MA 01701
Voice Telephone: (508) 879-7330; Toll-free: (800) 999-2673
Website: www.bose.com

Etymotic Research, Inc. (refer to the listing under Companion Mics in the Resources section for Chapter 9 for complete contact information [above])
Visit: www.etymotic.com

Shure Incorporated
5800 West Touhy Avenue
Niles, IL 60714-4608
Voice Telephone: (847) 600-2000; Toll-free: (800) 257-4873
Fax: (847) 600-1212
E-mail: info@shure.com
Website: www.shure.com

Sony Style, USA
Toll-free Voice Telephone: (877) 865-7669
Website: www.sonystyle.com

High-fidelity or Musician's Earplugs

Etymotic Research, Inc. (refer to the listing under Companion Mics in the Resources section for Chapter 9 for complete contact information [above])
Visit: www.etymotic.com

Westone Laboratories, Inc.
P.O. Box 15100
Colorado Springs, CO 80935
Voice Telephone: (719) 540-9333; Toll-free: (800) 525-5071
Fax: (719) 540-9183
E-mail: westone@westone.com
Website: www.westone.com

Campaigns Dedicated to Educating People about Hearing Loss and the Need to Protect Hearing

Dangerous Decibels
Oregon Health & Science University
3181 SW Sam Jackson Park Road NRC04
Portland, OR 97201-3098
Voice Telephone: (503) 494-0670
Fax: (503) 494-5656
E-mail: info@dangerousdecibels.org
Website: www.dangerousdecibels.org

Healthy Hearing 2010
Office of Health Communication and Public Liaison, NIDCD
31 Center Drive, MSC 2320
Bethesda, MD 20892-2320
Voice Telephone: (301) 496-7243; Toll-free: (800) 241-1044
Fax: (301) 402-0018
E-mail: nidcdinfo@nidcd.nih.gov
Website: www.nidcd.nih.gov/health/healthyhearing

Listen to Your Buds!
American Speech-Language-Hearing Association (ASHA)
10801 Rockville Pike
Rockville, MD 20852
Voice Telephone: (301) 897-5700; Toll-free: (800) 638-8255
TTY: (301) 897-0157
Fax: (301) 571-0457
E-mail: actioncenter@asha.org
Website: www.listentoyourbuds.org

Wise Ears!
NIDCD Information Clearinghouse
1 Communication Ave.
Bethesda, MD 20892-3456
Voice Telephone: (301) 496-7243; Toll-free: (800) 241-1044
Toll-free TTY: (800) 241-1055

E-mail: nidcdinfo@nidcd.nih.gov
Website: www.nidcd.nih.gov/health/wise

Organizations Dedicated to Reducing Noise Pollution and Noise-induced Hearing Loss

H.E.A.R. (A Non-Profit Hearing Information Source for Musicians and Music Lovers)
San Francisco, CA 94115
Voice Telephone: (415) 409-3277
Website: www.hearnet.com

Noise Center of the League for the Hard of Hearing
50 Broadway, 6th Floor
New York, NY 10004
Voice Telephone: (917) 305-7700
TTY: (917) 305-7999
Fax: (917) 305-7888
E-mail: info@lhh.org
Website: www.lhh.org/noise

Noise Free America
P.O. Box 1551
Madison, WI 53701
Voice Telephone: (877) 664-7366
E-mail: noisefree@hotmail.com
Website: www.noisefree.org

The Noise Pollution Clearinghouse
P.O. Box 1137
Montpelier, VT 05601-1137
Toll-free Voice Telephone: (888) 200-8332
Website: www.nonoise.org

The Right to Quiet Society
#359, 1985 Wallace Street
Vancouver, BC
Canada V6R 4H4
Voice Telephone: (604) 222-0207
E-mail: info@quiet.org
Website: www.quiet.org

APPENDICES

Electronic Drying Kits for Hearing Aids

Dry and Store
P.O. Box 1017

Johnson City, TN 37605
Voice Telephone: (423) 928-9060; Toll-free: (800) 327-8547
Fax: (423) 928-0515
E-mail: info@dryandstore.com
Website: www.dryandstore.com

Index

About the Author

SUSAN DALEBOUT is an audiologist with more than 30 years of experience. She has served as Associate Director and Associate Professor for the Communication Disorders Program at the University of Virginia and has also taught at Western Michigan University and The Ohio State University. She has published award-winning research papers in academic journals and served as Assistant Editor for the *Journal of the American Academy of Audiology*. Dr. Dalebout has mentored hundreds of audiology students who are now practicing clinicians. Currently, she is an administrator in the College of Education at Michigan State University.